CRC SERIES IN MODERN NUTRITION

Edited by Ira Wolinsky and James F. Hickson, Jr.

Published Titles

Manganese in Health and Disease, Dorothy J. Klimis-Za

Nutrition and AIDS: Effects and Treatments, Ronald R. W

Nutrition Care for HIV-Positive Persons: A Manual for Individuals and Thei
Saroj M. Bahl and James F. Hickson, Jr.

Calcium and Phosphorus in Health and Disease, John J.B. Anderson and Sanford C. Garner

Edited by Ira Wolinsky

Published Titles

Practical Handbook of Nutrition in Clinical Practice, Donald F. Kirby and Stanley J. Dudrick

Handbook of Dairy Foods and Nutrition, Gregory D. Miller, Judith K. Jarvis, and Lois D. McBean

Advanced Nutrition: Macronutrients, Carolyn D. Berdanier

Childhood Nutrition, Fima Lifschitz

Nutrition and Health: Topics and Controversies, Felix Bronner

Nutrition and Cancer Prevention, Ronald R. Watson and Siraj I. Mufti

Nutritional Concerns of Women, Second Edition, Ira Wolinsky and Dorothy J. Klimis-Zacas

Nutrients and Gene Expression: Clinical Aspects, Carolyn D. Berdanier

Antioxidants and Disease Prevention, Harinda S. Garewal

Advanced Nutrition: Micronutrients, Carolyn D. Berdanier

Nutrition and Women's Cancers, Barbara Pence and Dale M. Dunn

Nutrients and Foods in AIDS, Ronald R. Watson

Nutrition: Chemistry and Biology, Second Edition, Julian E. Spallholz, L. Mallory Boylan, and Judy A. Driskell

Melatonin in the Promotion of Health, Ronald R. Watson

Nutritional and Environmental Influences on the Eye, Allen Taylor

Laboratory Tests for the Assessment of Nutritional Status, Second Edition, H.E. Sauberlich

Advanced Human Nutrition, Robert E.C. Wildman and Denis M. Medeiros

Handbook of Dairy Foods and Nutrition, Second Edition, Gregory D. Miller, Judith K. Jarvis, and Lois D. McBean

Nutrition in Space Flight and Weightlessness Models, Helen W. Lane and Dale A. Schoeller

Eating Disorders in Women and Children: Prevention, Stress Management, and Treatment, Jacalyn J. Robert-McComb

Childhood Obesity: Prevention and Treatment, Jana Pařízková and Andrew Hills

Alcohol and Coffee Use in the Aging, Ronald R. Watson

Handbook of Nutrition in the Aged, Third Edition, Ronald R. Watson

Vegetables, Fruits, and Herbs in Health Promotion, Ronald R. Watson

Nutrition and AIDS, Second Edition, Ronald R. Watson

Advances in Isotope Methods for the Analysis of Trace Elements in Man, Nicola Lowe and Malcolm Jackson

Nutritional Anemias, Usha Ramakrishnan

Handbook of Nutraceuticals and Functional Foods, Robert E. C. Wildman

The Mediterranean Diet: Constituents and Health Promotion, Antonia-Leda Matalas, Antonis Zampelas, Vassilis Stavrinos, and Ira Wolinsky

Vegetarian Nutrition, Joan Sabaté

Nutrient–Gene Interactions in Health and Disease, Naïma Moustaïd-Moussa and Carolyn D. Berdanier

Micronutrients and HIV Infection, Henrik Friis

Tryptophan: Biochemicals and Health Implications, Herschel Sidransky

Nutritional Aspects and Clinical Management of Chronic Disorders and Diseases, Felix Bronner

Forthcoming Titles

Handbook of Nutraceuticals and Nutritional Supplements and Pharmaceuticals, Robert E. C. Wildman

Insulin and Oligofructose: Functional Food Ingredients, Marcel B. Roberfroid

NUTRITIONAL *and* ENVIRONMENTAL INFLUENCES *on the* EYE

Edited by

Allen Taylor, Ph.D.

Director of the Laboratory for Nutrition and Vision Research
USDA Jean Mayer Human Nutrition Research Center on Aging
Tufts University

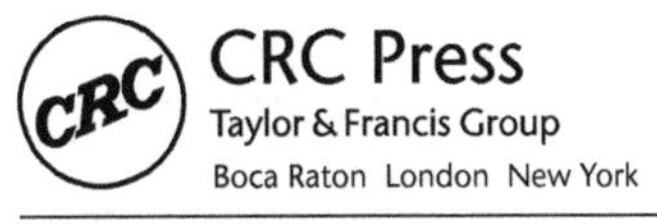

CRC Press is an imprint of the
Taylor & Francis Group, an informa business

CRC Press
Taylor & Francis Group
6000 Broken Sound Parkway NW, Suite 300
Boca Raton, FL 33487-2742

First issued in paperback 2019

ISBN-13: 978-0-8493-8565-0 (hbk)
ISBN-13: 978-0-367-39984-9 (pbk)

Library of Congress Card Number 98-49170

Library of Congress Cataloging-in-Publication Data

Nutritional and environmental influences on the eye / edited by Allen Taylor.
p. cm.—(Modern nutrition)
Includes bibliographical references and index.
ISBN 0-8493-8565-2 (alk. paper)
1. Eye—Pathophysiology, 2. Eye—Diseases—Nutritional aspects. 3. Eye—Diseases—Environmental aspects. 4. Cataract—Etiology. 5. Retina—Diseases—Etiology. I. Taylor, Allen, 1946—
II. Series: Modern nutrition (Boca Raton, FL.)
RE67.N88 1999
617.7′.071—dc21 98-49170
CIP

Visit the Taylor & Francis Web site at
http://www.taylorandfrancis.com

and the CRC Press Web site at
http://www.crcpress.com

SERIES PREFACE FOR MODERN NUTRITION

The CRC Series in Modern Nutrition is dedicated to providing the widest possible coverage of topics in nutrition. Nutrition is an interdisciplinary, interprofessional field par excellence. It is noted by its broad range and diversity. We trust the titles and authorship in this series will reflect that range and diversity.

Published for a scholarly audience, the volumes in the CRC Series in Modern Nutrition are designed to explain, review, and explore present knowledge and recent trends, developments, and advances in nutrition. As such, they will also appeal to the educated layman. The format for the series will vary with the needs of the author and the topic, including, but not limited to, edited volumes, monographs, handbooks, and texts.

Contributors from any bona fide area of nutrition, including the controversial, are welcome.

We welcome the contribution by Allen Taylor on nutrition, the environment, and the eye. It is a timely subject where much valuable new information has been obtained in recent years. It fills an important information gap.

Ira Wolinsky, Ph.D.
University of Houston
Series Editor

PREFACE

This book was designed to be of service to clinicians and basic vision scientists.

Several years ago the clouding of the lens–or cataract–was thought to be an inevitable consequence of aging, one only treatable by surgery. This is not surprising since cataract is the most frequently performed surgical technique, and costs associated with lens problems comprise the largest line item in the Medicare budget. Biochemists and other medical researchers thought of the lens as a remote, specialized organ with little relationship to many other organs in the body. Another reason for limited enthusiasm for lens research is that there is a widely successful procedure for removal of cataractous lenses. A recent explosion of biochemical, cell biological, physiological, and epidemiological information has changed that perspective.

The appreciation that lens molecules show age-related damage, and characterization of a majority of that damage as oxidatively induced, led researchers to ask if antioxidants could be used to diminish the risk for lens damage and function. The demand for this knowledge revealed a need for a better means to classify cataracts and more information regarding the nature of the damage.

Unlike the lens, which is made of only two cell types and is one of the slowest metabolizing tissues in the body, the retina is made of many different types of cells and is one of the fastest metabolizing tissues in the body. Despite these contrasts, recently acquired data indicate that the retina also suffers from oxidative damage. Thus, as in the lens, it appeared that retinal health might be prolonged with the use of antioxidants. Also required for such investigations were better means to define and characterize and quantify retinal change. In addition, knowledge regarding composition of these organs needed to be expanded.

For the first time this text presents in one place an organized compendium of the recently obtained information regarding theories of lens and retina aging, new data relating the composition of these tissues, documentation regarding the best means to characterize clinical appearance of lens and retina age-related changes, and summaries of correlations between nutrient antioxidant and cataract or retinopathy. Separate chapters also summarize correlations between environmental influences and visual capabilities. These include examination of the effects of smoking and light exposure for risk of cataract. The book concludes with two chapters that look toward the future with descriptions of non-invasive technologies to define eye tissue composition.

It is hoped that by compiling this information within one text, this compendium will make possible more rapid advances in the future and will lead to a new generation of studies which allow us to prolong visual function.

PREFACE

THE EDITOR

Allen Taylor, Ph.D., is the Director of the Laboratory for Nutrition and Vision Research at the Jean Mayer USDA Human Nutrition Research Center on Aging at Tufts University and Professor of Nutrition, Biochemistry, and Ophthalmology. He received his B.S. from The City College of the City University of New York and Ph.D. in organic chemistry from Rutgers University. He then did postdoctoral studies in biochemistry at the University of California at Berkeley. Research objectives in the Laboratory for Nutrition and Vision Research include elucidating relationships between oxidative stress protein turnover, aging, and antioxidant function. The laboratory has published over 100 articles, and Dr. Taylor edited this book, as well as a recent book on the Aminopeptidases. Dr. Taylor has been the recipient of a Guggenheim fellowship, a Fulbright Senior Scholar award, and grants from the National Institutes of Health, USDA, and other organizations. He has been the organizer of a FASEB summer conference on the Role of Antioxidants in Health and Disease and has been on the Program Planning Committee of the Association for Research in Vision and Ophthalmology.

CONTRIBUTORS

Ali H. Ali, B.Sc.
Ophthalmology Research
University of Maryland at Baltimore
School of Medicine
Baltimore, Maryland

Felix M. Barker, II
The Hafter Family Light and Laser Institute
The Pennsylvania College of Optometry
Philadelphia, Pennsylvania

George E. Brunce, Ph.D.
Department of Biochemistry & Nutrition
Virginia Polytechnic & State
University
Blacksburg, Virginia

William G. Christen, Sc.D.
Department of Medicine
Brigham & Women's Hospital
Boston, Massachusetts

Leo T. Chylack, Jr., M.D.
Division of Ophthalmology
Brigham & Women's Hospital
Boston, Massachusetts

John I. Clark, Ph.D.
Department of Biological Structure & Ophthalmology
University of Washington School of
Medicine
Seattle, Washington

Pierrette Dayhaw-Barker
The Hafter Family Light and Laser Institute
The Pennsylvania College of Optometry
Philadelphia, Pennsylvania

Palaniyandi S. Devamanoharan, Ph.D.
Ophthalmology Research
University of Maryland at Baltimore
School of Medicine
Baltimore, Maryland

Billy R. Hammond, Jr., Ph.D.
College of Arts & Sciences
Arizona State University, West Campus
Phoenix, Arizona

Toshihiko Hiraoka, M.D., Ph.D.
Department of Biological Structure
University of Washington School of
Medicine
Seattle, Washington

Ronald Klein, M.D.
Department of Ophthalmology
& Visual Sciences
University of Wisconsin
Madison, Wisconsin

Moshe Lahav, M.D.
Chief of Ophthalmology
NEEL Boston VA Medical Center
Boston, Massachusetts

Julie A. Mares-Perlman, Ph.D.
Department of Ophthalmology and
Visual Sciences
University of Wisconsin Medical
School
Madison, Wisconsin

Cathy McCarty, Ph.D., M.P.H., R.D.
The University of Melbourne
Department of Ophthalmology
The Royal Victorian Eye and Ear Hospital
East Melbourne, Australia

Wolfgang Schalch, Ph.D.
F. Hoffmann-La Roche Ltd.
Human Nutrition Research
Basel, Switzerland

D. Max Snodderly, Ph.D.
Schepens Eye Research Institute
Boston, Massachusetts

Allen Taylor, Ph.D.
Laboratory for Nutrition and Vision Research
Jean Mayer USDA Human Nutrition Research
Center on Aging at Tufts University
Boston, Massachusetts

Hugh R. Taylor, M.D., FRACO
The University of Melbourne
Department of Ophthalmology
The Royal Victorian Eye and Ear Hospital
East Melbourne, Australia

Shambhu D. Varma, Ph.D.
Ophthalmology Research
University of Maryland at Baltimore
School of Medicine
Baltimore, Maryland

Sheila K. West, Ph.D.
The Wilmer Institute
The Johns Hopkins University
School of Medicine
Baltimore, Maryland

DEDICATION

This book is dedicated to the friends and colleagues who supported me through the years of study. It is also dedicated to Jacob and Noa; may their future be as bright as the days of joy they have provided already. The book would not have occurred without the encouragement of Dr. Moshe Lahav. He always welcomed me to his clinic, to the operating room and to his enormous and broad base of knowledge. We owe our first successes in clinical/epidemiologic investigations to his personal and academic generosity. His recent passing leaves a gap that will be hard to fill. Finally, the tireless efforts of Esther Epstein, and the generous support of the Jean Mayer U.S.D.A. Human Nutrition Research Center on Aging at Tufts University, and other sources must be acknowledged.

DEDICATION

[illegible]

TABLE OF CONTENTS

NUTRITIONAL AND ENVIRONMENTAL INFLUENCES ON THE EYE

Chapter 1

LENS AND RETINA FUNCTION: INTRODUCTION AND CHALLENGE

Allen Taylor

Vision is one of the most valued senses. Proper vision is achieved by a series of eye tissues working in concert. In simplistic phenomenological terms, light is collected in the anterior portion of the eye by the cornea and lens. It passes to the posterior of the eye where, in the retina, the light energy is transduced first to biochemical signals and then converted to electrical impulses before being passed on to the brain. Since most eye debilities involve dysfunction in the lens or retina, this book focuses on studies which elucidate the etiologies of debilities which affect these organs.

The lens is an elegantly simple tissue. It is made of only two types of cells: epithelial cells, which have not yet completely differentiated and not yet elaborated the major gene products, and fiber cells, in which these processes have been initiated or even completed (see Fig. 2, Chapter 4). Like red blood cells, the lens synthesizes a restricted group of major gene products, called crystallins. The crystallins fill the fiber cells, and proper packing of the fiber cells and the molecules within the fibers results in a clear lens.

The retina is the thin, transparent, light-sensitive neural tissue that originates from central nervous system tissue during embryonic development (see Fig.1, Chapter 11). The macula is a structure near the center of the retina that contains the fovea. This specialized portion of the retina is responsible for the high-resolution vision that permits activities such as reading. This tissue contains photoreceptor cells (both rods and cones) and neurons that convert the light images into electrical signals. The retina depends on cells of the adjacent retinal pigment epithelium (RPE) for support of its metabolic functions. Surrounding these organs and within them there are many other biological and molecular players.

In order to perform its function, the lens must remain clear throughout life. Various insults, including photooxidation, result in alteration and crosslinking of the long-lived lens proteins. These eventually aggregate and precipitate out of the normally clear milieu. Such precipitates are involved in cataracts. From a functional perspective, cataract is an opacity of the eye's normally clear lens that interferes with vision. Cataract may develop at any time during life, although it is most often associated with advancing age. In addition to aging, cataract may be a consequence of diabetes and other metabolic disorders, trauma, exposure to ionizing radiation, or it may be inherited or congenital in nature.

The other major age-related lens problem, presbyopia, is the loss of the ability of the lens to focus from distant to near (known as accommodation), and involves rigidification of the lens. From a chemical and structural perspective, the modifications to lens proteins which result in cross-linking and thus, rigidification, are probably similar to changes involved in cataractogenenesis.

Photoreceptors in the retina, perhaps because of their huge energy requirements

0-8493-8565-2/99/$0.00+$.50

and highly differentiated state, are sensitive to a variety of genetic and environmental insults, many of which involve photooxidative stress. Thus, whereas the lens is avascular and the retina is highly vascularized and much more complex than the lens, the etiologies of these diseases may have much more in common than was previously thought.

The loss of central vision in macular degeneration (MD) is devastating. Degenerative changes to the macula (maculopathy) can occur at almost any time in life but are much more prevalent with advancing age. With growth in the aged population, age-related macular degeneration (AMD) will become a more prevalent cause of blindness than both diabetic retinopathy and glaucoma combined.

The inspiration for putting together this book was my conviction that we are on the verge of achieving a means to diminish the risk for cataract and AMD. In order to foster this process, I chose to focus attention on research areas that are required in order to achieve a delay in onset or progress of cataract or AMD. As a prerequisite it is important to devise uniform means to evaluate eye tissue change. This will allow more comparison of various studies than is currently possible. Thus, the sum will be greater than its parts. It is also hoped that this summary will be a harbinger of and inspiration for research to follow, research that will expand our understanding of lens and retinal dysfunction, and which will allow further progress in diminishing risk for onset and progress of these debilities. Diminishing risk for onset of these debilities is of obvious benefit. Diminishing risk for progress of these debilities will allow, for the first time, treatment for those persons with incipient disease.

Consideration of the problem on a personal level and from a public health perspective offers a compelling justification for this research. Worldwide, 50 percent of all blindness is due to cataract. Although cataract treatment in this country is one of the most successful procedures, the only treatment involves surgical removal of the natural lens and replacement with a plastic implant. Each year an estimated $3.4 billion is spent through the Medicare program alone on the ≈1.4 million procedures which are performed each year. It is estimated that there were almost 34 million Americans over the age of 65 in 1995, and, by the year 2030, this number will more than double, and medical costs due to cataract and AMD can be expected to consume an ever-increasing proportion of the Medicare budget. Clearly there would be major fiscal and personal benefits if a means to delay onset or progress of cataract or AMD could be achieved.

There have been several summaries of previous information about lens and retina function. These studies have been augmented by recent advances in methods to observe and document lens and retina function and composition, as well as by a myriad of laboratory investigations which provide more information regarding normal function of these tissues.

Many of the ideas presented in this book are based on contemporary studies and may be accordingly biased. For example, it is currently widely believed that dysfunction of the lens is due to age-related alterations to many lens molecules. Whereas the lens, when considered in its entirety, is probably one of the slowest metabolizing tissues and the retina is probably one of the fastest metabolizing tissues, these tissues are found within millimeters of each other. Evolving data indicate that the age-related alterations in the retina have common features with those described for the lens. The most common alteration is oxidative change. This is caused by the high-energy forms of oxygen or other oxidants (i.e., peroxynitrite) as well as the light to which the eye tissues are exposed. Proteins, lipids and carbohydrates all undergo oxidative changes. These changes beget further modification and result in dysfunction on the molecular level. Such changes may be compounded since the molecules which are responsible for repairing or removing damaged molecules may themselves also be damaged. Thus the aging eye is in multiple jeopardy. Both the original constituents are damaged and the repair machinery is also compromised in function. It should be noted that, whereas the phenomena are common to both tissues, the damaging moieties may not be identical.

Nutrients provide potent antioxidative influence and may be exploited to delay damage to these tissues. Eventually, pharmacological agents may also be designed to provide protection against the age-related stresses which these tissues must endure.

The book is roughly divided into two portions. The first portion emphasizes studies regarding the lens and the second gives more attention to the retina. However, since many phenomena which apply to one tissue also are relevant to the other, no clear delineation is intended and considerable effort was made to cross-reference the materials presented in each part of the text.

In order to present a contemporary overview of the field, the book starts in Chapter 2 with a theoretical explanation of oxidation and oxidative damage. This is followed in Chapter 3 by a description of the most modern means for evaluating lens opacity and changes in color. In Chapter 4 a summary is presented of many studies which describe age-related changes to the lens and the effects of nutrients on such changes in cell-free, *in vitro*, and whole animals. The chapter ends with a graphical summary of the clinical/epidemiological studies which seek to establish relationships between nutrition and risk for cataract in humans. Risk, in general, is given the most consideration, but risk for onset and progress of cataract is also discussed where possible. Various types of clinical studies are considered in this chapter. Accordingly, this chapter is followed in Chapter 5 by an evaluation of the value of various types of clinical studies. Most of the human studies had precedents in animal investigations, and these are documented briefly in Chapter 6. The advent of pharmacologicals to delay cataract onset or progress is on the horizon, and the means to evaluate such compounds and the results of some tests are summarized in Chapter 7.

In Chapters 8 and 9 the effects on age-related eye disease of light and smoking, respectively, are evaluated.

The focus of the text changes to the retina in Chapter 10. In this chapter various means to quantify retinal change are evaluated. This chapter is followed by a discussion of the etiology of age-related maculopathy and a summary of the clinical/epidemiological data regarding relationships between nutrition and risk for age-related maculopathy. Chapter 12 discusses the retinal carotenoids. New techniques are being developed to examine retinal constituents non-invasively, *in vivo,* in humans. A description of these very exciting developments concludes the book.

Chapter 2

OXYGEN RADICALS IN THE PATHOGENESIS OF CATARACTS– POSSIBILITIES FOR THERAPEUTIC INTERVENTION

Shambhu D. Varma, Ph.D., Palaniyandi S. Devamanoharan, Ph.D., and Ali H. Ali, B.Sc.

I. INTRODUCTION

Cataract is one of the major causes of visual impairment leading eventually to blindness. Fortunately, surgical removal of the cataract is successful in restoring adequate vision in most of the cases. However, the magnitude of the problem is so large that performing the surgery presents a significant public health burden. In the U.S.A. alone 1.35 million cataract extractions are performed every year. The problem is even much greater in the developing countries. Hence, studies on the pathogenesis of cataract and on development of pharmacological strategies to prevent its development have been very actively pursued over the last four decades. It is now well established that cataract formation is a multifactorial disease. This is apparent by the association of cataracts with a number of clinical conditions such as diabetes, galactosemia, hypoparathyroidism, myotonia, aminoaciduria, phenyl ketonuria, homocystinuria, mucopolysaccharidosis, premature aging syndromes and Wilson's disease, to name a few.[1-4] Cataract can also be induced by nutritional deficiency of certain amino acids such as tryptophan, proteins (hypoproteinemia) and hypovitaminosis-B_2.[5] Experimentally, it can also be induced by exposure to various wavelengths of ionizing as well as nonionizing radiations and certain heavy metals.[6,7] Most intriguingly, it develops simply as a function of age, irrespective of the presence or absence of any systemic disease. This category is usually classified as senile cataract or age dependent cataract. The maturation of this age dependent cataract, which is the most common cause of visual impairment, is indeed accelerated by some systemic diseases referred to above. Development of a common theory of age dependent cataract is therefore difficult. However some clues to common factors involved in the development of cataract can be derived from certain epidemiological studies. Sunlight has been suggested to be one such significant factor. A number of epidemiological studies have shown that the geographic incidence of cataract is positively correlated to the duration and intensity of sunlight.[8-10] The increased lens coloration and its brunescence with age have also been similarly correlated with sunlight. Since cataract-related damage also involves oxidation of lens constituents, it would appear that opacification and brunescence have common (photo) oxidative etiologies. In experimental animals as well as in human beings, opacification can also be induced by simple exposure to a high oxygen atmosphere.[11-12] These two findings led us to propose that light and oxygen constitute a synergistic pair in the onset of cataractogenic process associated with aging (senile), irrespective of any systemic disease.[13] In essence, it was proposed that a photochemical generation of certain reactive oxygen species (ROS) in the intraocular chambers surrounding the lens (aqueous humor, vitreous

0-8493-8565-2/99/$0.00+$.50

humor) as well as in the tissue itself could be a common factor in the genesis of the majority of cataracts. The significance of the reactive forms of oxygen in several other pathological manifestations associated with aging was first made obvious by studies from Harman et al.[14] Administration of 3-aminotriazole (an inhibitor of catalase) has also been reported to cause cataract formation in rabbits.[15] The significance of the proposal that an intraocular oxyradical generation might be a causative factor in the genesis of cataracts is now well supported by several experimental as well as epidemiological studies.

A. OXYGEN AND OXYRADICAL TOXICITY

That oxygen can become toxic was realized soon by its discoverer himself (Priestley, 1775), wherein it was observed that life processes burn too fast in the event if ambient oxygen is replaced by pure oxygen, apparently on account of its relatively high oxidizing power. This is the most electro-negative element after fluorine. The high reactivity of oxygen ($E^\circ=+0.82V$) was subsequently explained at a molecular level by Newman[16] and Pauling.[17]

Pauling's studies on the physical properties of oxygen demonstrated that the substance is paramagnetic. The paramagnetism of oxygen was explained on the basis of an unusual distribution of electrons in the various suborbitals.

As shown in Fig. 1, molecular oxygen (dioxygen) is exceptional in having the two electrons in the p^x2p antibonding orbitals in a parallel spin orientation. Quantum rules (Paulis' exclusion principle) of electron addition, according to which no two electrons in an atom or a molecule can have the same set of quantum numbers, impose a spin restriction for a direct divalent reduction of oxygen at ambient temperatures incapable of causing spin inversion. Hence the reduction of oxygen in most biochemical processes, associated with metabolic or chemical oxidation of oxidizable substrates, must proceed through univalent steps of electron addition. The availability of a pair of electrons in most reducing molecules with parallel spins and with orientations opposite to that in dioxygen is not known. Hence the first product derived from oxygen in the process of its reduction to water, hydrogen peroxide, carbon dioxide or other oxygenation reactions is superoxide radical ($O_2^{\cdot-}$). Hence a relatively less reactive oxygen molecule is converted to superoxide, a more highly reactive free radical, capable of oxidizing other substances by acting as a potent acceptor of reducing equivalents as the superoxide is further reduced to the peroxide di-anion. In addition, superoxide can act as a reductant as it reverts to molecular oxygen. Both the phenomena can cause tissue toxicity. The superoxide anion undergoes prompt self dismutation with the production of hydrogen peroxide (H_2O_2) and water ($O_2^{\cdot-} + O_2^{\cdot-} + 2H^+ \rightarrow H_2O_2 + O2$, $\Delta E^\circ = 0.64$ volts, $\Delta G^\circ = -29.3$ k.cal mole^{-1} deg^{-1}). Although the dismutation process is thermodynamically very favorable, the rate of dismutation is increased severalfold by superoxide dismutases, enzymes known to be present in most tissues including that in the lens (Fig. 2).

The presence of the enzyme in the lens was described simultaneously from three laboratories including the author's laboratory.[18-20] Hence this enzyme offers the first line of defense against oxygen radical damage in the lens as in other body

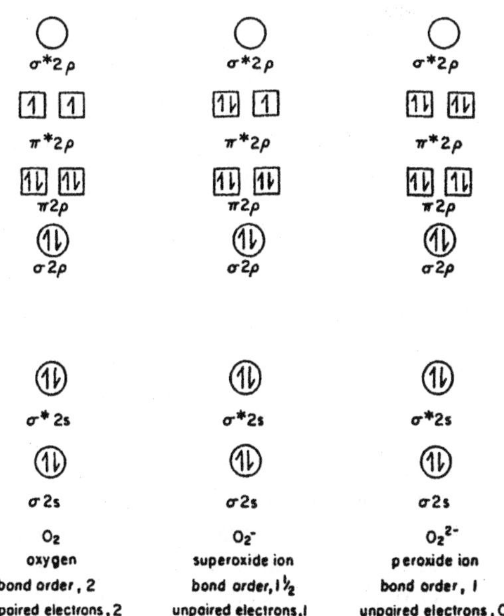

Figure 1. Molecular Orbital Energy Level Diagrams for Oxygen, Superoxide Anion, and the Peroxide Anion: Note the presence of unpaired electrons in π*2p orbitals of oxygen and its sequential filling up during conversion to superoxide (O_2^{-}) and peroxide (O_2^{2-}) anions. Electrons only with principal quantum number 2 have been shown. From Varma, S.D. et al., *Curr. Eye Res.*, 3, 35-57, 1984. With permission.

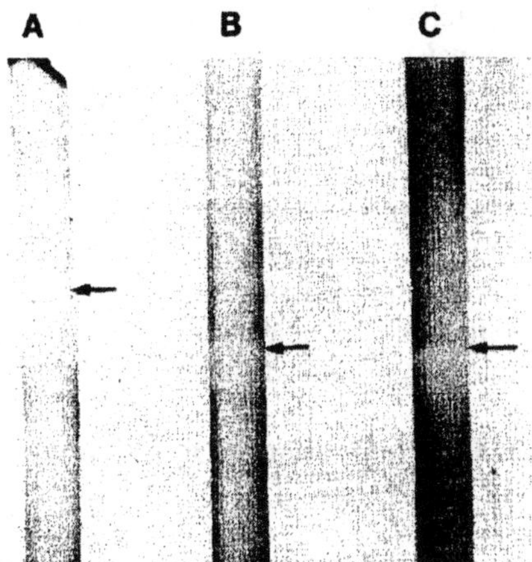

Figure 2. Identification of superoxide dismutase in lens: An aqueous extract of lens protein (200 μg) prepared by homogenization of rat lens in water and centrifugation at 17,000 x g was applied to 10% polyacrylamide gel and electrophoresed. The enzyme activity was localized by successive immersion of the gel in buffers containing nitroblue tetrazolium and riboflavin with TEMED and exposure to light. The enzyme activity was discerned by the appearance of achromatic bands. A = Sigma Bovine. SOD; B = Human Lens; C = Rat Lens. From Varma S.D. et al., *Curr. Eye Res.*, 3, 35-57, 1984. With permission.

tissues. Akin to most other lens enzymes, superoxide dismutase is localized in the epithelial and cortical fibers of the tissue, the nuclear fibers being unprotected.

The H_2O_2 formed by $O_2^{\cdot-}$ dismutation, although a relatively weak oxidant, can become highly toxic by generating $OH^{\cdot}$, especially in the presence of multivalent metal ions. The reaction is commonly referred to as Fenton's-Haber Weiss reaction,[21,22] and is represented as follows.

$$Fe^{+++} + O_2^{\cdot -} \rightarrow Fe^{++} + O_2$$
$$Fe^{++} + H_2O_2 \rightarrow Fe^{+++} + OH^- + OH^{\cdot}$$

$$O_2^{\cdot -} + H_2O_2 \rightarrow OH^{\cdot} + OH^- + O_2$$

The toxicity due to H_2O_2 is preventable by catalase as well as glutathione peroxidase. Both the enzymes are known to be present in the epithelium and cortical fibers.[23,24] In addition, the lens contains a very high concentration of GSH, required as a co-substrate for glutathione peroxidase.[25] Other related protective enzymes are the enzymes of the HMP shunt involved in the maintenance of GSH levels.

B. OXYRADICAL DAMAGE AND CATARACT FORMATION

Based on the higher incidence of cataracts in populations exposed to excessive sunlight, coupled with the experimental findings on lens damage due to exposure to excessive oxygen, the possibility of oxyradical involvement in the pathogenesis of cataracts and other age related eye diseases appears more highly relevant.[13,26-28] By virtue of the transparency of the cornea, aqueous, lens and retina, the eye offers a unique situation for an incessant *in vivo* (intraocular) photochemical generation of oxy-radicals in its component tissues as well as in the bathing extracellular fluids (aqueous and vitreous), at least during long periods of photopic vision. Increasing intensity of light would apparently increase the cataractogenic insult. The amount of oxyradicals produced in the eye by photochemical reactions would be additive to that produced under ambient dark conditions by non-photochemical reactions. The continuous generation of $O_2^{\cdot -}$, and its derivatives H_2O_2 and $OH^{\cdot}$, can be explained by the following set of redox reactions catalyzed by light.

Photochemical Generation of $O_2^{\cdot -}$ and its Derivatives
Cyclic Production of Active Oxygen

$$Rb \xrightarrow{hv} Rb^*$$
$$Rb^* + 2H^+ + 2e^- \rightarrow RbH_2$$
$$RbH_2 + O_2 \quad Rb + O_2^{\cdot -} + 2H^+$$
$$2O_2^{\cdot -} + 2H+ \quad H_2O_2 + O_2$$
$$H_2O_2 + O_2^{\cdot -} \quad OH^- + OH^{\cdot} + O2$$

The cyclic nature of reaction is emphasized. Rb: Photosensitizer

As indicated above, a small amount of a photosensitizer, if present in any ocular fluid or tissues such as in the aqueous and the lens, can lead to a continuous generation of $O_2^{\cdot-}$ and its derivatives such as H_2O_2 and $OH^{\cdot}$, as long as the person's eyes are open, light is penetrating through, and oxygen and reducing equivalents are present in situ. The superoxide radical and its derivatives would be generated repeatedly through the above cyclic series of reactions. While the tissues supposedly detoxify the oxyradicals enzymatically, these enzymes are normally not present in the aqueous. Hence reactive forms of oxygen would not be adequately scavenged. It is also known that in most cataracts the pathological process is triggered by an initial damage to the epithelial cell membranes, exposed directly to the aqueous environ, by the ROS generated in the aqueous medium. This has been shown to be the case by several *in vitro* lens culture experiments.[29-33]

As summarized in Table 1, culture of rat lenses in the presence of light in a medium containing μM quantities of riboflavin acting as a photosensitizer leads to severe physiological damage. That this is due primarily to an initial membrane damage is evidenced by a decrease in its ability to transport rubidium ions (surrogate to K^+) against an electrochemical gradient as summarized in Table 1. The decreased transport is apparent by a lowering of the distribution ratio of the cation between lens water and the medium of incubation attained after an overnight (18 hr) culture. That the observed decrease is due to the damaging effects of the

TABLE 1
Uptake of ^{86}Rb by the Rat Lens Incubated in Light in Medium Containing Riboflavin: Effect of Various Scavengers

Conditions	n	CL/CM	E/C x 100
Blank control	20	22.0 ± 3.0	
-SOD (control)	20	5.06 ± 2.27	
+8 units Mn SOD	9	9.19 ± 2.98	166.9 ± 26.9*
+20 units Mn SOD	11	10.04 ± 2.75	198.2 ± 34.8*
-Catalase (control)	20	6.5 ± 2.5	
+4 units catalase	10	20.0 ± 3.00	307.0 ± 80.0*
+16 units catalase	10	21.0 ± 2.00	323.0 ± 80.0*
-$Na_3Fe(CN)_6$ (control)	16	7.44 ± 1.43	
+5 μM $Na_3Fe(CN)_6$	8	20.44 ± 2.35	213.2 ± 39.8*
+10 μM $Na_3Fe(CN)_6$	8	20.88 ± 3.97	280.2 ± 18.4*
-$Na_4Fe(CN)_6$	10	7.00 ± 1.47	
+5 μM $Na_4Fe(CN)_6$	5	19.55 ± 2.00	
+10 μM $Na_4Fe(CN)_6$	5	19.97 ± 3.86	223.3 ± 15.1*
-Mannitol (control)	7	6.02 ± 3.20	
+100 μM mannitol	8	11.05 ± 3.00	138.9 ± 34.5*
+$FeSO_4$ (5 μM)(control)	8	8.33 ± 2.19	
+$FeSO_4$ (5 μM) + 100 μM mannitol	10	12.09 ± 3.07	156.6 ± 31.3*

Note: The blank control consisted of lenses incubated in the dark in medium containing 50 μM riboflavin. In other cases, the controls and corresponding experimentals were incubated in light for a period of 18 to 20 h and CL/CM determined. The values have been expressed as mean ± SD. An asterisk indicates that the values are significantly different from the contralateral controls; $p<0.001$. CL - concentration of ^{86}Rb in the initial medium of incubation. From Varma, S.D. and Mooney, *J., Free Radic. Biol. Med.*, 57-62, 1986. With permission.

reactive forms of oxygen has been ascertained by the preventive effect of several oxygen radical scavengers as indicated in the table.[24]

C. ASCORBATE IN LENS PHYSIOLOGY

It is interesting to find that such a lens damage does occur, despite the fact that tissue contains all the components of the battery of protective enzymes that are found in other cells. However, the cell membranes which are exposed to the aqueous environ are not enzymatically protected. The long latent period required for cataract-development *in vivo* suggests that in the natural condition there are additional factors involved in protecting the cell membranes from oxidative damage. It is highly likely that the high concentration of ascorbate present in the primate aqueous may perform such a function.[35-37] This hypothesis is supported by several observations.

As summarized in Tables 2 and 3, the concentration of ascorbic acid in most of the ocular tissue is substantially higher in comparison to other tissues. This is so especially when one compares the extracellular fluid such as the cerebrospinal fluid. The aqueous humor concentration is hence one of the highest. This high concentration is maintained by an active transport of ascorbate from the plasma to the aqueous across the blood aqueous barrier, maintaining an approximately 20x higher concentration in the latter.

TABLE 2
Ascorbic Acid Content of Certain Mammalian Tissues

Brain	110		
Pancreas	95		
Liver	64		
Spleen	81		
Kidney	47		
Lung	45		
Heart	21		
Thymus	45		
White Blood Cells & Platelets	250		
Epididymis	140		
Ovary (S Corpus Luteum)	280		
Adrenal	220		
Cornea	240		
Lens	250	Saliva	1
Aqueous Humor	200	Seminal Vesicle Secretion	50
Vitreous	360	Urine	2-25
Retina (dog)	115	Blood' s WBC & Platelets	10 mg
Choroid (dog)	250	Serum	10 mg
Ciliary Body (dog)	90	CSF	10 mg
Sclera (rabbit)	140		

Values are collected from literature[35-37] and have been expressed as mg/kg of the wet tissue weight or mg/L in case of liquids. Adapted from: Bessey O.A. and King, *C.G., J. Biol. Chem*:, 1933; Long, C., *Biochemists Handbook*, 1961; and Taylor, A. et al., *Curr. Eye Res.*, 1997.

TABLE 3
Levels of Vitamin C in Lens and Aqueous Humor[36]

Animal	Aqueous Humor mmol/L	Lens mmol/kg wet weight
Man	1.00 ± 0.20	1.25 ± 0.45
Monkey	1.00 ± 0.10	Unknown
Horse	1.20 ± 0.20	3.02 ± 0.20
Ox	1.08 ± 0.20	2.04 ± 0.45
Rabbit	1.70 ± 0.60	0.74 ± 0.34
Sheep	1.20 ± 0.20	1.81 ± 0.60
Guinea pig	0.75 ± 0.50	0.65 ± 0.10
Pig	0.57 ± 0.03	1.20 ± 0.35
Dog	0.31 ± 0.03	0.20 ± 0.10
Cat	0.07 ± 0.04	-
Galago	0.03 ± 0.02	-
Rat	0	0.08 ± 0.08

x ± SEM. Adapted from Long, C.,[36] *Biochemists Handbook*, 1961. Also see Chapter 4.

Thus the ascorbate concentration is higher in the diurnal animals in comparison to nocturnal and arrhythmic animals and can be construed as an evolutionary response to the diurnal life where photo-oxidative stress in the eye is much greater in comparison to the nocturnal animals. Supporting this hypothesis is the low concentration of ascorbate in the eye, in utero.

Thermodynamically, ascorbate reacts with most of the reactive oxygen species, albeit with different efficacy.

The rate constants of its reactivity with various ROS have been summarized in Table 4.[38-40] Ascorbate is maximally active with $OH^{\cdot}$, one of the most potent oxidants.[39] Hence it was proposed that the function of a high concentration of ascorbate in human aqueous and lens is to protect it against the oxidative damage induced by reactive oxygen and thereby participate in prolonging the clarity of the lens in humans and other diurnal animals.[13,29] However, in view of the fact that it can under certain conditions also act as an oxidant, further experimental verification of the above hypothesis is considered crucial. This was initially accomplished in the lens organ culture system wherein lenses were cultured in medium-199, containing the full complement of the ingredients present in the normal aqueous, and containing riboflavin (50 μM) as a photosensitizer.

As summarized in Fig. 3, the transport of rubidium ion is greatly inhibited in the lens incubated in light (150 ft candle-white daylight) for 18 hours. But, such an inhibition is substantially attenuated when the physiological level of ascorbate was incorporated into the riboflavin medium. Hence, this was the first demonstration in support of the hypothesis that one of the main functions of ascorbate in the aqueous is to protect the lens membranes from undergoing oxidative damage.[29]

This was proven further by culture experiments in the dark, wherein the oxy-radicals were generated by the addition of xanthine and xanthine oxidase to the medium.

TABLE 4
The Energetics of Ascorbate Reaction with Xanthine: Oxygen Interaction Products Catalyzed by Xanthine Oxidase[38-40]

	nΔEo′ (V)	ΔGo′ (kJ mol^{-1})	Rate constant
$HA^- \longrightarrow A + H^+ + 2e$	−0·108		
$H_2O_2 + 2H^+ + 2e \longrightarrow 2H_2O$	+2·640		
*$HA^- + H_2O_2 + H^+ \longrightarrow A + 2H_2O$	2·532	−245	8 $M^{-1}s^{-1}$
$HA^- \longrightarrow A^{\cdot -} + H^+ + e$	−0·282		
$OH^{\cdot} + H^+ + e \longrightarrow H_2O$	+2·180		
†$HA^- + OH^{\cdot} \longrightarrow H_2O + A^{\cdot -}$		−184	$1{\cdot}3 \times 10^{10} M^{-1}s^{-1}$
‡$HA^- + O_2^- \longrightarrow$ Products		−64	$5 \times 10^4 M^{-1}s^{-1}$

*Determined from the initial rate of ascorbate and H_2O_2 disappearance from the medium on incubation.[38]
†Farhataziz and Ross (1977).
‡Cabelli and Bielski.
§Assuming that H_2O_2 and $A^{\cdot}$ are the products.
From Varma S.D. et al., *Exp. Eye Res.*, 43, 1067-1076, 1986. With permission.

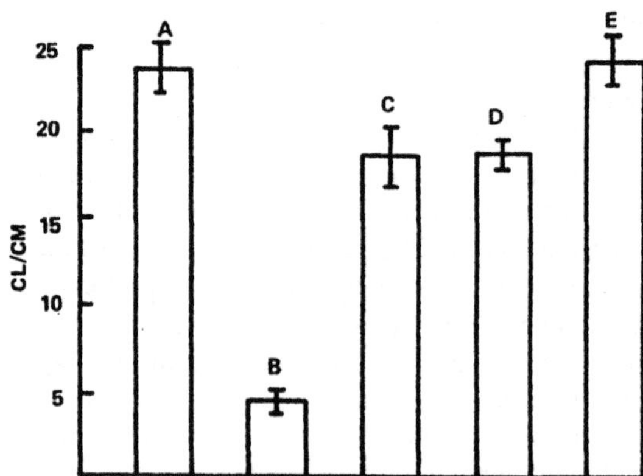

Figure 3. Effect of riboflavin phosphate and light on the uptake of Rb^+ by rat lens in organ culture. A) Control with riboflavin phosphate in dark; B) With riboflavin phosphate, 50 μm in light; C) With riboflavin phosphate and SOD, ≈4 units/ml in light; D) With ascorbic acid, 2.5 mm in light; E) With catalase, ≈4 units/ml in light. Adapted from Varma, S.D., *Red Blood Cell and Metabolism*, Srivastava, S.K., Ed., Elsevier, No. Holland, 1980.

Again, as summarized in Table 5, the inhibition of the rubidium pump resulting from oxy-radical damage is preventable by the addition of physiological concentrations of ascorbate. The secondary active transport process as determined by α-aminoisobutric acid translocation is also fully protected.[38] Taylor et al. demonstrated that dietary ascorbate can prevent photochemically induced deactivation of the enzyme leucine aminopeptidase.[41] The brown color development on lenses incubated in UV light is also preventable by ascorbate.[42,43]

TABLE 5
Lens Damage by Xanthine-Xanthine Oxidase: Preventive Effect of Ascorbate

Additions to the medium	CL/CM	E/C x 100 (n)
	Rubidium Uptake	
C None (6)	21 ± 5	
E Na ascorbate 1.0 mM (2)	21 ± 2.0	100
E Na ascorbate 2.0 mM (3)	21.5 ± 0.5	102
C XA, 1 mM	19 ± 1.5	
E XA + XO, 0.1 unit (6)	4.5 ± 1.0	24
C XA + XO, 0.1 unit	5.2 ± 0.5	
E XA + XO, 0.1 unit + Na ascorbate, 2 mM (10)	10.4 ± 0.4	200
C XA + XO, 0.1 unit	4.54 ± 0.4	
E XA + XO, 0.1 unit + DHA, 2.5 mM (5)	4.78 ± 0.28	105
	AIB Uptake	
XA (4)	5.5 ± 0.5	
C XA + XO, 0.1 unit	1.48 ± 0.38	
E XA + XO, 0.1 unit + (7) Na ascorbate, 2 mM	3.0 ± 0.47	203
C XA + XO, 0.1 unit	0.92 ± 0.31	
E XA + XO, 0.1 unit + DHA, 2.5 mM (5)	1.0 ± 0.5	108

Note: Paired lenses were incubated as C and E in the medium with additions indicated above. Rubidium and AIB were used as ^{86}RbCl and ^{14}C AIB, respectively. XA, xanthine; XO, xanthine oxidase; n, number of contralateral pairs used in each group of experiments; AIB, alpha aminoisobutyric acid; C, control; E, contralateral lenses incubated as experimental.[42,43] From Varma, S.D. et al., *Exp. Eye Res.*, 43, 1067-1076, 1986.

D. *IN VIVO* EFFECT OF ASCORBATE

One of the most difficult problems, however, has been to verify and establish the anticataractogenic effect of ascorbate *in vivo*. The most suitable animal for experiments on ascorbate deficiency is the guinea pig. However, these animals do not develop cataract when ascorbate deficiency is induced. Nevertheless, studies from this laboratory have demonstrated that lenses of such animals when fed simultaneously with a 30% galactose diet are more susceptible to membrane damage, when compared to animals fed with an ascorbate-sufficient diet containing 30% galactose, as evident by a greater leakage of ^{51}Cr in the former case. These findings demonstrate that vitamin C deficiency indeed contributes to the overall cataractogenic process. The matter, however, needs further resolution.

Recently, a more clear in vivo demonstration of the anti-cataractogenic effect of ascorbate has now been accomplished by the use of a sodium selenite model of cataracts in young rats.[44] An intraperitoneal injection of 0.5 micromole of sodium selenite to rat pups by the 10th day postnatally leads to a very reproducible formation of nuclear cataracts by the 5th day after injection.[32] The incidence of cataract in these animals is about 95% or greater.

As shown in Fig. 4, a simultaneous treatment with ascorbate leads to a substantial prevention of cataracts.[45] The incidence of cataracts in the ascorbate-treated group is only about 20-30%. Additionally, the preventive effect is also reflected by the biochemical parameters.

At least six lenses were analyzed in each case, except when MDA was determined. Values of ATP, GSH and soluble protein were obtained from analyses of single lenses. MDA determination was done on a homogenate derived from a pool of at least four lenses (from four animals), the contralateral lens being used in other experiments. Figures have been expressed as mean $\pm$ SD: A) data from normal pups; B) the pups were treated with sodium selenite on the 10th day postnatally; C&D) the pups received vitamin C intraperitoneally starting at postnatal day 8 until the termination on the 21st day. They also received sodium

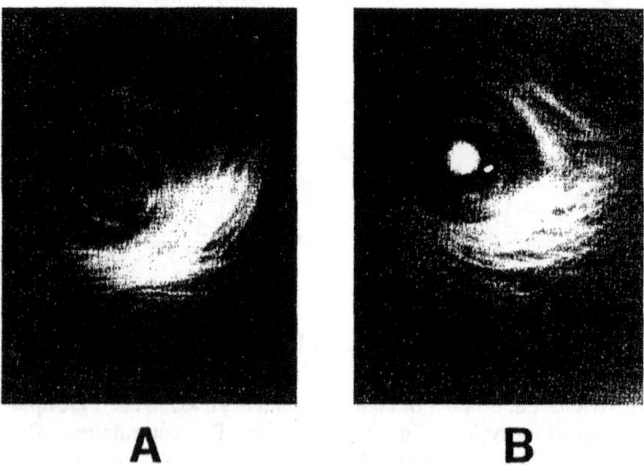

Figure 4. Pictures of the eyes of representative animals from the control (A) and experimental (B) groups. The white rim in both the cases represents the reflection of the circular light tube adjusted to a proper height as described in methods. The photographs were taken using a Zeiss operating microscope attached with a Polaroid camera, using a black and white film. The pictures were taken at x 25 magnification with an exposure time of approximately 1/30 sec. From Devamanoharan, P.S. et al., *Exp. Eye Res.* 52, 563-568, 1991. With permission.

selenite as in group B on the 10th day. Animals in group C had cataracts while those in group D did not. The starting weight of the pups was 20 ± 3 g. Final weight of the pups in all groups was 35 ± 5 g. Lenses were analyzed on the 21st day postnatally. Values marked with asterisks in groups C and D are significantly different from that in group B. *P<0.001; **P<0.05.[45]

As summarized in Table 6, the level of ATP in the lenses of selenite-injected pups was only ≈500 nmoles/gm lens, as compared to ≈1800 nmoles/gm lens in rats of the control group. However, treatment of the selenite-group with ascorbate protected against this fall in ATP, even in the small percentage of rats that developed cataracts despite ascorbate treatment. The involvement of oxidation in cataract formation was however more apparent from the significant decrease of GSH observed in the lenses of rats injected with selenite. The antioxidant effect of ascorbate is evident by a better maintenance of GSH levels in the lenses of selenite-rats treated with ascorbate. Simultaneously, ascorbate was shown to prevent buthionine sulfoximine-induced cataracts in mice as well.[46] This compound has been shown to cause cataracts by inhibiting GSH synthesis.[47] It is interesting to note that sodium selenite also depletes the tissue GSH levels, presumably due to oxidation.[48,49]

Additionally, ascorbate administration prevented against the increased lipid peroxidation observed in the lenses of selenite-treated rats, demonstrating once again the potential antioxidant and anticataractogenic nature of this important nutrient.

TABLE 6
ATP, GSH, Soluble Protein, and Malonaldehyde Contents of Rat Lenses

	Group of Animals			
	A	**B**	**C**	**D**
	untreated	selenite	ascorbate	ascorbate
ATP (nmol g^{-1} lens)	1759 ± 330	583 ± 235	1138 ± 209*	1616 ± 210*
GSH (μmol g^{-1} lens)	5.4 ± 0.5	1.6 ± 0.6	3.5 ± 0.5*	3.7 ± 0.2*
Soluble protein (mg g^{-1} lens)	380 ± 45	255 ± 33	320 ± 41**	334 ± 17*
MDA (nmol g^{-1} lens)	5 ± 1.0	17.6 ± 1.8	6.7 ± 3.0*	7.0 ± 0.9*

From Devamanoharan, P.S. et al., *Exp. Eye Res.* 52, 563-568, 1991. With permission.

E. ROLE OF PYRUVATE IN CATARACT PREVENTION

As noted above, the main endogenous antioxidants of the cells consist of the battery of oxyradical scavenging enzymes such as superoxide dismutase, catalase and glutathione peroxidase, along with some secondary participating enzymes like glucose-6-phosphate dehydrogenase, glutathione reductase and glutathione-s-transferase. However the distribution of these enzymes in the cell is not uniform, being mostly cytosolic. In addition, they are unable to prevent buried site-specific oxidation. The effect of antioxidants such as ascorbate may also become self-limiting due to the poor dietary intake and the decreased activity of the blood-aqueous barrier with aging. In view of these limitations, we have undertaken a study on the possibility of preventing oxidative stress and cataract formation by certain low molecular weight endogenous compounds of metabolic origin, such that they may not be toxic to the tissues. We propose that pyruvate, an α-keto acid, produced as the end product of glycolysis, and present in the cytosol and in the mitochondria as well as in the extracellular fluids, could perform the role of an effective antioxidant. These studies are based on original findings of Holleman (1904) who demonstrated that it can scavenge hydrogen peroxide via peroxidative decarboxylation, producing acetic acid, water and carbon dioxide, all being harmless.[50] Subsequently, it has been shown to prevent certain bacterial strains against oxygen toxicity.[51] In addition, we have demonstrated that it can scavenge superoxide radical as well,[52] thus ultimately preventing the formation of the potent $OH^{\cdot}$. These radical-scavenging properties of pyruvate prompted us to study in detail its possible anticataractogenic function in the lens. Initially, we studied this possibility through *in vitro* experiments using a rat lens organ culture system generating oxyradicals enzymatically.[33] Hence, lenses were cultured in medium-199, containing xanthine/xanthine oxidase; its ability to accumulate rubidium ions against a concentration gradient measured in the absence or presence of pyruvate. Lenses were cultured in basal medium with or without pyruvate. Similar experiments were also performed by direct addition of hydrogen peroxide to the medium in the absence or presence of pyruvate.[33]

As shown in Table 7, pyruvate prevented the *in vitro* oxyradical damage to the lens cation pump induced by xanthine/xanthine oxidase, as well as by direct peroxide addition to the medium. It also prevents against the simultaneous loss of ATP (Fig. 5), GSH (Fig. 6) and soluble proteins (Table 8).

TABLE 7
Effect of Pyruvate (PY) on the Uptake of Rubidium by Rat Lens from Medium to which H_2O_2 was Added Directly

	CL/CM	E/C x 100	% of blank control
A: Blank control(xanthine 0.5 mM)	10.1 ± 0.5		
B: A + PY (5 mM)		11.5 ± 0.8	114 ± 5
C: A + Xanthine oxidase		6.1 ± 0.6	
D: C + PY (5 mM)		10 ± 1.0	164 ± 16
99*			
E: Blank control (TC 199)		8.9 ± 0.5	
F: E + PY (5 mM)		9.6 ± 0.4	108 ± 10
G: E+ H_2O_2 (0.2 mM)		5.4 ± 1.2	
H: G + PY (5 mM)		11 ± 0.5	204 ± 24
124*			

Lenses were incubated in 4 ml of TC 199 medium for 3.5 h with additions indicated above. The results are expressed as mean ± SD. The values marked with an asterisk are significant P<0.001. CL-concentration of ^{86}Rb in lens water, CM-concentration of ^{86}Rb in the initial medium of incubation. From Varma, S.D. and Morris, S.M., *Free Radic. Res. Commun.*, 4, 283-290, 1988. With permission.

Pyruvate was also effective in protecting the lens gainst oxidative stress caused by the photochemical system, as apparent from the results summarized in Table 9, demonstrating that it can protect the lens against oxyradicals generated either ambiently or photochemically.[53]

As suggested earlier, in these *in vitro* models, catarctogenesis is induced primarily by an initial membrane damage, followed by subsequent intracellular

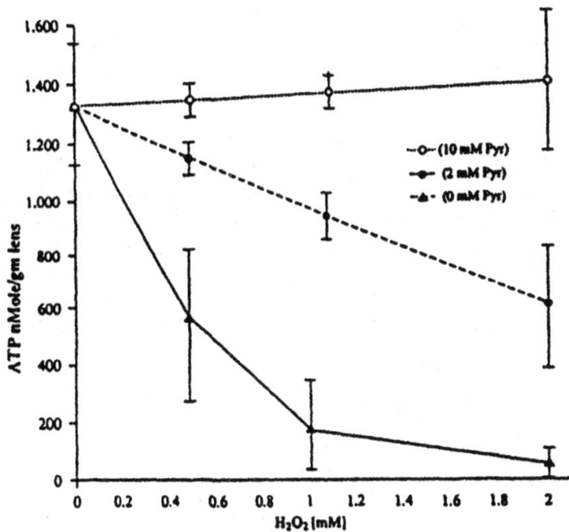

Figure 5. Depletion of ATP by H_2O_2: Effect of Pyruvate. From Varma, S.D. et al., *Curr. Eye Res.*, 14, 643-649. With permission.

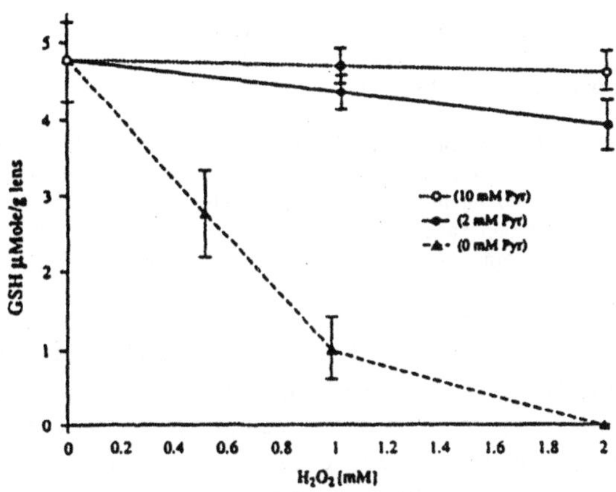

Figure 6. Depletion of GSH by H_2O_2: Effect of Pyruvate. From Varma, S.D, et al., *Curr. Eye Res.*, 14, 643-649. With permission.

TABLE 8
Insoluble Protein Generation by H_2O_2: Effect of Pyruvate

	(A) H_2O_2 concentration (mM)	(B) Pyruvate (mM)	(C) WS protein (mg/g)	(D) US protein (mg/g)	(E) WS/US
1	0	-	373* ± 6	24* ± 4	15.5
2	0.5	-	368 ± 8	28 ± 6	13.5
3	1.0	-	346 ± 12	41 ± 8	8.5
4	2.0	-	281* ± 17	92* ± 8	3.05
5	2.0	5.0	348 ± 17	38 ± 13	9.15
6	2.0	10	370* ± 12	26* ± 8	14.2
7	0	10	372 ± 5	23 ± 5	16.2

Rat lenses weighing 16 mg were used. Two lenses were incubated in 4 ml of TC 199 medium at 37°C in an atmosphere of 95:5 air/CO_2 mixture for 16 hours, with additions described above. Soluble (WS) and insoluble fractions were separated by centrifugation at 6000 x g. The insoluble pellet was washed twice with phosphate buffered saline (PBS), mixed in 300 µl of 7M urea containing 0.05M Tris, pH 7.4 and microfuged to obtain the supernatant representing the urea soluble fraction (US). Protein was then determined on both the fractions. The values are described as mean ± S.D. The $n \geq 4$, P values between 1 & 4 and 6 & 4, columns C & D are <0.001. These values are marked with an asterisk. From Varma, S.D. et al., *Curr. Eye Res.*, 14, 643-649, 1995.

TABLE 9
Uptake of Rubidium: Effect of Light and Pyruvate

Incubation period	Incubation condition	CL/CM	E/C x 100
4 h	Dark	10.3 ± 1.3	100
	Dark + pyruvate	12.5 ± 1.0	121*
	Light	4.0 ± 1.0	39
	Light + pyruvate	8.1 ± 2.5	202*
16 h	Dark	19.0 ± 2.0	100
	Dark + pyruvate	22.0 ± 2.0	114
	Light	5.4 ± 1.1	28
	Light + pyruvate	13 ± 5.3	233*

Rat lenses were incubated for 4 to 16 hours in TC 199 medium containing 150 µM riboflavin, in the absence and presence of daylight. The concentration of pyruvate when used was 10 mM. The results are expressed as the ratio of ^{86}Rb counts in lens water to that in the initial medium (mean ± SD). The number of experiments in each group was at least six. Values marked with an asterisk are statistically significant with P<0.01.53. From Varma, S.D. et al., *Exp. Eye Res.*, 50, 805-812, 1990. With permission.

changes. Moreover, the radicals are generated and scavenged in the medium outside the lens, simulating an *in vivo* situation where the lens is bathed in the aqueous and vitreous. Hence, in order to assess the efficacy of pyruvate in preventing intracellular damage, we have recently developed a new *in vitro* system using the quinone menadione, which generates oxyradicals by redox-cycling. Pyruvate, as well as its ester, was found to protect the lens against quinone-mediated damage as evident from the results summarized in Table 10.

TABLE 10
Menadione-Induced Damage to Lens: Prevention by Pyruvate and its Ester

	ATP nmole/gm	GSSG µmol/gm	GSH µmol/gm	water insoluble protein mg/lens
A Menadione (40 µM)	222 ± 95	0.65 ± .034	1.04 ± 0.13	55.83 ± 5.9
B Pyruvate(5mM)	533 ± 289	0.332 ± .07	0.97 ± 0.3	47.83 ± 12.7
C Pyruvate ester (5 mM)	1216 ± 388	0.388 ± .034	2.10 ± 0.58	41.05 ± 1.6
D Blank control	2147 ± 274	0.201 ± 0.02	3.68 ± 1.0	36.01 ± 8.7

The number of lenses used in determining each of these parameters was 6 in each case. The results are expressed as Mean ± Standard Deviation. P values are as follows:
ATP: Between A&D ≤.001, A&B ≤.001, A&C <.001
Water insoluble: Between A&D ≤ .005, A&B N.S., A&C = .05
GSH: Between A&D ≤.001, A&B ≤N.S., A&C <.001.
From Varma, S.D. et al., *Free Radic. Res.*, 28, 131-135, 1998. With permission.

It is interesting to see that the ester form is more effective than pyruvate, possibly due to its better penetration into the lens.[54] Finally, it has also been shown to prevent the formation of cataracts *in vivo* in the selenite model, as well as in the sugar model. In the selenite model, 0.5 mmoles of pyruvate was administered intraperitoneally to the rats that received 0.5 micromole of selenite on the 10th day postnatally. This dose of pyruvate prevented the cataract formation as apparent from Fig. 7.[55]

In the case of the sugar model, topical application of pyruvate as eye drops (10% and 15%) was tested using rats fed a 30% galactose-containing diet. In the group of rats that received 15% pyruvate eye drops, cataract formation was almost completely inhibited, as apparent from the pictures of the representative eyes from various groups (Fig. 8).[56] In this case, the preventive effect is probably related to a competitive inhibition of polyol formation, as well as to the inhibition of an oxidative stress.

The inhibition of polyol formation by pyruvate is attributed to its ability to divert the reducing equivalents (NADPH) required for aldose reductase catalyzed reduction of galactose to dulcitol, towards its reduction to lactate catalyzed by lactate dehydrogenase. This dual mode of action of pyruvate, coupled with its ability to support the tissue in providing the energy source[57] through the citric acid cycle and its possible non-toxic nature, have prompted us to pursue more actively on the use of other keto acids and their derivatives in the development of a possible pharmacological treatment against cataractogenesis.

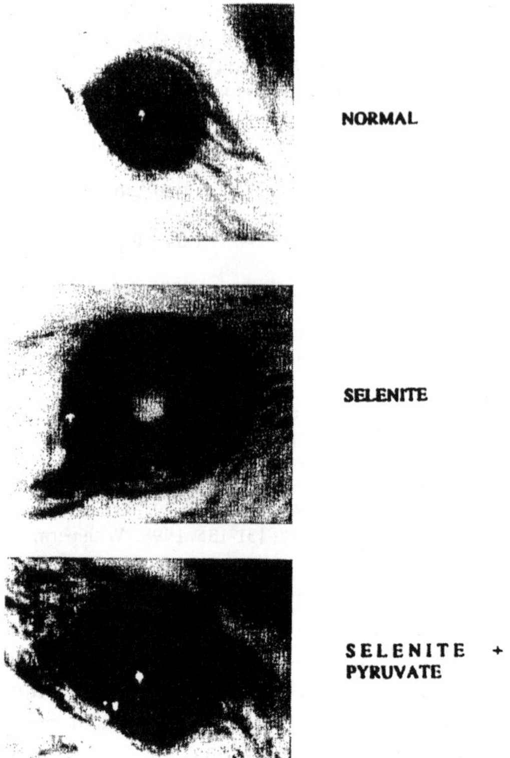

Figure 7. Photographs of the eyes of representative normal, selenite, and selenite plus pyruvate treated rat pups. The weight of the animals at this stage was 35 ± 5 gm. Photographs were taken with a video digital system and copied with normal photography. The pictures were taken 25 days postnatally and 15 days after selenite injection. The total number of animals in each group was at least 8. The experiments were repeated 3 times. 85 ± 5 percent of the animals in the pyruvate treated group did not develop central opacity against a similar percentage of animals in the selenite alone group who developed cataracts as shown in the photograph. From Varma, S.D. et al., *Curr. Eye Res.*, 14, 643-649, 1995. With permission.

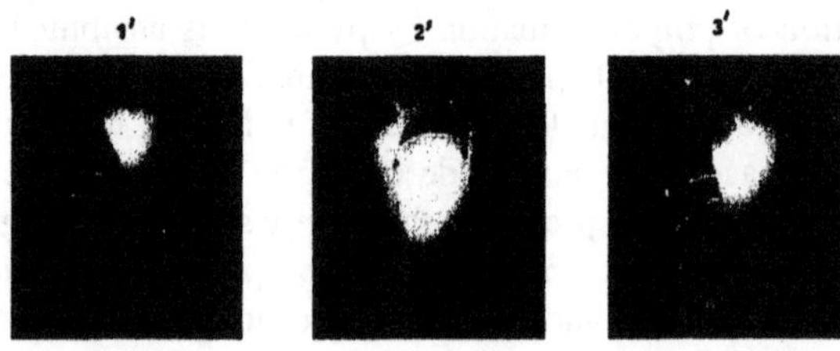

Figure 8. Prevention of galactose cataract by pyruvate. Slitlamp pictures of the eyes of representative animals. The animals were anesthetized with 100 μl of 10% ketamine H Cl for handling during photography. Pictures 1,2,3 represent eyes of normal, galactose-fed, and galactose-fed rats with 15% topical pyruvate eye drops, respectively. Pictures were taken with a Schiempflug camera, 48 days after the start of the experiment. All the animals in group 2 appeared fully cataractous even at 28 days, while in group 3 the appearance of cataract was mild even after 48 days. Cataract could not be discerned by visual inspection in this group.[56] From Henein, M. et al., *Lens Eye Toxicity Res.*, 25-36, 1982. With permission.

REFERENCES

1. **Kirby, D.B.**, Cataract and diabetes, *Arch. Ophthalmol.*, 9, 966-973, 1933.
2. **United States Department of Health, Education and Welfare,** Public Health Service, Division of Chronic Diseases, in *Diabetes Source Book* (PHS Publication No. 1168). Washington, DC. Government Printing Office, 1964.
3. **Kinoshita, J.H.**, Cataracts in galactosemia, *Invest. Ophthalmol. Vis. Sci.*, 4, 786-799, 1965.
4. **Brooks, M.H.**, Lenticular abnormalities in endocrine dysfunction, in *Cataract and Abnormalities of the Lens*, Bellows, J.G., Ed., Grune & Stratton, Inc., New York, 1975, pp. 285-301.
5. **McLaren, D.S., Halasa, A.**, Nutritional and metabolic cataract, in *Cataract and Abnormalities of the Lens,* Bellows, J.G., Ed., Grune and Stratton, Inc., New York, 1975, pp. 255-264.
6. **Hanna, C.**, Cataract of toxic etiology; A: Radiation cataract, in *Cataract and Abnormalities of the Lens*, Bellows, J.G., Ed., Grune & Stratton, Inc., New York, 1975, pp. 217-224.
7. **Hollwich, F., Boateng, A., Kolck, B.**, Toxic cataract, in *Cataract and Abnormalities of the Lens*, Bellows, J.G., Ed., Grune & Stratton, Inc., New York, 1975, pp. 230-243.
8. **Brilliant, L.B., Grasset, N.C., Pokhvel, R.P., Kolstad, A., Lepkowski, J.M., Bradhant, G., Hocks, W.N., Pararajasegrom, R.**, Association among cataract prevalence, sunlight hours, and altitude in the Himalayas, *Am. J. Epidemiol.*, 118, 250-264, 1983.
9. **Chatterjee, A., Milton, R.C., Thyal, S.**, Prevalence and etiology of cataracts in Punjab, *Brit. J. Ophthalmol.*, 66, 35-42, 1982.
10. **Varma, S.D., Morris, S.M., Bauer, S.A., Koppenol, W.H.**, In vitro damage to rat lens by xanthine-xanthine oxidase: Protection by ascorbate, *Exp. Eye Res.*, 43, 1067-1076, 1986.
11. **Schocket, S.D., Esterson, J., Bradford, B., Michaelis, M., Richards, R.D.**, Induction of cataracts in mice by exposure to oxygen, *Israel J. Med. Sci.*, 8, 1596-1601, 1972.
12. **Palmquist, B., Phillipson, B., Bar, P.**, Nuclear cataract and myopia during hyperbaric oxygen therapy, *Br. J. Ophthalmol.*, 68, 113-117, 1984.
13. **Varma, S.D., Chand, D., Sharma, Y.R., Kuck, J.F., Richards, R.D.**, Oxidative stress on lens and cataract formation: role of light and oxygen, *Curr. Eye Res.*, 3, 35-57, 1984.
14. **Harman, D.**, Free radical theory of aging: Effect of free radical reaction inhibitors on the mortality rate of male LAF mice, *J. Gerontol.*, 23, 476-482, 1968.
15. **Bhuyan, K.C., Bhuyan, D.K., Katzen, H.M.**, Amizol induced cataract. Inhibition of lens catalase in rabbit, *Ophthalmol. Res.*, 5, 236-247, 1973.
16. **Newman, E.W.**, Potassium superoxide and the three electron bond, *J. Chem. Phys.*, 2, 31-33, 1932.

17. **Pauling, L.,** The nature of the chemical bond. The one electron bond and the three electron bond, *J. Am. Chem. Soc.*, 53, 3225-3230, 1931.
18. **Varma, S.D., Ets, T., Richards, R.D.,** Protection against superoxide radicals in rat lens, *Ophthalmic Res.*, 9, 421-431, 1977.
19. **Kuck, J.F., Jr.,** Activity of superoxide dismutase in rat lens epithelium and in fiber, *Invest. Ophthalmol. Vis. Sci.*, 16 (ARVO suppl), 15, 1977.
20. **Bhuyan, D.K., Bhuyan, K.C.,** Superoxide dismutase of calf lens, *Invest. Ophthalmol. Vis. Sci.*, 16 (ARVO suppl), 15, 1997.
21. **Haber, F., Weiss, J.,** The catalytic decomposition of H_2O_2 by iron salts, *Proc. Royal Soc., (London), Series A,* 147, 332-351, 1934.
22. **Fenton, H.J.H., Jackson, H.,** The oxidation of polyhydric alcohols in the presence of iron, *J. Chem. Soc. (London),* 75, 1-22, 1899.
23. **Zeller, E.A.,** Contributions to the enzymology of the normal and cataractous lens. III. On the catalase of the crystalline lens, *Am. J. Ophthalmol.*, 36, 51-63, 1953.
24. **Pirie, A.,** Glutathione Peroxidase in lens and a source of H_2O_2 in the aqueous humor, *Biochem. J.*, 96, 244-253, 1965.
25. **Reddy, V.N.,** Glutathione and its function in the lens - an overview, *Exp. Eye Res.,* 50, 771-778, 1980.
26. **Mares-Perlman, J.A., Brady, W.E., Klein, B.E.K., Klein, R., Palta, M., Bowen, P., Stacewicz-Sapuntzakis, M.,** Serum carotenoids and tocopherols and severity of nuclear and cortical opacities, *Invest. Ophthalmol. Vis. Sci.*, 36, 276-288, 1995.
27. **Mares-Perlman, J.A., Brady, W.E., Klein, B.E.K., Klein R., Hans, G.J., Palta, M., Ritter, L.L., Shoft, S.M.,** Diet and nuclear lens opacities, *Am. J. Epidemiol.*, 141, 322-334, 1995.
28. **Taylor, A., Jaques, P.F.,** Relationship between aging, antioxidant status and cataract, *Am. J. Clinical Nutr.*, 62, 1439S-1447S, 1995.
29. **Varma, S.D., Kumar, S., Richards, R.D.,** Light-induced damage to ocular lens cation pump: Prevention by vitamin C, *Proc. Natl. Acad. Sci. USA*, 76, 3504-3506, 1979.
30. **Fukui, H.N.,** The effect of H_2O_2 on the rubidium transport of the rat lens, *Exp. Eye Res.*, 23, 595-599, 1976.
31. **Zigler, J.S., Jr., Goosey, J.D.,** Singlet oxygen as a possible factor in human senile nuclear cataract development, *Curr. Eye Res.*, 3, 39-45, 1984.
32. **Jernigan, H.M., Fukui, H.N., Goosey, J.D., Kinoshita, J.H.,** Photodynamic effects of rose bengal or riboflavin on carrier-mediated transport systems in rat lens, *Exp. Eye Res.,* 32, 461-466, 1981.
33. **Varma, S.D., Morris, S.M.,** Peroxide damage to the eye lens in vitro: Prevention by pyruvate, *Free Radic. Res. Commun.,* 4, 283-290, 1988.
34. **Varma, S.D., Mooney, J.M.,** Photodamage to lens in vitro. Implications of Haber-Weiss reaction, *J. Free Radic. Biol. Med.,* 2, 57-62, 1986.
35. **Bessey, O.A., King, C.G.,** The distribution of vitamin C in plant and animal tissues, and its determination, *J. Biol. Chem.,* 103, 687-698, 1933.

36. **Long, C.,** *Biochemists Handbook*, Van Nostrand Publishers, Princeton, New Jersey, 1961.
37. **Taylor, A., Jaques, P., Nowell, T., Jr., Perrone, G., Nadler, D., Joswiak, B.,** Vitamin C in human and guinea pig aqueous, lens and plasma in relation to intake, *Curr. Eye Res.*, 16, 857-864, 1997.
38. **Varma, S.D., Morris, S.M., Bauer, S.A., Koppenol, W.H.,** In vitro damage to rat lens by xanthine-xanthine oxidase: protection by ascorbate, *Exp. Eye Res.*, 43, 1067-1076, 1986.
39. **Farhataziz, F., Ross, A.B.,** Selected specific rates of reactions transients from water in the aqueous solution. III. Hydroxyl radical and their ions, *N.S.R.D.S. - N.B.S.*, Washington, DC, 1977.
40. **Cabelli, D.E., Bielski, J.H.,** Kinetics and mechanism of oxidation of ascorbate by H_2O_2/O_2 radicals. A pulse radioisotope and stopped flow study, *J. Phys. Chem.*, 87, 1809-1832, 1983.
41. **Blondin, J., Taylor, A.,** Measure of leucine aminopeptidase can be used to anticipate UV-induced age-related damage to lens proteins: ascorbate can delay this damage, *Mech. Ageing Dev.*, 41, 39-46, 1987.
42. **Blondin, J., Baragi, V.J., Schwartz, E., Sadowski, J., Taylor, A.,** Delay of UV-induced eye lens protein damage in guinea pigs by dietary ascorbate, *Free Radic. Biol. Med.*, 2, 275-281, 1986.
43. **Blondin, J., Baragi, V.J., Schwartz, E., Sadowski, J., Taylor, A.,** Dietary vitamin C delays UV-induced age-related eye lens protein damage, *Ann. NY Acad. Sci.*, 498, 460-463, 1987.
44. **Ostadalova, I., Babicyk, A., Obenberger, J.,** Cataract-induced by administration of a single dose of sodium selenite to suckling rats, *Experientia*, 34, 222-223, 1978.
45. **Devamanoharan, Pl.S., Henein, M., Morris, S.M., Ramachandran, S., Richards, R.D., Varma, S.D.,** Prevention of selenite cataract by vitamin C, *Exp. Eye Res.*, 52, 563-568, 1991.
46. **Martenson, J., Meister, A.,** Glutathione deficiency decreases tissue ascorbate levels in newborn rats. Ascorbate spares and protects, *Proc. Natl. Acad. Sci.*, 88, 4656-4661, 1991.
47. **Calvin, H.I., Medvedosky, C., Worgul, B.W.,** Near glutathione depletion and age specific cataracts induced by buthionine sulfoximine in mice, *Science*, 233, 523-525, 1986.
48. **Bhuyan, K.C., Bhuyan, D.K., Podos, S.M.,** Cataract induced by selenium in rat. I. Effect on the lenticular proteins and thiols, *IRCS Med. Sci.*, 9, 194, 1981.
49. **Bhuyan, K.C., Bhuyan, D.K., Podos, S.M.,** Cataract induced by selenium in rat. II. Increased lipid peroxidation and impairment of enzymatic defense against oxidative damage, *IRCS Med. Sci.*, 9, 195-196, 1981.
50. **Holleman, M.A.F.,** Note on the action of oxygenated water on alpha ketoacids and 1,2, diacetones, *Recl. Trav. Chi. Pays-bas Belg.*, 23, 169-172, 1904.

51. **Sevag, M.G., Maiweg, L.,** The respiration mechanism of pneumococcus, *J. Exp. Med.,* 60, 95-105, 1934.
52. **Varma, S.D., Devamanoharan, P.S., Morris, S.M.,** Prevention of cataracts by nutritional and metabolic antioxidants, *Crit. Rev. Food Sci. Nutr.,* 35, (1x2), 111-129, 1995.
53. **Varma, S.D., Devamanoharan, P.S., Morris, S.M.,** Photoinduction of cataracts in rat lens. Preventive effect of pyruvate, *Exp. Eye Res.*, 50, 805-812, 1990.
54. **Ali, A.H., Devamanoharan, P.S., Varma, S.D.,** Effectiveness of pyruvate and pyruvate-ester against in vitro cataracts, *Invest. Ophthalmol. Vis. Sci.*, 38, S1025, 1997.
55. **Varma, S.D., Ramachandran, S., Devamanoharan, P.S., Morris, S.M., Ali, A.H.,** Prevention of oxidative damage to rat lens by pyruvate in vitro: possible attenuation in vivo, *Curr. Eye Res.*, 14, 643-649, 1995.
56. **Henein, M., Devamanoharan, P.S., Ramachandran, S., Varma, S.D.,** Prevention of galactose cataract by pyruvate, *Lens Eye Toxicity Res.*, 9, 25-36, 1992.
57. **Devamanoharan, P.S., Varma, S.D.,** Effect of metabolic inhibitors and anaerobiosis on rat lens, *Curr. Eye Res.,* 12, 55-60, 1993.

Chapter 3

FUNCTION OF THE LENS AND METHODS OF QUANTIFYING CATARACT

Leo T. Chylack, Jr.

I. INTRODUCTION

A. PURPOSE

1. Overview of our expanded understanding of lens function

In the human eye two optical lenses, the cornea and the crystalline lens, focus images on the retina. The focal distance of the cornea is fixed. The focal distance of the young crystalline lens is variable. By contracting the ciliary muscle, varying the tension on the zonules, and rounding up the lens, a young person may vary the focal point of his eye. This variable focus is called "accommodation". It decreases with age, and by the late forties is lost. Then an individual is left with a more-or-less fixed-focus optical system which may be focused on infinity (emmetropia), at a point closer than infinity (myopia), or at a virtual point (hyperopia). To see at different distances, however, an individual needs bi- or trifocal spectacle lenses.

As long as the lens and cornea are clear, and the eye is either naturally emmetropic or corrected to emmetropia with spectacle lenses, the image on the retina is sharply focused. When the clarity of the lens diminishes, as in cataract, the retinal image becomes blurred, the contrast between the image and its surround diminishes, and the ability of the eye's optical system to resolve two small targets is lost. The degradation of the retinal image with a mature cataract may be complete, and in this situation the eye is cataract-blind. On a worldwide basis, cataract is the leading cause of blindness. [1]

In addition to the ability of the lens to focus an image on the retina, there are pigments in the lens which modify light transmission. They selectively absorb near UV and short-wavelength visible light, increase in number and concentration in older individuals, and thereby, spare the retina a certain amount of photooxidative stress (see Chapter 4).

The lens also serves as a structural barrier between the anterior and posterior segments. The importance of this barrier is most apparent after extracapsular cataract extraction when the lens capsule has been removed or opened; then the risk of macular edema and retinal detachment is increased severalfold.

In addition, new research indicates that the lens influences, if not directs, the embryological development of the anterior segment of the eye.

2. Overview of evolution of cataract quantification

Until recently there has been no pressing need to accurately quantify the size density or rates of growth of different forms of cataract. The rate of cataract progression is measured in years; it is a very slow process! During the past twenty years it has become important to precisely define, not only whether a cataract is

0-8493-8565-2/99/$0.00+$.50

cortical, nuclear, posterior subcapsular, or mixed, but also how rapidly the cataract is growing (see Fig. 1). Such precision enabled epidemiologists to define many risk factors associated with age-related cataract. [2,3] Initially efforts to quantitate the severity of cataract took the form of accurately imaging the cataract and then measuring the area or density of the cataract in these images. Scheimpflug optics, which provided an in-focus view from the front of the eye to the back of the lens, enabled in-focus slit photography of the nuclear region of the lens. Retroillumination optics, used to visualize cortical and posterior subcapsular cataracts, improved with the addition of polarizing filters. These eliminated bothersome light reflexes and enabled nearly artefact-free retroillumination images.

The human eye also has proved to be a very effective tool to measure cataract severity, and several "subjective" (as contrasted to the "objective" or machine-based) methods have been developed to classify cataract at the slitlamp.

The method of choice will always depend on the goal of the project. For example, if one wishes to separate eligible individuals into cases and controls, only a coarse scale of cataract severity is needed. If, however, one wishes to determine which of two anti-cataract drugs is more effective in slowing the rate of cataract progression, then a very precise method is needed.

This chapter will present a detailed overview of the different techniques of cataract quantitation which are available and in use in 1998.

3. Detailed discussion of individual methods of cataract quantitation

This chapter will cover several of the newer quantitative systems for measuring the light-scattering properties of the lens. These will include "subjective" and "objective" cataract quantitation systems. "Subjective" systems rely on visual inspection of the lens or its image and a comparison of this image to a set of standard images. "Objective" systems rely on machine-based processing of either film-based or digital images obtained with Scheimpflug or retroillumination optics.

B. SCOPE

The focus of this chapter is on the human lens, and the scope is limited to the topic of age-related cataract. Congenital cataract, drug-induced cataract, traumatic cataract, etc. will not be covered. Animal models of the cataractogenic process and basic studies of animal lenses are treated in other chapters.

C. AUDIENCE

This chapter is intended for use by students and scientists interested in cataract quantitation, and clinical scientists responsible for selecting appropriate quantitative methods for particular clinical research projects. References will be provided for detailed information about individual topics.

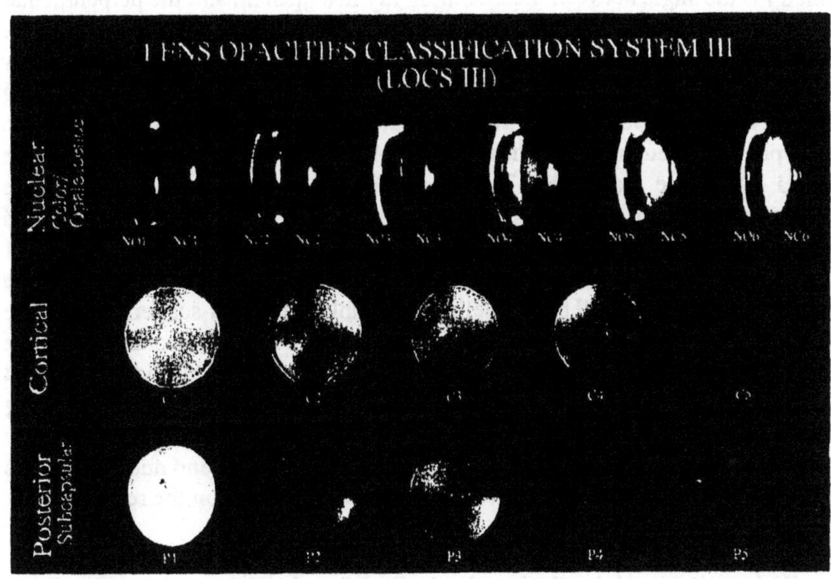

Figure 1.
Lens Opacities Classification System, Version III
Adapted from Chylack et al., *Arch Ophthalmol.*, 111, 1993.
Top row: standard images for grading nuclear opalescence (cataract) and nuclear color (brunescene); Middle row: standard image for grading cortical cataract; Bottom row; standard images for gradi posterior subcapsular cataract. The grades for each standard are indicated by the letter and number co beneath the image.

II. FUNCTIONS OF THE LENS

A. OPTICAL

1. Focusing

a. Index of Refraction (n)

The index of refraction is a measure of the degree to which light is bent on passing from one material into another. It is a ratio defined as (n) = sin I / sin r in which I is the angle between the incoming ray in a medium and the perpendicular to the surface of the medium (normal), and r is the angle of refraction (angle between the ray in the medium and the normal). It is also the ratio of the velocity of light in a vacuum to the velocity of light in the medium. [4] Light passing through media whose indices of refraction are very similar will not be bent much. Light passing through media whose indices of refraction are very different will be bent a lot (hence scattered). This occurs in cortical cataracts at the interface between a lens fiber cell (whose cytoplasm has a high protein concentration) and an interfibrillar lacuna (which has a low protein concentration).

In a slit image of the lens, one can easily see the lens epithelium, but not the underlying lens fibers. The epithelium is visible because it scatters light. The refractive indices of intracellular organelles are very different from those of the surrounding cytoplasm, and at the interface of an organelle and the cytoplasm, light is scattered. Since organelles are absent in the normal lens fiber cell, light falling on a fiber is transmitted, not scattered. In a transparent lens, where there are only gradual changes in the indices of refraction across the cortex and nucleus, light is efficiently transmitted through the lens and sharply focused on the retina.

b. Transparency

For someone studying the lens for the first time, the highly developed order of lens fiber structure is truly marvelous. The uniform cytoplasm is most apparent in cross section; a hexagonal cell membrane surrounds a nearly organelle-free cytoplasm. Scanning electron microscopy reveals the uniform structures of the neatly "stacked" fibers. In young lenses cortical and nuclear fibers have very similar sizes and shapes. In older clear lenses, cortical fibers retain nearly identical size and shape, but nuclear fibers, while similar in size, have very complex and varying surface shapes. The cellular uniformity and the regular layering of the individual fibers creates a transparent structure in which there are only gradual variations of the indices of refraction across cortical and nuclear cells.

The index of refraction of the peripheral parts of the lens is approximately 1.38; it increases in the center of the nucleus to about 1.50. [5-7] Even though the nucleus is a stronger lens than the cortex, the young lens produces a sharply focussed image on the retina. In juvenile nuclear cataract the disparity in the power of the nuclear and cortical lenses may produce a size diplopia with a larger image superimposed on a smaller one. One of the two images is usually clearer than the other.

It is interesting that the protein concentration in the lens is the highest in the body. If cytoplasmic proteins from other cells in the body were concentrated to those levels found in the lens, the solution would be opaque. The great heterogeneity among proteins and their indices of refraction would create many light scattering interfaces. The lens fiber contains a less heterogenous population of proteins; there are three major groups of crystallin proteins, and the cytoskeletal proteins. When there are large fluctuations in the concentration of cytoplasmic proteins and their indices of refraction, such as occurs when high molecular weight aggregates form in the cytoplasm, opacification results. [8-10]

c. Opacification

The process of opacification of the lens begins with the disorganization of the spatial uniformity of the intracellular cytoplasm (formation of high molecular weight aggregates of lens proteins), and the disorganization of the uniform macromolecular structure (formation of interfibrillar lacunae). The biochemical and biophysical processes which underlie these transitions are dealt with in Chapters 3, 4, and 6.

Until recently there were no standardized methods for documenting and specifying the severity of human age-related lens opacification. With the improvement in epidemiological techniques, it became possible to determine specific risk factors of cataractogenesis, and means to specify the type and severity of cataract were needed. Routine clinical techniques of assessing the lens were not adequate. In a slitlamp assessment of the lens, an infinite number of views is possible. This variety in itself was a problem. Simply by specifying certain conventions for the examination of the lens, rapid progress in cataract classification was possible. For example, by specifying that retroillumination images should be the only views used to grade cortical and posterior subcapsular cataract, it was possible to create a standard view. Also by emphasizing that a two-dimensional image of a cataract is a good approximation of the three-dimensional object, it was possible to simplify the object to be graded. [11].

In the case of nuclear cataract there was agreement that a slit view was the appropriate view in which to grade the opacity, but there was controversy as to whether brunescence and opalescence were separate features of the opaque zone. If so, should they be graded separately or together? The traditional term "nuclear sclerosis" referred in a non-quantitative way to both brunescence and opacification. Although these two processes often change in the same direction, there are cases in which there is no opalescence and intense brunescence, and vice versa. It proved easier to grade them separately, and now in most classification systems, they are graded separately.

The measure of opalescence or opacification in a slit image of a nuclear cataract had to be determined. The increased light scattering from the nucleus was obvious, but how to measure it was less obvious. As Scheimpflug photography emerged as an accepted method of documenting nuclear cataract, densitometry of a standardized film image was recommended as a measure of nuclear cataract. There was some debate as to whether a linear scan through the nucleus, or a scan of a defined area of the nucleus, was a better sample. There was little difference in the results obtained from these two approaches, and both are now widely used.

d. Aberrations

The ability of the lens to sharply focus an image on the retina is reduced by spherical aberration. This aberration occurs when one region of the lens has a different focal point from another portion of the lens. For example, the focal point of the cortical portion of the lens might be on the retina. The focal point of the nucleus, because of its higher index of refraction, might fall on a point anterior to the retina. This spherical aberration prevents the whole lens from sharply focusing an object at any one point.

In any lens system the refractive power is wavelength dependent; therefore in polychromatic light, there will be different focal points for each wavelength. This is called chromatic aberration; it results in shorter wavelength blue light being focused 1.5 diopters in front of the longer wavelength red light. [12] In fact this has little effect in human vision because of the narrow spectral sensitivities of cones and the lack of blue cones in the human fovea.

Aberration color perception results from the gradually increasing brunescence of the human lens nucleus. As the nucleus becomes more and more brunescent, it absorbs increasing amounts of blue light; this reduces the ability of individuals with brunescent lenses to discriminate accurately among blue hues.

2. Accommodation

Accommodation is the process by which the lens moves its focal point from infinity to somewhere in the near range. It is the focusing of the eye that enables a young adult to see clearly at infinity and at near without glasses. It is the loss of focusing or accommodative amplitude in an older adult with clear distance vision that leads to the use of reading glasses to see clearly at near. Accommodation involves the contraction of the circular ciliary muscle, a relaxation of the zonules, and a rounding up of the lens, as the zonular forces on both the elastic capsule and the vitreous body are relaxed. The lens moves anteriorly during the accommodative effort. The exact balance of these forces and the identification of each of the major forces responsible for accommodation are now better understood. [13]

3. Filtering of Light by Lens Chromophores

The newborn primate lens is faintly yellow; as the lens ages, this yellow color intensifies. In old age the color may be orange, brown, or black. This process is called brunescence, or nuclear sclerosis, and is due to the accumulation of glycated proteins, oxidation products of the amino acid tryptophan, and numerous fluorescent proteins. Brunescence may be an adaptive process allowing better vision by absorbing long wavelength UV light and blue visible light, both of which cause photooxidative damage. Brunescent pigments also reduce the overall intensity of polychromatic light; this may be a help in bright light or a hindrance in dim light.

Lenticular pigments complicate the process of grading nuclear cataract by absorbing some of the light scattered by nuclear opacities. In a brunescent lens the amount of light scattered from the nucleus appears less than in a non-brunescent lens with the same cataract. This is less important when grading the area involved with cortical and posterior subcapsular cataract, because in a retroillumination image, there is usually still enough light leaving the eye to create high contrast between the opacity and the clear lens. If brunescence reduces the contrast between clear and opaque regions of the lens, it may be more difficult to identify the boundaries of a cortical or posterior subcapsular cataract.

B. MECHANICAL

The lens also serves a purely mechanical barrier function between the anterior chamber and the vitreous body. The significance of this function is more evident when absent than when present. When the entire lens is removed, as in intracapsular cataract extraction, the vitreous body can move into the anterior chamber. This anterior displacement can increase traction on the retina and result in retinal detachment. Intracapsular cataract extraction has been replaced largely by extracapsular extraction or phacoemulsification, in part because these newer techniques leave the posterior capsule intact. Even with an intact capsular bag containing an intraocular lens, however, there is more opportunity for vitreous movement and a slightly increased risk of retinal detachment.

Many ophthalmologists consider the posterior capsule to be a barrier to diffusion of harmful substances from the anterior segment into the posterior segment and vice versa. There is little experimental evidence for this, but the occurrence of retinal problems (cystoid macular edema, retinal degeneration, and breaks) and elevated intraocular pressure following YAG laser capsulotomy is cited as support for this assumption.

C. CONTROL OF EMBRYOLOGICAL DEVELOPMENT OF THE ANTERIOR SEGMENT

In recent work [14-16] there is strong evidence that the embryonic lens influences, and perhaps controls, the development of many anterior segment structures. The factors responsible for this have not yet been identified, but some of them must come from the epithelial layer. When the position of the epithelium is changed in the embryonic eye, the development of the adjacent structures is abnormal.

D. ANTIGENIC SUBSTANCES PRODUCED BY LENS

1. Immune mechanisms of lens epithelial cell death

For many years there has been speculation that autoimmune factors may be involved in cataract formation. Angunawela [17] in 1987 demonstrated a cataractogenic effect of an antibody to a 35,000-40,000 kDa lens protein. A more recent investigation [18] revealed that autoantibodies against β-crystallins, when transfused into an immunologically naive mouse, induced lens epithelial cell damage and cataract formation. The latter study was the first to show that an antibody to a lens protein, not derived from a "leaking" cataract, is capable of injuring the lens epithelial cell and causing cataract.

There had been considerable resistance to the idea that cataract was primarily an autoimmune phenomenon. This was not unreasonable skepticism, since lens proteins in a clear lens are isolated from the immune system and are not regarded by the immune system as "self". If, as a result of cataract formation, lens proteins leak into the anterior chamber, eventually enter the circulation, and act as foreign antigens, "anti-lens antibodies" would be produced. These antibodies would be epiphenomena or secondary phenomena, since they were not the cause of the primary damage to the lens. More work on the autoimmune aspects of human cataract formation is underway.

III. METHODS FOR QUANTIFYING CATARACT

A. INDIRECT

1. High Contrast Visual Acuity

a. Snellen Acuity

The Snellen chart was introduced as a measure of vision shortly prior to 1866. Its use to measure visual acuity and assist in refraction was promoted by Donders. [19] Its design was based on the principle that the arms of the rectangular chart letters subtended one minute of arc at a distance of one meter. It contained high-contrast targets–jet black letters on a snow white background. It was the standard measure of visual function from its introduction until the late 1960s.

Snellen acuity was used with some success for many years as an indirect measure of cataract severity. When cataract surgery carried a moderately high risk of complications and post-operative morbidity, there was little demand from patients for early surgery. Most patients put off the five-seven day hospitalization and the need for thick aphakic glasses as long as possible. A reduction in Snellen acuity in an otherwise healthy eye could be attributed to cataract, and there was some correlation between the cataract's maturity and the loss of Snellen acuity. Clinicians were aware, however, that it was possible to have advanced cataract and good Snellen acuity. This was particularly true of cortical cataracts, which could obliterate a good part of the pupillary space and not cause much visual dysfunction.

When cataract surgery could be done rapidly in an out-patient setting, and when contact lenses and intraocular lenses replaced aphakic spectacles, cataract surgery was sought eagerly by individuals seeking visual rehabilitation. The demand for cataract surgery greatly increased. Often patients with little loss of Snellen acuity energetically sought cataract surgery. There was an increasing awareness by patients and clinicians that the Snellen measure of visual function was not an accurate measure of the impact of a cataract on a patient's visual function.

Concurrently, as the benefits of laser treatment of diabetic retinopathy became more well known, there was a demand for measures of acuity that better reflected the true visual potential of the eye and were less affected by imperfections of the Snellen measure. The letters on the Snellen chart are not all equally difficult or equally easy to identify; some letters are more easily guessed than others. The change in vision associated with a drop in Snellen acuity from 20/20 to 20/30 (two lines) is not the same as the change from 20/40 to 20/80 (also two lines). Also the number of letters on each line of the Snellen chart is not constant; the big "E" at the top of the chart (the 20/400) line stands alone, while the 20/20 line has six letters. The "big E" could be guessed correctly even by people with far less than 20/400 vision, just because they knew that the Snellen chart started with the "big E".

In 1980 new recommendations for measuring visual acuity were made by the NAS-NRC Committee on Vision. [20] New logarithmic measures of visual acuity were soon forthcoming; these charts overcame many of the limitations of the Snellen chart.

b. LogMAR (Bailey-Lovie) Visual Acuity

The logMAR charts (separate ones for the right and left eyes) developed by Drs. Bailey and Lovie have been identified by several names: the "Bailey-Lovie charts" is perhaps the most common. Synonymous are the "LogMAR charts," standing for logarithm of the minimal angle of resolution, and the "ETDRS charts," an acronym for the Early Treatment Diabetic Retinopathy Study charts. These charts contain high contrast targets (black letters on a white background) which are to be presented to the patient under conditions of standardized illumination. There are the same number of letters on each line, and the letters are all equally easy or difficult to identify. The change in vision is the same for any two lines, because the size of the letters is based on a logarithmic scale. The logMAR measures of acuity correspond to Snellen acuities according to Table 1, but no one makes the conversion; they use the LogMAR score directly. The clinical significance of a logMAR score of 0.2 might be easier to understand as an approximate Snellen score, but the conversion of logMAR to Snellen scores serves no other significant purpose (see Fig. 2).

LogMAR acuity is not a better measure of cataract-related visual loss than Snellen acuity; it is just a better (more accurate and more informative) measure of vision. As a measure of high contrast acuity, it suffers from the same disadvantages as the Snellen measure. The explanation for why patients with cataract and normal Snellen or logMAR acuities still complained of abnormal vision stimulated a study of the relationship of cataract to other measures of acuity, such as contrast sensitivity. In these tests targets that were grey on white or dark grey on light grey proved more sensitive to the adverse effects of early cataract than high contrast targets, and several tests of contrast sensitivity function were developed and applied the assessment of cataract-related visual dysfunction. [21]

A particularly good study of the basis for visual dysfunction in early cataracts was done by Elliott et al., [22] in which they simulated cataract and then tested face recognition, reading speed, mobility orientation and other aspects of "real world" visual function. They found that large amounts of wide angle (forward and/or backward) light scatter are partially responsible for visual disability in cataract patients with good high-contrast acuity.

The effect of light scattering on retinal images was studied also by Beckman et al., [23] with the scanning laser ophthalmoscope. They were able to document the degradation of retinal image detail in patients with cataract.

Table 1.
Correspondence of LogMAR and Snellen Visual Acuities

LogMAR Acuity	Snellen Acuity (equivalent)
-0.3	20/10
-0.1	20/16
0.0	20/20
0.1	20/25
0.3	20/40
0.4	20/50
0.5	20/63
0.6	20/80
0.7	20/100
0.8	20/125
0.9	20/160
1.0	20/200

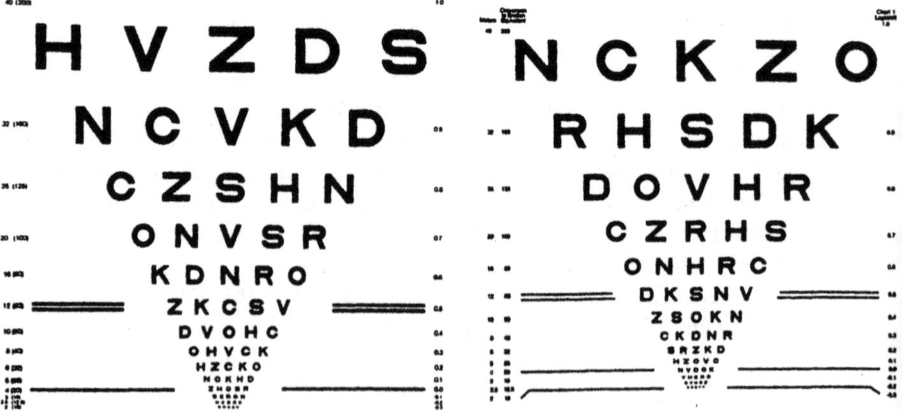

Figure 2. LogMAR Acuity (Chart adapted from Ferris F, Kassoff A, Bresnick GH et al.: New visual acuity charts for clinical research. *Am. J. Ophthalmol.*, 94:97, 1988)

c. Contrast Sensitivity Function

When high contrast is retained in a retinal image (as that of a white object on a black surround), one can infer that the optical media of the eye (cornea, aqueous, lens, and vitreous) are clear. When light from an object is transmitted through cloudy media, the contrast in the image is greatly reduced; an observer with cloudy media might see a black object against a white background as a dark grey image on a lighter grey background. Diminished contrast perception may occur with the development of cataract, corneal edema, anterior or posterior uveitis, and other ocular diseases which increase backscatter of incident light (see Fig. 3).

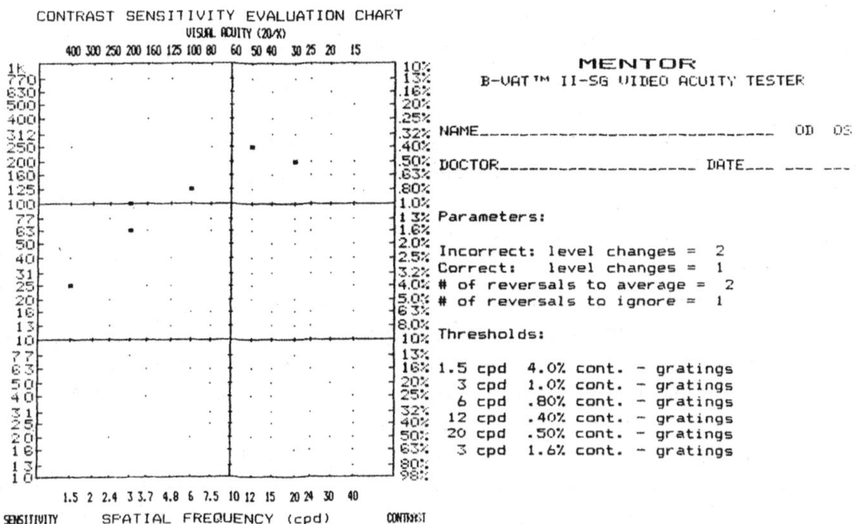

Figure 3. Contrast sensitivity plot of contrast versus spatial frequency. Adapted from Mentor O & O, Inc. manual.

Recognizing that this loss of contrast sensitivity might be a useful measure of cataract-related visual loss, many clinical investigators tried to measure the degree to which cloudy media reduced the contrast of the image on the retina.

i. Mentor O and O, Inc. developed the "B-VAT" [24] device to measure the contrast sensitivity function (CSF) by presenting on a television monitor a series of sine waves in which the frequency (cycles per degree: cpd), the tilt of the wave (left, right, or straight up or down), and the contrast between the waves (black alternates with white, or dark grey alternates with light grey) vary. The subject is presented with a forced choice task in which s/he must identify only the orientation of the wave. If the answer is correct, the contrast between the waves is further reduced. If the answer is incorrect, the contrast between the waves is increased. When the subject identifies (or misses) 50% of the targets incorrectly, the test at that frequency is over. The tester then presents a similar set of tests at a different frequency. The complete test usually involves testing at five different spatial frequencies. The results are plotted as the contrast sensitivity function, and the plot for the subject is compared to a normal plot or range of values derived from a set of individuals with no eye disease.

ii. Vistech developed a similar test in which a series of sine wave patterns are depicted on a large chart. There are several rows of images containing patterns of different contrast and different spatial frequency. [25] The subject identifies the tilt of the wave pattern reading from left to right and proceeds from top to bottom moving from high to lower contrast sets. A contrast sensitivity function graph similar to that from the Mentor B-VAT is derived from the test results.

iii. The Pelli-Robson test of CSF is another widely used test of CSF. [26] On a 3'x4' matte white plastic background are presented sets of three letters. Each of the letters in the set has the same contrast, but as one moves from left to right and from top to bottom of the chart the contrast between the letters and the background diminishes until it is no longer possible to correctly identify the letters in the set. The end of the test is when the subject fails to identify the sets of letters.

d. Glare Testing

Patients with cataract or corneal haze often complain of "glare", a decrease in vision when the ambient light intensity increases. Glare may occur gradually, as on a summer day when the sun rises higher in the sky and the overall light intensity increases, or it may be sudden, as occurs when an individual walks from a darkened movie theater into bright sunlight, or at night, when high beams from an oncoming automobile are suddenly directed into one's eyes. In an attempt to approximate and measure the glare which patients experience, vision scientists have added a means of increasing the ambient luminance to standard tests of contrast sensitivity function. The first of these tests was the Miller-Nadler Glare Tester. [27]

i. In the Miller-Nadler test a subject views the screen of a rear projection slide projector. Letters are presented on a background of varying brightness. As the contrast between the letters and the background decreases, the difficulty of correctly identifying the letter increases. In this manner it was possible to derive a measure of the effects of brightness on the ability to correctly identify the target letters. This led to a "glare score". It was not strictly a measure of contrast sensitivity.

ii. After the introduction of the Miller-Nadler test, glare sources were added to standard tests of contrast sensitivity. One such test is Mentor's "B-VAT" Glare testing device. [24] In this device a hand-held, battery-powered glare source is held in front of the eye being tested with the B-VAT CSF test. The hand-held device comprises a white hemisphere with a hole in its center through which the subject can view the monitor. The white hemisphere is diffusely illuminated by a lamp whose intensity can be varied from low to intermediate to high. The subject is given the standard CSF test, and then the test is repeated with the glare source in place. The difference between the test results is a measure of the glare effect.

In another study Maraini et al., [28] studied the influence of cataract on visual acuity and CSF. They studied 1076 eyes with cataracts classified by the Lens Opacities Classification System, Version II (LOCS II), and measures of logMAR acuity and Pelli-Robson CSF. In age-adjusted analyses, increasing severity of nuclear, cortical, and posterior subcapsular cataract was associated with progressively poorer logMAR acuities and lower CSF scores. The effect was greatest for nuclear and least for cortical cataract. When their analyses were adjusted for both age and logMAR acuity, there was no longer any association between cataract severity and CSF. These results suggest that little additional information (in addition to that in the logMAR measure of acuity) about cataract-related visual dysfunction is found in the measure of CSF. They also showed that there is a strong correlation between cataract severity and logMAR and CSF measures of visual function. These results were similar to those obtained by Hirvela et al., [29] showing that, in the elderly, CSF does not add much additional information to that obtained from logMAR acuity alone.

e. Displacement Threshold Hyperacuity (DTH) or Vernier Acuity

Measurements are tests of visual acuity based on the ability of the eye to align two or more targets, much like one aligns the lines on a vernier scale. Because the minimal angle of discrimination in the normal eye, namely 0.15' arc, is less than the diameter of the photoreceptor element that is responsible for fine discrimination (0.5' arc for foveal cones), the test is also referred to as "hyperacuity". The test is much less sensitive to imperfections in the ocular media, so it is often used to measure potential postoperative acuity in patients with cataract or other surgically remediable diseases of the ocular media. One of these hyperacuity tests has been developed by Bueno and Hurst. [30] They tested the ability of this technique to predict visual outcome in 45 patients with cataract and macular disease awaiting cataract surgery. They found that DTH was sensitive to decreased macular function but was relatively unaffected by the severity of cataract. DTH sensitivity and specificity for decreased macular function was 1.00 and 0.8, respectively. They were able to conclude that, if preoperative DTH is 50 seconds of arc or lower, the subject will achieve postoperative logMAR acuity better than 0.3 (Snellen equivalent of 20/40). This test has proven useful when one is assessing visual acuity in populations in which there may be cataract-related and macular disease-related visual loss. One can measure separately the cataract and macular components of the visual loss.

f. Visual Function Questionnaires

As the results of extracapsular cataract extraction and the quality of intraocular lens implants improved, there was increased demand for cataract surgery. This came from patients who were increasingly aware of the benefits and reduced risks of this ever-improving operation. It was even difficult at times for ophthalmologists to convince some patients that there were any risks at all to this procedure, so eager were they for surgery. Not unexpectedly, this steadily increasing demand for surgical care led to a concurrent increase in the cost of care–most of which was paid for by Medicare or private insurance. These payers soon demanded some means of deciding, not who wanted cataract surgery, but who needed cataract surgery. Neither Snellen nor Bailey-Lovie high-contrast acuity tests, nor any of several tests of contrast sensitivity, successfully detected those patients with serious cataract-related visual dysfunction. At the outset visual dysfunction was not clearly defined, so it was not surprising that it could not be measured. However, in response to some excellent work by Mangione [31] and investigators at the National Eye Institute and Rand Corporation [32], standardized questionnaires were developed which did measure in practical terms a patient's visual disability. These questionnaires could be self-administered or administered by an interviewer. They contained questions about one's age and general health and questions about visual function such as: "How much time do you worry about your eyesight?" "How much does pain or discomfort in and around your eyes, for example, burning, itching, or aching, keep you from doing what you'd like to be doing? Would you say: "None of the time," "Some of the time," "About half the time," "Most of the time," or "All of the time?" "How much difficulty do you have doing work, or hobbies that require you to see well up close, such as cooking, sewing, fixing things around the house, or using hand tools?" "Because of your eyesight, how much difficulty do you have playing cards or games like bingo or Monopoly?" The questionnaire developed by the NEI and Rand Corporation was called the "NEI-VFQ" questionnaire. These questionnaires have provided considerable insight into the nature of the relationship between cataract and cataract-related visual dysfunction and the impact of cataract surgery on the daily activities of patients undergoing this operation.

Adamsons et al., [33] using a task-oriented questionnaire, logMAR measures of visual acuity, CSF and glare testing on patients pre-and post-cataract/IOL surgery, demonstrated a resolution or improvement in subjective symptoms (as measured by the questionnaire) and improvement in objective test criteria (logMAR acuity and CSF, but not glare testing) following uncomplicated cataract surgery. There was also a strong association between the degree of preoperative objective impairment in visual function and the subjective improvement in visual function. Their study supported the decision to intervene surgically in patients with subjective impairment in vision and the use of CSF to assess preoperative visual impairment.

B. DIRECT

1. Ordinal Classification

The need for a more direct classification and specification of cataract type and severity led clinicians away from their traditional methods of categorizing severity in such terms as immature, mature, and hypermature or 1+, 2+, 3+, etc. These terms were never standardized or clearly defined, and their meaning to individual clinicians often changed with time.

Alternative methods of classifying cataract in terms of etiology (traumatic, x-ray, steroid cataract, etc.) were no better, because they also lacked standardized definitions.

In the mid 1970s in the American lens research community, there was a shift in emphasis from animal to human lens research. Increasingly there was a need to accurately classify the type and severity of age-related cataract in intracapsularly extracted specimens. The Cooperative Cataract Research Group (CCRG) method was devised and used widely for about five years. [34] Fundamental to the CCRG system was the principle of amalgamating disparate sections of clear and opaque cortex into a binary lens containing clear cortex and opaque cortex. For example, if there were opaque spokes in the superonasal, superotemporal, and inferotemporal cortex, each of which involved less than a whole quadrant, the classifier would mentally combine the separate opaque zones into one opaque zone and grade it in terms of its size (equaling ≤1 quadrant, >1 quadrant but ≤2 quadrants, >2 quadrants but ≤3 quadrants, etc). The grades would be I, II, and III respectively, and the zone of the opacity would be specified as anterior cortex (CXA), equatorial cortex (CXE), or posterior cortex (CXP).

Posterior subcapsular cataract severity was graded in terms of area of the posterior capsule involved, and nuclear opacity was graded in terms of the intensity of nuclear opalescence on an ordinal scale with standardized definitions of opalescence 1+, 2+, 3+, etc.). These fundamental principles of grading were incorporated more or less intact in later systems of *in vivo* cataract classification.

A major problem facing scientists working with intracapsularly extracted cataracts was what to use as the control for the measures they obtained. There was never a clear contralateral lens extracted from the same patient at the time of cataract surgery. When both lenses were obtained from cadaver eyes, both were often clear or cataractous, and the lack of control tissue led scientists to try the difficult microdissection of a whole lens into clear and opaque sections. Although this was successful occasionally, it was never completely satisfactory.

When the intracapsular cataract extraction was replaced by the extracapsular technique as the method of choice, the ready supply of whole human cataractous lenses was eliminated, and so was the need for *in vitro* systems of cataract classification.

a. LOCS I and II

In 1988 the Lens Opacities Classification System (so-called LOCS I) was published (35). It had been developed for use in a cross-sectional case-control study of risk factors associated with pure types of age-related cataract. Approximately 1350 patients were enrolled in the original LOCS study. The system was based on a set of photographic standards containing a single slit image of an immature nuclear cataract, a single retroillumination image of a clear lens (to illustrate the type of artefacts that are seen in Neitz-CTR retroillumination images), two Neitz-CTR retroillumination images of cortical cataracts, one very immature, and the second moderately immature, and a single retroillumination image of a small posterior subcapsular cataract. By viewing the eye of a subject at a slitlamp under standardized viewing conditions, and comparing the severity of the subject's cataract to the set of standards, it was possible to grade consistently the severity of nuclear cortical and posterior subcapsular cataracts.

Shortly after publishing LOCS I, the opportunity to follow a subset of the original LOCS population appeared, and the need arose for a system of cataract classification capable of detecting and specifying change in the severity of the cataract. The small number of standards in LOCS I made this system in its original form unsuitable for this task. This was the stimulus for the development of LOCS II–a similar system in which there were four nuclear standards for grading opalescence, one nuclear standard for grading brunescence, five retroillumination standards for grading cortical cataract, and four retroillumination standards for grading posterior subcapsular cataract. In this system the grading was still ordinal, because the intervals between the standards were not equal, and the numerical designations were not intended as exact amounts of cataract. [36] This system could be used at the slitlamp to grade cataract *in vivo*, or it could be used to grade lens photographs of images obtained with standardized retroillumination and slit cameras. This system has been used in epidemiological studies around the world in the past several years.

b. Wilmer System

At about the time the original LOCS system was introduced, Dr. Hugh Taylor, Dr. Sheila West and their collaborators at The Wilmer Ophthalmological Institute in Baltimore, MD, published a system of cataract classification that they had designed for use in the Chesapeake Bay Watermen Study–a study of the risk factors for age-related cataract in a population of watermen. [37,38] Their system employed a set of four colored standards for grading nuclear cataract. Their standards did not have separate scales for grading nuclear opalescence and brunescence, as is done in the LOCS systems of classification, and in their original grading rules, there were visual acuity criteria for each grade.

To grade cortical cataract one estimated the number of opaque pie-shaped sectors (up to eight) using rules for estimating the circumferential extent of the opacity.

To grade the extent of PSC one measured the height and width of a PSC using the vernier scale of the slitlamp. This ordinal system of cataract classification has been used in several studies of the Chesapeake Bay Watermen and in several similar studies in Australia. [39] It is an ordinal system of cataract classification. It does not offer a separate scale for grading brunescence. It is suitable for grading cataracts at the slitlamp or images of cataracts in standardized photos.

c. Oxford System

Dr. John Sparrow and his colleagues at Oxford University, Oxford, UK developed the Oxford Cataract Classification System, which is also designed to be used at the slitlamp. [40] It specifies several features of cortical cataract (spokes, flecks, retrodots, vacuoles, and others), standards for grading white nuclear scatter, and separate Munsell color chips for grading nuclear brunescence. It has scales for grading each feature. It is a considerably more complex system than either the LOCS I or II, or the Wilmer systems. It has been used by the authors in their epidemiologic research.

d. The Wisconsin Cataract Grading System (WCGS)

Drs. Ronald and Barbara Klein and their associates in Madison, WI developed a system of grading cataract type and severity from standardized lens photographs obtained from specialized retroillumination and slitlamp cameras. [41] Their system uses a set of nuclear standards and rules for grading the extent of cortical and PSC which are similar to those in the Wilmer system. The system has been used in the Beaver Dam Eye studies and is being used in the NEI-sponsored Age-related Eye Disease Study (AREDS). It is not a system that can be applied at the slitlamp for *in vivo* grading.

2. Continuous Cataract Classification Scales

a. LOCS III

See Fig. 1 for the set of LOCS III standards. With increasing use of the LOCS II classification system, it became apparent that there were certain deficiencies that could be improved. Ian Bailey suggested that using a continuous decimalized grading scale, rather than an ordinal scale, would increase the sensitivity of the system to small changes in cataract severity. The LOCS III system was designed to allow continuous decimalized grading of cataract severity. In addition to the increased sensitivity of this scale, additional statistical power is afforded by the continuous nature of the classification data. There was a need for an expanded set of nuclear standards to allow finer grading of the early stages of opalescence and a much broader scale of nuclear brunescence. There was also a need for an expanded scale for grading PSC cataract. This led to the development of the LOCS III cataract [42] classification system.

In LOCS III there are six standards for grading nuclear opalescence and color, five standards for grading cortical cataract, and six standards for grading PSC. The images for the standard sets were selected from a large library of lens photos after obtaining quantitative measures of the intensity of the opalescent or color change and the area of cortical and PSC change. The standards were selected, so that the intervals between the nuclear standards were equal, and the intervals between the cortical and PSC standards created a monotonic sequence. With these standards and intervals, it was possible to use a decimalized scale in which there was a specifiable quantitative relationship between different grades. For example, a grade 4.0 nuclear cataract could be viewed as twice as advanced as a grade 2.0 nuclear cataract.

In testing the reproducibility of LOCS III, some part of a set of 150 quality control slides representing all types and grades of cataract was introduced into each set of unknowns. Graders, masked as to the identity of the standards and unknowns, supplied replicate grades of these quality control images several times during a six-month grading session. Since the grades of the quality control slides should be constant, the variation in grades actually obtained in the grading of the slides yielded a measure of the noise of the classification system–a so-called 95% tolerance interval. This interval represented the difference in grades that could be attributed to the inconsistency of classifiers in applying the rules of the system. If a change in cataract grade was less than the 95% tolerance interval, no significant change in cataract severity had occurred. If the change in LOCS III grades was more than the 95% tolerance interval, there was less than a 5% chance that this amount of change could have occurred on the basis of chance alone. In other words, there had been a significant change in cataract severity.

b. WHO Simplified Cataract Grading System

In 1996 the World Health Organization (WHO) convened a meeting of investigators who had developed validated systems of cataract grading and classification. [43] The purpose of the meeting was to develop a new cataract classification system that would incorporate the advantages of the individual systems of classification and yet serve the needs of the WHO. A major responsibility of the WHO is estimating the prevalence and incidence of blinding diseases around the world. Age-related cataract is the leading cause of blindness worldwide. The cataract classification systems available to the WHO, prior to its developing its own system, were well suited to assessing cataract in the developed countries of the world where most cataracts being extracted were not mature or hypermature. In many of the developing countries, cataracts were mature or hypermature, and available systems were not well suited to grading these opacities. Among extant systems, moreover, there were differences in the techniques of grading cortical and subcapsular cataracts; some used a simple estimate of overall area of opacification, and others used a measure of the circumference to express the extent of involvement. Also in the grading of posterior subcapsular cataract, some techniques used an areal approach, and others used measurements of vertical and horizontal height of the opacity in mm. It was possible to arrive at a compromise in which some of the features of the most widely used systems were incorporated into the new WHO system. The WHO system uses:

(a) three standards to grade nuclear opalescence
(b) a circumferential approach to grade cortical cataract, and
(c) a measurement of height and width to grade posterior subcapsular cataract.

c. Scheimpflug Imaging

Scheimpflug optics were introduced at the turn of the century to facilitate aerial photography. In 1979 these optics were incorporated into a special camera for slit photography of the lens nucleus by Hockwin and Dragomirescu. [44] By tilting the film plane in a slitlamp camera, one is able to obtain a focused slit image from the anterior pole to the posterior pole of the lens. This had not been possible with the conventional slitlamp cameras which had a limited (1-2 mm) depth of focus, which when applied to the lens yielded a clear image of the central nucleus, but a blurred image of the regions anterior and posterior to this central zone. The blurred zones of the lens (both cortex and nucleus) were regarded as unsuitable for grading cataract severity or applying densitometric techniques to quantitate nuclear light scatter. In a Scheimpflug image the entire nucleus was in focus and could be graded subjectively or objectively. In fact, there is a considerable literature from the 1960s and 1970s in which fine points of linear densitometry are presented and debated.

Topcon Instruments in collaboration with Professor Otto Hockwin and Mr.

Viorel Dragomirescu developed the SL 45 series of slit cameras with Scheimpflug optics and film imaging. [44,45] These were rugged, marvelously engineered cameras, maintained and updated largely by Mr. Dragomirescu. In the SL-45 camera the angle between the camera and the visual axis of the eye was fixed; one had to use a set of x-y-z controls to position the slit in the pupil and at the proper antero-posterior position. A device using the position of the corneal light reflex to identify the proper position of the slit gave a pleasant beeping sound when the x-y-z orientation was correct. Then the exposure was taken. The flash intensity was standardized and nearly constant during the lifetime of the bulb, and there was a grey scale step wedge incorporated into each image so that a linear densitometer scanning the nuclear image would also pass over a grey scale step wedge, thereby affording a means of calibrating the measurement. These images had all the components needed to get a valid, sensitive, objective measure of the change in nuclear light scatter with time.

At this time there was general consensus among clinical investigators that machine-derived measures of nuclear light scattering (nuclear cataract) were better than measures obtained from visual inspection of images. Accordingly, the Topcon SL-45 and SL-45B (a later version) were the workhorses of the lens research community through much of the 1960s and 1970s. Since they were film-based devices, it was necessary to obtain all of the film for one trial at one time, keep the film refrigerated, warm the film before use, and then use standardized film development techniques before analyzing the image.

Linear densitometry of Scheimpflug images [44] was the first method used to generate a number representing the intensity of nuclear light scatter. A scan across the lens from the anterior to posterior poles and across the grey scale step wedge was made. The analyst assumed that intensity of the corneal light reflex was constant over time and used this to normalize the baseline of a set of different images. The grey scale step wedge could then be used to adjust other levels of grey in the black-white image that might fall outside the linear response range of the film. With these calibration methods, it was possible to document the change in nuclear light scatter with age and during the course of nuclear cataractogenesis.

In 1988 [46,47] a different approach to assessing nuclear light scattering was introduced by Chylack. In this approach, a large oval mask was placed around the part of the nuclear image corresponding to the adult nucleus. The average pixel density in this area was calculated and reported as representing the degree of nuclear cataract. By sampling a larger area, it was believed that some of the inherent variation in the linear sample was avoided. Both approaches were used. The more modern digital Scheimpflug cameras offer both approaches to image analysis of the nuclear image (see below).

The Scheimpflug SL-45 instrument also allowed one to measure sizes and distances in the anterior segment. After correcting the Scheimpflug image for the geometrical distortion (not blur) caused by the optics, it was possible to get accurate measures of the thickness of the cornea, the depth of the anterior chamber, the curvatures and thickness of the lens, and the size of the anterior chamber angle. This feature of the camera has been incorporated into all of the newer versions of the Scheimpflug camera, and it has been used to study changes in the eye with age, changes in the anterior segment associated with accommodation, and different orientation properties of intraocular lenses.

d. Retroillumination Imaging

Retroillumination images were used to image cortical and posterior subcapsular cataracts, but until Kawara's and Obazawa's seminal publication [48], these images were taken only with a conventional photoslitlamp with the slit beam entering the lens near one edge of the pupil. This approach generated a bright retroillumination image of the opposite half of the pupil, but the half of the pupil through which the light entered contained a mix of bright light reflexes and shadow, but little clearly visible lens or cataract. To avoid using two images for each cataract, some investigators recommended taking two such photographs with the light entering on opposite sides of the pupil, then discarding the bad side of each image, and constructing a composite from the two remaining good sides. This was not an efficient alternative, and was not widely adopted.

In a separate effort to image cortical and posterior subcapsular cataracts, Professor Otto Hockwin and his colleagues in Bonn, Germany, recommended rotating Scheimpflug photography. [44] By rotating the Scheimpflug camera around the optical axis, and taking images at each point, it was possible to collect a series of slit images that could be used to reconstruct a cortical cataract. This was a very labor-intensive effort in an era predating sophisticated 3-D computerized reconstruction techniques and, not surprisingly, was not widely used.

Kawara and Obazawa introduced the technique that is used today in most retroillumination cameras and solved most of the problems with standard retroillumination slitlamp photography. They placed polarizing filters oriented 90 degrees apart in the light paths. One was located in front of the illuminating beam, and the second was located in front of the beam entering the camera. Thus light polarized in one plane could pass into the central pupil along the optical axis and light leaving the eye would be polarized in a second plane. The polarizing filters removed most of the specular reflections that obscured the view of the cataract in these images. These retroillumination images filled the entire pupil and were nearly artifact free. With one or two images one could record the extent of most cortical and posterior subcapsular cataracts. This photographic system had a limited depth of focus which created a small problem. In an image of an anterior cortical cataract, in which the focal point had to be at the plane of the pupil in order to clearly image the anterior features of this cataract, some of the cortical or posterior subcapsular cataract was out of focus. This problem was overcome by taking two retroillumination images, one focused on the anterior surface of the lens at the plane of the pupil, and a second image focused at the plane of the posterior capsule. Even though many of the most troubling artefacts were obviated by the polarizing filters, there were some new artifacts in these images. There was a small faint rectangular light reflex in the center of the field, a cruciate artifact over the entire image due to the birefringence from the cornea, and in a widely dilated pupil a visible boundary between the edge of the pupil and the edge of the cone of light entering the eye. But overall, this retroillumination image was one that could be classified accurately and consistently with either objective or subjective techniques.

The same approach was used to photograph the posterior subcapsular region, and in fact, the posteriorly focused member of the pair was ideal for capturing the type and extent of most posterior subcapsular cataracts.

The first commercially available retroillumination camera with polarizing filters was the Neitz-CTR. It used film (color or B/W) and a bright white, polychromatic flash. Considerable skill and training was needed to get excellent photographs, because the photographer had to locate the optic nerve (the brightest reflector in the eye) to obtain a bright, high-contrast retro image of the lens. Failure to locate the optic nerve as a reflector often yielded low contrast, underexposed lens images. Also the patient had to endure at least four bright flashes while the photographer endeavored to capture anteriorly and posteriorly focused images of both eyes. Often additional exposures were needed to get optimized images. These 35 mm images were kept in a standard 2"x 2" slide format and graded either subjectively with a classification system or subjected to a number of image analysis techniques (see below).

More recently Nidek Co., Ltd. [49] and Marcher Industries [50] introduced digital versions of the retroillumination and Scheimpflug cameras that used either infrared light or lower polychromatic light intensities. These cameras were much more user- and patient-friendly and are the standard imaging devices used today. They are well-engineered and suitable for use in an office setting. They may not be suitable for use in rugged terrain such as in eye camps, etc.

e. *Fast Spectral Scanning Colorimetry*

In 1993 Chylack [51] and his colleagues applied fast spectral scanning colorimetry to an objective quantitation of nuclear color as a means of studying the biological process of nuclear brunescence. In conventional and even Scheimpflug color images of the lens nucleus, careful inspection of the nuclear region reveals a broad spectrum of colors in the areas characterized clinically as brunescent. There are greens and blues in the anterior nucleus, increasing yellow in the mid nucleus, and brown-red tones in the posterior nucleus. In the specular reflex off the posterior capsule in such an image, there is a fairly homogenous area of color which may be used to specify the clinical grade of brunescence. Occasionally, even in this zone, however, there can be peculiar variations in color–pinks and browns showing up in lenses in which there is little brunescence. Notwithstanding the occasional anomalous colorations of this region, it was possible to grade most lens brunescence by focusing on the specular reflex from the posterior capsule.

Color quantitation is a science in itself, but, in brief, it is possible to specify a color with three quantities: hue (spectral wavelength), luminosity (brightness), and value (saturation). [52,53] The fast spectral scanning colorimeter (FSSC) gives these quantities when it is applied to a particular region of interest. By measuring these quantities in the area of the specular reflex in Kodak Ektachrome, ASA 200, color transparencies of the nucleus, it was possible to derive an objective measure of nuclear color. These slit images were obtained either with conventional slit or Scheimpflug photography. Using commercially available software, it was possible to subtract the FSSC values for the retroilluminating light source alone, from the values of the lens image plus the light source, and obtain three values describing the nuclear color. The hue of the color could be expressed in terms of its C.I.E. (Commision Internationelle d'Eclairage) chromaticity coordinates: C.I.E.-X or C.I.E.-Y. [54] These data were collected from several hundred images of the human lens nucleus, and it was determined that the LOCS III grade of nuclear color (LOCS III NC) was most highly correlated to the C.I.E.-X chromaticity coordinate. In this manner it was possible to identify risk factors associated with nuclear brunescence and dissect out the relative importance of color change and opalescence in nuclear cataract-derived visual loss.

f. Image Analysis Used in "Objective" Systems of Cataract Grading

The specification of the intensity of nuclear light scatter as evident in Scheimpflug film images as mentioned above was done with standardized linear densitometry along the optical axis of the lens or with areal densitometry of the adult nuclear zone. These techniques are used today in the Nidek EAS 1000 digital instrument, and both are generally accepted as measures of nuclear cataract.

None of the current digital instruments affords the opportunity to do objective color assessment of the nucleus.

The algorithms used for quantitating the severity of cortical and posterior subcapsular cataracts documented in retroillumination images are still controversial. A technique introduced by Chylack, Wolfe et al., [54] to estimate the area of opacification in film images of cortical and posterior subcapsular cataracts is called "OPAC." This program divides the retroillumination image into 93 sectors, and, within each sector the image, subjects the image to tests of criteria of opacification which include: absolute pixel density, presence of boundaries, and the gradient across boundaries. Based on the results of this assessment, the sector is designated either clear or opaque. This same process is applied to all sectors, and then the number of opaque sectors x 100 / 93 = % area opaque. This percentage is then used as the measure of cortical or subcapsular cataract.

To enable specification of "% area opaque" in a longitudinal study in which there are inevitable variations in a patient's pupil size from visit to visit, at each visit OPAC analyses are done within each of several concentric circles fitting within the pupil. In OPAC there is not just one size for the mask in which the analysis is done; rather there are ten masks, each a concentric circle of specified size. At the end of a study when the sizes of the pupils in all of the images from a particular patient can be assessed, the largest circle which will fit within all the pupils for a given patient is chosen, and the data from the OPAC analyses with that mask are chosen to characterize the progress of the opacity for that patient during the trial.

OPAC does not differentiate between posterior subcapsular and cortical cataract. The analyst may limit the analysis to a particular region of the image, so that if a posterior subcapsular cataract is seen in the central region of the image, an estimate of the area of this opacity will be very accurate, but if the entire pupil is filled with cortical and posterior subcapsular cataract, OPAC will give a measure of their aggregate area. This system has been applied in several clinical studies and has worked well.

In another approach to designating the size of cortical and posterior subcapsular cataracts in retro images, the instrument automatically binarizes the retro image into zones of "clear" and "opaque" lens. The threshold pixel density separating clear from opaque lens is selected automatically by the instrument. The Nidek EAS 1000 allows the operator to override this binarization procedure and select a different threshold, if the automatic binarization creates an image that is inconsistent with the original image of the lens. This may be necessary when there are significant birefringent artifacts in the image. In any retroillumination image taken with crossed polarizers, there are cruciate shaped artifactual shadows in the image. These shadows may be read by the computer operator as cataract rather than artifact, and if this occurs the binarized image of a small cataract and a large artifactual shadow will be read out as a large cataract. In such a case both the true cataract and the artifact are presented as cataract–an exaggeration of the amount of cataract. When the operator overrides the automatic thresholding of the binarization protocol, one must rely on the skill and experience of the operator to select a threshold that creates a binary image that resembles the true cataract in the unbinarized image. Such an operator must be able to recognize the wide varieties of cataract and the several artifacts which occur in these images. Once an operator designates a threshold, then this should be applied throughout the study to all the images from this patient, but occasionally the subsequent images manifest different artifacts than those which were present in the original image, and the operator must again select a biologically plausible threshold. This threshold may not be the same as the one chosen originally, and when these differences occur, the longitudinal analysis of the images is complicated. At present there is no completely satisfactory solution to this problem.

Marcher Industries has produced a digital instrument combining retroillumination and Scheimpflug optics. In their device, the Scheimpflug and retroillumination cameras are separately mounted on a single base, and the operator takes the two images separately. In contrast, in the Nidek EAS 1000 both the Scheimpflug and retroillumination images are obtained in a single exposure. The Marcher Industries instrument offers essentially the same analytical approach as the Nidek EAS 1000.

3. Light Scattering

Light scattering is the most fundamental manifestation of cataract. It is the scattering of light onto the peripheral retina that reduces the perceived contrast of an image, and it is the light scattered out of the eye by the nuclear region that creates the slitlamp image of the nuclear cataract. One may quantitate the intensity and angle of scattered light and use these measures as indices of the severity of cataract formation. There are two basic measures of light scattering–static and dynamic. They are presented below.

a. *Static*

Over the years different photometric devices have been introduced to measure the static-light scattering properties of the lens. None of these has been widely used clinically, but simple photometers have been used extensively by Siew and Bettelheim [55,56] to study the light-scattering properties of whole human cataractous lenses extracted intracapsularly.

b. *Dynamic (Quasielastic)*

Dynamic or quasielastic light scattering (QLS) derives from the autocorrelation function of the intensity of light scattered vs. time, a measure of the average diffusion coefficient of the molecules scattering light. [57] Since the diffusion coefficient is inversely correlated with the size of the molecule scattering the light, the diffusion coefficient allows an estimate of the molecular size of the scatterers.

QLS has been applied to rabbit lenses in vivo, and an increase in the size of the scatterers occurs with increasing age. [58] There have been a few human studies with prototype instruments in which there has been an increase in the size of the scattering species with age and nuclear cataract formation.

Recently Nidek Instruments has developed a clinically applicable version of the QLS device, and this is currently being assessed in two American centers and in Japan. It is not yet ready for wider application, but assuming that the validation protocols will be successful, it is likely that this instrument will prove to be a very sensitive means of detecting small changes in light scattering in the human lens and possibly identify individuals with early predisposition to cataract formation.

IV. CONCLUSIONS

We have arrived at an era in which it is possible to accurately and precisely quantitate the type, severity, and rate of growth of age-related cataracts. We are prepared to move into prospective, randomized, placebo-controlled, double-masked clinical trials of anti-cataract medications or nutritional supplements. When, and if, they are developed these trials may involve as few as 200-300 patients per group and last only 1-2 years. It is now quite feasible to measure the slow pace of age-related cataractogenesis and the efficacy of anti-cataract drugs in slowing this rate.

We also have well-validated cataract classification systems to apply in cross-sectional studies of the prevalence or incidence of blinding age-related cataract. Some of these systems also may be applied to measure the longitudinal change in cataract status in a population and identify the risk factors associated with certain types of cataract.

These techniques of cataract quantitation may be useful to the WHO and the World Bank as they work with national programs of blindness prevention. Recently the WHO has shifted its strategy from treating patients with bilateral cataract blindness to treating patients with unilateral cataract blindness. It is likely that this shift will lead to increased demand for cataract surgery from patients who perceive themselves as functionally blind. Means of grading cataract severity and assessing visual function will be needed to assist public health officials to expeditiously allocate their limited health resources.

V. REFERENCES

1. **Thylefors B, Negrel AD, Pararajasegaram Dadzie KY,** Available data on blindness (update 1994), *Ophthalmic Epidemiol.*, 2, 5-39, 1995.
2. **Leske MC, Chylack LT Jr, Wu S-Y,** The Lens Opacities Case-Control Study. Risk factors for cataract, *Arch. Ophthalmol.*, 109, 244-251, 1991.
3. **Maraini G, Pasquini P, Sperduto RD, Rosmini F, Bonacini M, Tomba MC, Corona R,** Distribution of lens opacities in the Italian-American Case-Control Study of Age-related cataract. The Italian-American Study Group. *Ophthalmology*, 97, 752-756, 1990.
4. *Encyclopedia Britannica*, CD-ROM Version, Category: Index of refraction, 1997.
5. **Kleberger E, Plohn HJ, Simonsohn G,** On the distribution of the index of refraction in the lens of the eye, *Albrecht Von Graefes Arch. Klin. Exp. Ophthalmol.*, 176, 155-159, 1968.
6. **Bettelheim FA and Wang TJY,** Topographic distribution of refractive indices in bovine lenses, *Exp. Eye Res.*, 18, 351-356,1974.
7. **Campbell MCW,** Measurement of refractive index in an intact crystalline lens, *Vision Res.*, 24, 409-415, 1984.
8. **Benedek GB, Chylack LT Jr, Libondi T, Magnante P, Pennett M,** Quantitative detection of the molecular changes associated with early cataractogenesis in the living human lens using quasielastic light scattering, *Curr. Eye Res.*, 6, 1421-1432, 1987.
9. **Jedziniak JA, Kinoshita JH, Yates EM, Hocker LO, Benedek GB,** On the presence and mechanism of formation of heavy molecular weight aggregates in human normal and cataractous lenses, *Exp. Eye Res.*, 15, 185-192, 1973.
10. **Benedek GB,** Cataract as a protein condensation disease. The Proctor Lecture, *Invest. Ophthalmol. Vis. Sci.*, 38, 1911-1921, 1997.
11. **Chylack LT Jr**, Classification of human cataracts, *Arch. Ophthalmol.*, 96, 888-892, 1978.
12. *Encyclopedia Britannica*, CD-ROM Version, Topic: chromatic aberration, 1997.
13. **Koretz J and Handelman GH**, Model of the accommodative mechanism in the human eye, *Vision Res.*, 22, 917-927,1982.
14. **Hyatt GA and Beebe DC**, Regulation of lens cell growth and polarity by an embryo-specific growth factor and by inhibitors of lens cell proliferation and differentiation, *Development*, 117, 701-709, 1993.
15. **Bassnett S and Beebe DC,** Coincident loss of mitochondria and nuclei during lens fiber cell differentiation, *Dev. Dyn.*, 194, 85-93,1993.
16. **Beebe DC,** *Alcon Research Institute Award Lecture*, 1997.
17. **Angunawela II,** The role of autoimmune phenomena in the pathogenesis of cataract, *Immunology*, 61, 363-368, 1987.
18. **Singh DP, Guru SC, Kikuchi T, Abe T, and Shinohara T,** Autoantibodies against β-crystallins induce lens epithelial cell damage and cataract formation in mice, *J. Immunol.*, 155, 993-999, 1995.

19. **Donders FC,** *Refraction und Accommodation des Auges*, Braumüller, Wien, 1866.
20. **NAS-NRC Committee on Vision, Working Group 39,** Recommended standard procedures for the clinical measurement and specification of visual acuity, *Adv. Ophthalmol.*, 41, 103-148, 1980.
21. **Chylack LT Jr, Padhye N, Khu PM, Wehner C, Wolfe J, McCarthy D, Rosner B, Friend J,** Loss of contrast sensitivity in diabetic patients with LOCS II classified cataracts, *Br. J. Ophthalmol.*, 77, 7-11, 1993.
22. **Elliott DB, Bullimore MA, Patla AE, Whitaker D,** Effect of a cataract simulation on clinical and real world vision, *Br. J. Ophthalmol.* 80, 799-804, 1996.
23. **Beckman C, Bond-Taylor L, Lindblom B, Sjostrand J,** Confocal fundus imaging with a scanning laser ophthalmoscope in eyes with cataract, *Br. J. Ophthalmol.*, 79, 900-904, 1995.
24. *Mentor O & O, Inc. B-VAT-SG Video Acuity Tester, Model 32-4850*, Norwell, MA.
25. **Salomao SR and Ventura DF,** Large sample population age norms for visual acuities obtained with Vistech-Teller Acuity Cards, *Invest. Ophthalmol. Vis. Sci.*, 36, 686-691, 1995.
26. **Pelli DG, Robson JG, Wilkins AJ,** The design of a new letter chart for measuring contrast sensitivity, *Clin. Vision Sci.*, 2, 187-199, 1988.
27. **Hirsch RP, Nadler MP, Miller D,** Clinical performance of a disability glare tester, *Arch. Ophthalmol.*, 102, 1633-1636, 1984.
28. **Maraini G, Rormini F, Graziosi P, Tomba MC, Bonacini M, Cotichini R, Pasquini P, and Sperduto R,** Influence of type and severity of pure forms of age-related cataract on visual acuity and contrast sensitivity. Italian American Cataract Study Group. *Invest. Ophthalmol. Vis. Sci.*, 35, 262-367, 1994.
29. **Hirvela H, Koskela P, Laatikainen L,** Visual acuity and contrast sensitivity in the elderly, *Acta Ophthalmol. Scand.*, 73, 111-115, 1995.
30. **Bueno G, Hurst MA,** Displacement threshold hyperacuity as a predictor of postsurgical visual performance in patients with cataract, *Invest. Ophthalmol. Vis. Sci.*, 36, 686-691,1995.
31. **Mangione CM, Orav EJ, Lawrence MG, Phillips RS, Seddon JM, Goldman L,** Prediction of visual function after cataract surgery. A prospectively validated model, *Arch. Ophthalmol.*, 113, 1305-1311, 1995.
32. See *Measuring Visual Functioning: Test Version of the NEI-VFQ*, NEI-VFQ Phase I Development Team, Santa Monica, CA, RAND MR-609-NEI/IMES, 1995.
33. **Adamsons IA, Vitale S, Stark WJ, Rubin GS,** The association of postoperative subjective visual function with acuity, glare, and contrast sensitivity in patients with early cataract, *Arch. Ophthalmol.*, 114, 529-536, 1996.
34. **Chylack LT Jr,** Classification of human cataractous change by the American Cooperative Cataract Research Group method, *Ciba Foundation Symp.*, 106, 3-24, 1984.
35. **Chylack LT Jr, Leske MC, Sperduto R, Khu P, McCarthy D, the LOCS Research Group,** Lens Opacities Classification System. *Arch. Ophthalmol.*,

106, 330-334, 1988.
36, **Chylack LT Jr, Leske MC, McCarthy D, Khu P, Kashiwagi T, Sperduto R,** Lens Opacities Classification System II (LOCS II). *Arch. Ophthalmol.,* 107, 991-997, 1989.
37. **West SK, Rosenthal F, Newland HS, Taylor HR,** Use of photographic techniques to grade nuclear cataracts, *Invest. Ophthalmol. Vis. Sci.,* 29, 73-77, 1988.
38. **West S, Muñoz B, Emmett EA, Taylor HR,** Cigarette smoking and risk of nuclear cataracts, *Arch. Ophthalmol.* 107, 1166-1169, 1989.
39. **Taylor HR, West S, Muñoz B, Rosenthal FS, Bressler SB, Bressler NM,** The long-term effects of visible light on the eye, *Arch. Ophthalmol.,* 110, 99-104,1992
40. **Sparrow JM, Bron AJ, Brown NAP, Ayliffe W, Hill AR,** The Oxford clinical cataract classification and grading system, *Int. Ophthalmol.,* 9, 207-225, 1986.
41. **Klein BEK, Magli YL, Neider MW, Klein R,** *Wisconsin System for Classification of Cataracts from Photographs,* National Technical Information Service, Springfield, Va, 1989.
42. **Chylack LT Jr, Wolfe JK, Singer DM, Leske MC, Bullimore MA, Bailey IL, Friend J, McCarthy D, Wu S-Y,** The Lens Opacities Classification System III. The Longitudinal Study of Cataract Study Group, *Arch. Ophthalmol.,* 111, 831-836, 1993.
43. **Thylefors B, Chylack LT Jr, Konyamia K, Sasaki K, Sperduto R, Taylor HR, West S,** A simplified cataract grading system - The WHO Cataract Grading Group, WHO/PBD, WHO, Geneva, Switzerland, 1997.
44. **Hockwin O, Dragomirescu V, Koch HR,** Photographic documentation of disturbances of the lens transparency during aging with a Scheimpflug camera system, *Ophthalmic Res.,* 11, 405, 1979.
45. **Dragomirescu V, Hockwin O, Koch HR, Sasaki K,** Development of a new equipment for rotating slit image photography according to Scheimpflug's principle, in *Gerontological Aspects of Eye Research*, Hockwin, O., Ed., Karger, Basel, 1978, p. 118-130.
46. **Chylack LT Jr, McCarthy D, Khu P,** Use of Topcon SL-45 Scheimpflug slit photography to measure longitudinal growth of nuclear cataracts *in vivo*, *Lens Res.*, 5, 83, 1988.
47. **Chylack LT Jr, Rosner B, White O, Tung WH, Sher LD,** Standardization and analysis of digitized photographic data in the longitudinal documentation of cataractous growth, *Curr. Eye Res.,* 7, 223-235, 1988.
48. **Kawara T, Obazawa H,** A new method for retroillumination photography of cataractous lens opacities, *Am. J. Ophthalmol.,* 90, 186-189, 1980.
49. *Anterior Eye Segment Analysis System, EAS-1000*, Operators Manual, Nidek Co., Ltd., Nov. 19, 1990.
50. **Sparrow JM, Brown NAP, Shun-Shin GA, Bron AJ,** The Oxford Modular Cataract Image Analysis System, *Eye,* 4, 638-648, 1990.
51. **Chylack, LT Jr, Mantell G, Wolfe JK, Friend J, Rosner B,** Monitoring cataract with LOCS II and counterpart objective measures. Lovastatin and the

human lens, *Optom. Vis. Sci.,* 70, 937-943, 1993.

52. **Pauli H,** Proposed extension to the CIE recommendation on uniform color spaces, color difference equations, and metric color terms, *J. Opt. Soc. Am.,* 66, 866-867, 1976.
53. **Birren F,** Color identification and nomenclature: A history, *Color. Res. Appl.,* 4, 14-18, 1969.
54. **Chylack, LT Jr, Wolfe JK, Friend J, Khu PM, Singer DM, McCarthy D, del Carmen J, Rosner B,** Quantitating cataract and nuclear brunescence, The Harvard and LOCS Systems, *Optom. Vis. Sci.,* 70, 886-895, 1993.
55. **Siew EL, Bettelheim FA, Chylack LT Jr, Tung WH,** Studies on human cataracts II. Correlation between the clinical description and the light scattering parameters of human cataracts, *Invest. Ophthalmol. Vis. Sci.,* 20, 334-347, 1981.
56. **Bettelheim FA, Siew EL, Chylack LT Jr,** Studies on human cataracts III. Structural elements in nuclear cataracts and their contribution to the turbidity, *Invest. Ophthalmol. Vis. Sci.,* 20, 348-354, 1981.
57. **Tanaka T and Benedek GB,** Observation of protein diffusivity in intact human and bovine lenses with application to cataract, *Invest. Ophthalmol. Vis. Sci.,* 14, 449-456, 1975.
58. **Libondi T, Magnante P, Chylack LT Jr, Benedek GB,** *In vivo* measurement of the aging rabbit lens using quasielastic light scattering, *Curr. Eye Res.,* 5, 411-419,1986.

Chapter 4

NUTRITIONAL AND ENVIRONMENTAL INFLUENCES ON RISK FOR CATARACT

Allen Taylor

I. INTRODUCTION

The number of associations between nutriture and eye lens cataract has burgeoned in the last decade, inspired in part by early studies regarding antioxidant properties of nutrients.[1] Such studies include laboratory, clinical, and epidemiological investigations, as well as human intervention trials. Since this volume has as its focus relationships between nutritional and environmental influences on risk for age-related eye diseases, data regarding associations between nutriture and eye health are given the most thorough treatment. For a review of data regarding animal or cell free studies, readers can refer to other recent summaries and the rich body of pioneering work which is, of necessity, given limited coverage here. [2-11]

A. CATARACT AS A PUBLIC HEALTH ISSUE

Cataract is one of the major causes of blindness throughout the world. [12-14] In the United States, the prevalence of visually significant cataract increases from approximately 5% at age 65 to about 50% for persons older than 75 years. [15-17] In the U.S. and much of the developed world, cataract surgery, albeit costly, is readily available and routinely successful in restoring sight. In less-developed countries, such as India [18], China [19], and Kenya [20], cataracts are more common and develop earlier in life than in more-developed countries. For example, by age 60, cataract with low vision or aphakia (i.e., absence of the lens, which is usually the result of cataract extraction) is approximately five times more common in India than in the U.S. [17,18] The impact of cataract on impaired vision is much greater in less-developed countries, where more than 90% of the cases of blindness and visual impairment are found [14, 21-25] and where there is a dearth of ophthalmologists to perform lens extractions.

Given both the extent of disability caused by age-related cataract and its costs, \$5-6 billion/yr[1] [26] in the U.S., it is urgent that we elucidate causes of cataract and identify strategies to slow the development of this disorder. It is estimated that a delay in cataract formation of about 10 years would reduce the prevalence of visually disabling cataract by about 45%. [12] Such a delay would enhance the quality of life for much of the world's older population and substantially reduce the economic burden due to cataract-related disability and cataract surgery. It is such data which provide the impetus for this research.

[1]Congressional Testimony of S.J. Ryan, May 5, 1993.

0-8493-8565-2/99/\$0.00+\$.50

B. AGE-RELATED CHANGES IN LENS FUNCTION

The primary function of the eye lens is to collect and focus light on the retina (Figs. 1 and 2a). To do so it must remain clear throughout life. The lens is located posterior to the cornea and iris and receives nutriture from the aqueous humor. Although the clarity of the lens is frequently interpreted as indicative of an absence of structure, the lens is exquisitely organized. A single layer of epithelial cells is found directly under the anterior surface of the collagenous membrane in which it is encapsulated (Fig. 2b). The epithelial cells at the germinative region divide, migrate posteriorly, and differentiate into lens fibers. As their primary gene products, the fibers elaborate the predominant proteins of the lens, called crystallins. They also lose their organelles. New cells are formed throughout life, but older cells are usually not lost. Instead, they are compressed into the center or nucleus of the lens. There is a coincident dehydration of the proteins and of the lens itself. Consequently, protein concentrations rise to hundreds of mg/ml. [27] Together with other age-related modifications of the protein (noted below) and other constituents, these changes result in a less flexible lens with limited accommodative capability.

In addition, as the lens ages, the proteins are photooxidatively damaged, aggregate, and accumulate in lens opacities. Dysfunction of the lens due to opacification is called cataract. The term "age-related cataract" is used to distinguish lens opacification associated with old age from opacification associated with other causes, such as congenital and metabolic disorders or trauma. [28]

C. CLINICAL FEATURES IN CATARACT

There are several systems for evaluating and grading cataracts. Most of these employ an assessment of extent, or density, and location of the opacity [29] (see Chapter 3). Usually evaluated are opacities in the posterior subcapsular, nuclear, cortical, and multiple (mixed) locations (Fig. 2b). However, it is not established that cataract at each location has completely different etiology. Coloration or brunescence is also quantified, since these diminish visual function (Figs. 2c-e). [30,31]

II. HIGH-ENERGY RADIATION, OXIDATION, SMOKING AND FAILURE OF PRIMARY AND SECONDARY DEFENSE SYSTEMS

Only a brief introduction to some of these topics is offered here.

Associations between risk for cataract and light exposure or smoking are each covered in relevant chapters (Chapters 8 and 9, respectively). The solid mass of the lens is about 98% protein. These proteins undergo minimal turnover as the lens ages. Accordingly, upon aging they are subject to the chronic stresses of exposure to light or other high-energy radiation and oxygen. Several, if not all of these insults, cause oxidative damage to lens constituents, and this damage is thought to be causally related to cataractogenesis. A schematic summary of insults and protective species, along with a proposal of their interactions, is indicated in Fig. 3.

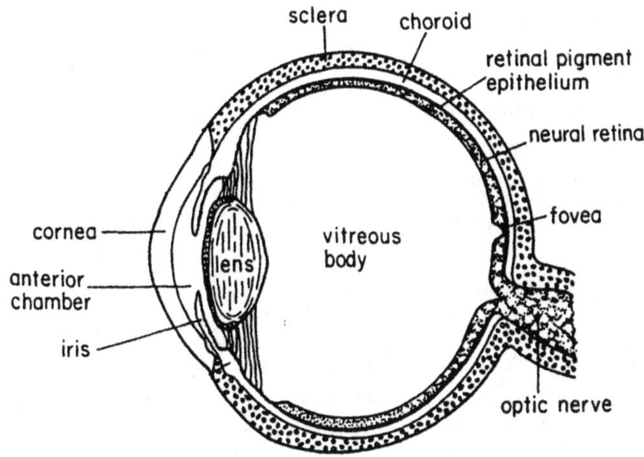

Figure 1.
Cross section of the eye. From Taylor, A., Dorey, C.K., and Nowell, T. *Vitamin C in Health and Disease,* Packer, L. and Fuchs, J., Eds., Marcel Dekker, Inc., New York, 1997. With permission.

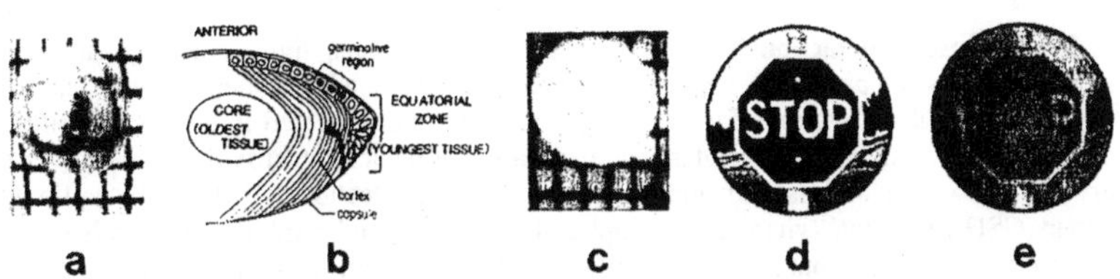

Figure 2. Clear and cataractous lens. a) Clear lens allows an unobstructed view of the wire grid placed behind it. b) Cartoon of the structure of the lens. The anterior surface of the lens has a unicellular layer of epithelial cells (youngest tissue). Cells at the anterior equatorial region divide and migrate to the cortex as they are overlaid by less mature cells. These cells produce a majority of the crystallins. As development and maturation proceed, the cells denucleate and elongate. Tissue originally found in the embryonic lens is found in the core or nucleus (oldest tissue). c) The cataractous lens prohibits viewing the wire grid behind it. d) Artist's view through a clear uncolored young lens. The image is clear and crisp. e) Artist's view through a lens with developing cataract. The image is partially obscured, and the field is darkened due to browning of the lens which accompanies aging. From Taylor, A., Dorey, C.K., and Nowell, T. *Vitamin C in Health and Disease,* Packer, L. and Fuchs, J., Eds., Marcel Dekker, Inc., New York, 1997. With permission.

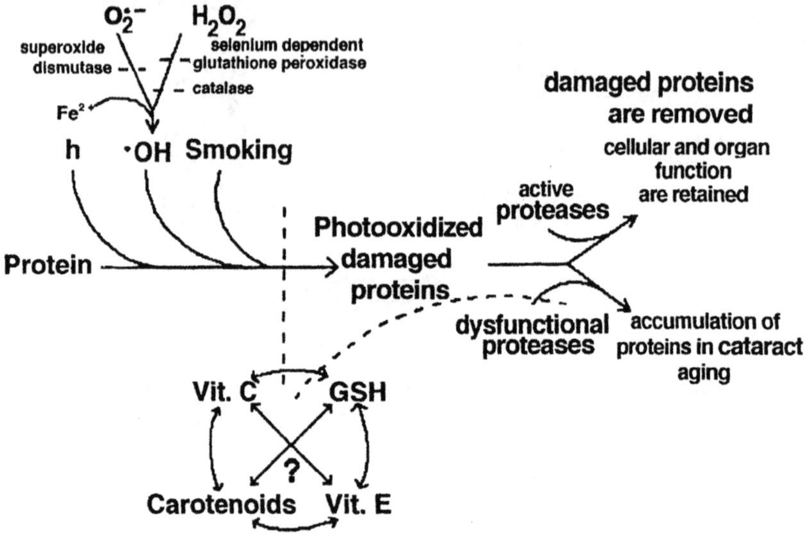

Figure 3. Proposed interaction between lens proteins, oxidants, light, smoking, antioxidants, antioxidant enzymes and proteases. Lens proteins are extremely long lived. Lens proteins are subject to alteration by light and various forms of oxygen. They are protected indirectly by antioxidant enzymes: superoxide dismutase, catalase, and glutathione reductase/peroxidase. These enzymes convert active oxygen to less damaging species. Direct protection is offered by antioxidants: glutathione (GSH), ascorbate (vitamin C), tocopherol (vitamin E), and carotenoids. Levels of reduced and oxidized forms of some, but perhaps not all (?), of these molecules are determined by interaction between the three and with the environment. [166-171] Proteins which are damaged may accumulate and precipitate in cataract if there is insufficient proteolytic capability. When the proteolytic capability is sufficient, obsolete and damaged proteins may be reduced to their constituent amino acids. Upon aging some of the eye antioxidant supplies are diminished, antioxidant enzymes inactivated, and proteases less active. This appears to be related to the accumulation, aggregation, and eventual precipitation in cataractous opacities of damaged proteins. From Taylor, A., Dorey, C.K., and Nowell, T. *Vitamin C in Health and Disease,* Packer, L. and Fuchs, J., Eds., Marcel Dekker, Inc., New York, 1997. With permission.

A. LIGHT EXPOSURE AS A RISK FACTOR FOR CATARACT

Various epidemiological studies show associations between elevated risk of various forms of cataract and exposure to higher intensities of incident and/or reflected ultraviolet light (Table 1). [15,32-40] Greater light exposure was (weakly) associated with an increased risk for cortical opacity in Chesapeake Bay watermen [32] and in men (but not women) in Wisconsin. [36] Light-related risk for cataract was also increased among Italians but not among residents of Massachusetts. [37] Risk for posterior subcapsular cataract was weakly related to light exposure in Chesapeake Bay watermen and (nonsignificantly) in residents of Wisconsin. Other studies (Massachusetts and Italy) did not find associations between posterior subcapsular cataract risk and light exposure. Nuclear cataract appears unrelated to risk for cataract in most studies.

Geographical data provide some support for purported relationships between light exposure and cataract risk. [41] Persons living closer to the equator [42] and living at higher elevations, appear to have an elevated risk of various forms of cataract. [35,38-41,43] Indeed, one of the strongest predictors of cataract surgery likelihood in a Medicare beneficiary is a person's latitude of residence. [40] Although not a uniform observation [2,44,45], these epidemiological data have been corroborated or anticipated by exposure of squirrels to ultraviolet light *in vivo* [46] and in many experiments *in vitro* [6-8,42,47-52], and references cited within. As an aggregate, the latter references indicate that exposure of lens constituents to various wavelengths of light results in alterations which are quite similar to those found in cataract.

B. HIGH ENERGY RADIATION AS A RISK FACTOR FOR CATARACT

Cataractogenesis is also clearly related to exposure to high-energy radiation. Taylor et al. showed a dose-response relationship between x-irradiation and risk for cataract in rats. [53] In a study with 99 patients, the 89 who received whole body irradiation (10 g) developed cataract in <4 years. [54] The 10 patients who were treated for aplastic anemia and did not receive radiation treatment did not show evidence of cataractogenesis.

C. EXPOSURE TO HIGH LEVELS OF OXYGEN AS A RISK FACTOR FOR CATARACT

Perhaps the clearest causal association between oxidative stress and cataract comes from experiences involving elevated levels of oxygen. Nuclear cataract was observed in patients treated with hyperbaric oxygen therapy [55], and markedly elevated levels of mature cataract were observed in mice that survived exposure to 100% oxygen twice weekly for 3h. [56] A decline in glutathione (GSH) and an increase in glutathione disulfide (oxidative changes normally related to aging or cataract) were also noted. A higher incidence of cataract was noted in lenses exposed to hyperbaric oxygen *in vitro* [57] and Giblin also noted very early stages of cataract in guinea pigs exposed to hyperbaric oxygen. [58] However, there was difficulty in repeating these results (Taylor et al., unpublished). Oxidative damage to membrane lipids in fiber cells is also associated with lens opacities. [59]

Table 1
Selected Correlations between Risk for Cataract and Extent of Light Exposure[a]

Study and Location	Exposure	Prevalence Ratio[b]	95%CI
USA-35 areas NHANES survey data[c] [157]	Daily hours of sunlight in area ages 65-74		
	<6.6 h	1.0	
	7.1-7.7 h	1.7	1.2-2.7
	>8.2	2.7	1.6-4.6
Australia [158]	Daily hours of sunlight in area		
	8 or less	1.0	
	8.5-9	2.9	0.6-13.2
	9.5 or more	4.2	0.9-18.9
	Average mean erythemal dose of area		
	2000	1.0	
	2500	1.3	0.8-2.3
	3000	1.8	1.0-3.4
Nepal [43]	Average hours of sunlight		
	low (7-9 h)	1.0	
	medium (10-11 h)	1.2	0.9-1.4
	high (12+h)	2.5	2.1-3.0

[a]Adapted from Dolin, 1995. [41]
[b]The prevalence ratios and 95% confidence intervals in this table were calculated from the published data.
[c]These data were originally reported as annual light exposure. To obtain daily exposure, the annual light exposure (<2400 h, 2600-2800 h, >3000 h, for each of the three prevalence groups) was divided by 365.

D. SMOKING AS A RISK FACTOR FOR CATARACT

Smoking and tobacco chewing appear to induce oxidative stress and have been associated with both diminished levels of antioxidants, ascorbate, and carotenoids [60-65] and with enhanced cataract at a younger age [66-69]; (also see Chapter 9). Of interest are recent observations that 1) for male smokers there appears to be an inverse relationship between serum levels of α-carotene, ß-cryptoxanthin, lutein, and severity of nuclear sclerosis [70] (but the reverse may be true for women), and 2) there is diminished risk for cataract in smokers who use multivitamins. [25]

E. CELLULAR ANTIOXIDANTS AS PRIMARY DEFENSES AGAINST LENS DAMAGE

Protection against photooxidative insult can be conceived as due to two interrelated processes. Primary defenses offer protection of proteins and other constituents by lens antioxidants and antioxidant enzymes (Fig. 3). Secondary defenses include proteolytic and repair processes, which degrade and eliminate damaged proteins and other biomolecules in a timely fashion. [71]

The major aqueous antioxidants in the lens are ascorbate [72] and GSH. [3,73-75] Both are present in the lens at mM concentrations. [76-78]

Ascorbate is probably the most effective, least toxic antioxidant identified in mammalian systems. [79,80] Interest in the function of ascorbate in the lens was prompted by teleological arguments, which suggested age-related compromises in ascorbate and compromises in lens function might be related. Thus, it was observed that: 1) the lens and aqueous concentrate ascorbate >10 fold the level found in guinea pig and human plasma [72,73,81,82] (Fig. 4a-d); 2) in the lens core (Fig. 2b), the oldest part of the lens and the region involved in much senile cataract, the concentration of ascorbate is only 25% of the surrounding cortex [83]; 3) lens ascorbate concentrations are lower in cataract than in the normal lens [84]; and 4) ascorbate levels in the lens are significantly lower in old guinea pigs than in young animals with the same dietary intake of ascorbate. [72,81] The same pertains in Emory mice. [78] These data suggest either that there is age-related depletion of ascorbate in the lens or that the bioavailability of this compound changes with age. Enthusiasm for nutrient antioxidants has been fueled by observations that ocular levels of ascorbate are related to dietary intake in humans and animals that require exogenous ascorbate (Fig. 4). [72, 81,82] Thus, the concentration of vitamin C in the lens was increased with dietary supplements beyond levels achieved in persons who already consumed more than two times the RDA (60 mg/day) for vitamin C. [72,73]

Feeding elevated ascorbate delayed progress of, or prevented: galactose cataract in guinea pigs [85] and rats [86], selenite-induced cataracts in rats [87], lens opacification in GSH-depleted chick embryos [88], and delayed UV-induced protein and protease damage in guinea pig lenses. [7-9,89] Increasing lens ascorbate concentrations by only twofold is associated with protection against cataract-like damage. [8]

Since ascorbate is a carbohydrate, it is biochemically plausible that vitamin C induces damage in the lens *in vivo*. [90,91] However, presently there are no data to support this as a medical concern. Mice fed 8% of the weight of their diet as ascorbate did not develop cataract. [92] In the event that glycation induces pathological lens damage, antiglycating agents such as phenacylthiazoliums may be useful. [93] It is interesting that comparable compounds have been tried as anticataractogens and were assumed to act as reducing cysteine prodrug agents. [94]

GSH levels are severalfold the levels found in whole blood and orders of magnitude greater than the concentration observed in the plasma. GSH levels also diminish in the older and cataractous lens. [74] There have been several attempts to exploit the reducing capabilities of GSH (see also chapter 6). Injection of GSH-OMe was associated with delayed buthionine sulfoxamine induced [95] and naphthalene cataract. [74,96,97] Preliminary evidence from studies with galactose-induced cataract also indicates some advantage of maintaining elevated GSH status in rats. [76] However, it is not clear that feeding GSH is associated with higher ocular levels of this antioxidant. [76] Other compounds, such as pantetheine, which also include sulfhydryls, are under investigation as anticataractogenic agents.

[98] However, the effficacy of this compound in later life cataract remains to be established. [99]

Pharmacological opportunities are suggested by observations that incorporating the industrial antioxidant 0.4% butylated hydroxytoluene in diets of galactose-fed (50% of diet) rats diminished prevalence of cataract. [100]

Tocopherols and carotenoids are lipid-soluble antioxidants [101,102] with probable roles in maintaining membrane integrity [103] and GSH recycling. [104] Concentrations of tocopherol in the whole lens are in the μM range [105] (Table 2), but it appears that lens and dietary levels of tocopherol levels are unrelated. [106] Since most of the compound is found in the membranes, particularly in the younger tissues (Taylor et al., unpublished), the concentrations can be orders of magnitude higher. Age-related changes in levels of tocopherol and carotenoids have not been documented. Tocopherol is reported to be effective in delaying a variety of induced cataracts in animals, including galactose [28,107,108] and aminotriazole-induced cataracts in rabbits. [109]

Elevated carotenoid intake is frequently associated with health benefits. However, little experimental work has been done regarding lens changes in response to variations in levels of this nutrient. It is intriguing that β-carotene levels in the human lenses are limited. [105] (Table 2) Instead, major lens carotenoids are lutein/zeaxanthin. These are also the major carotenoids in the macula. [110] Also present are retinol and retinol ester, and tocopherols. In beef, β-carotene was occasionally observed in lenses. This apparent quixotic appearance of the β-carotene appears to be due to seasonal and dietary availability.

The lens also contains antioxidant enzymes: glutathione peroxidase/ reductase, catalase, and superoxidase dismutase and enzymes of the glutathione redox cycle. [47,48,96,111,112] These interact via the forms of oxygen, as well as with the antioxidants, i.e., GSH is a substrate for glutathione peroxidase. The activities of many antioxidant enzymes are compromised upon development, aging, and cataract formation. [59]

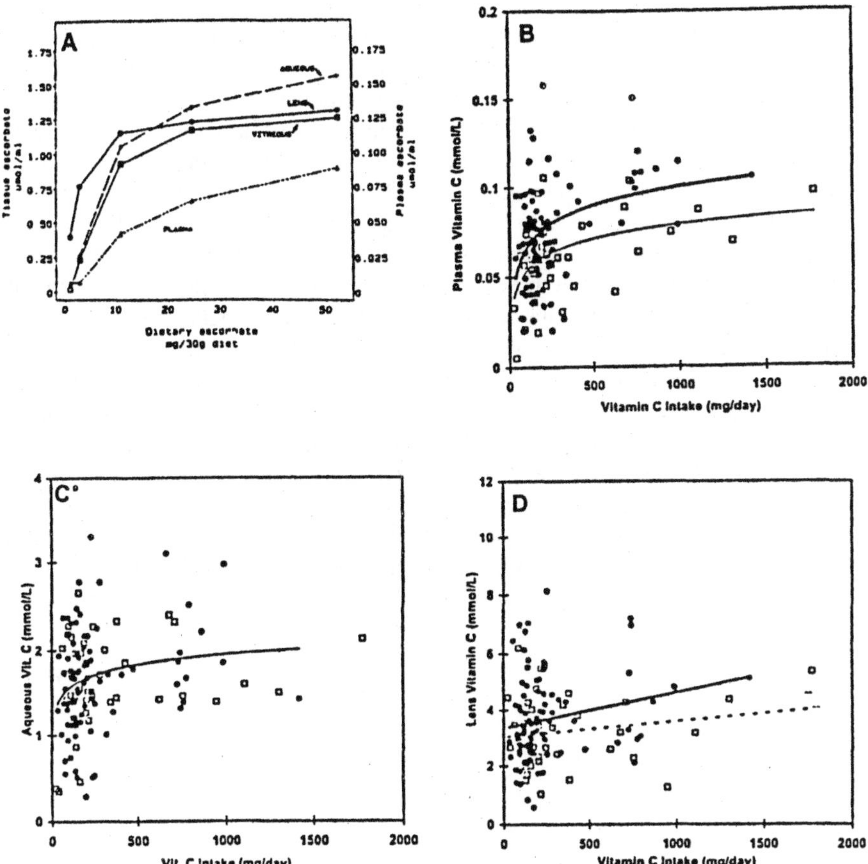

Figure 4. Tissue or plasma ascorbate versus ascorbate intake. a) guinea pig, b) plasma ascorbate versus ascorbate intake in men (light line and square symbols) and women (bold line and filled circles), c) aqueous ascorbate versus ascorbate intake in men (open squares) and women (filled circles), and d) lens ascorbate versus ascorbate intake in men (dashed lines and open squares) and women (solid line and filled circles). Panel a is adapted from Berger et al., *Curr. Eye Res.*, 1988. Panels b-d are adapted from Taylor et al., *Curr. Eye Res.*, 1997.

F. PROTEASES AS SECONDARY DEFENSES

Proteolytic systems can be considered secondary defense capabilities which remove cytotoxic damaged or obsolete proteins from lenses and other eye tissues. [2,71,85,113-124] Such proteolytic systems exist in young lens tissue, and damaged proteins are usually maintained at harmless levels by primary and secondary defense systems in younger lenses and in younger lens tissues within older lenses.

Two studies indicate interactions between primary and secondary defense systems. A direct sparing effect of ascorbate on a photooxidatively induced compromise of proteolytic function has been demonstrated. [7] GSH also spares activity of enzymes involved in the conjugation of ubiquitin to substrates. [115,122] Ubiquitin conjugation is required for selective targeting of substrates for degradation. However, upon aging or oxidative stress, most of these enzymatic capabilities are found in a state of reduced activity. [71] (Table 3) The observed accumulation of oxidized (and/or otherwise modified) proteins in older lenses is consistent with the failure of these protective systems to keep pace with the insults that damage lens proteins. This occurs in part because, like bulk proteins, enzymes that comprise some of the protective systems are damaged by photooxidation. [2,7,122,115,125] From these data it is clear that the young lens has significant primary and secondary protection. However, age-related compromises in the activity of antioxidant enzymes, concentrations of the antioxidants, and activities of secondary defenses may lead to diminished protection against oxidative insults. [123] This diminished protection leaves the long-lived proteins and other constituents vulnerable. Lens opacities develop as the damaged proteins aggregate and precipitate. [2] Current data predict that elevated antioxidant intake can be exploited to extend the function of some of these proteolytic capabilities.

Table 2
Endogenous Concentrations (ng/g wet wt) of Carotenoids, Retinoids, and Tocopherols in Human Lenses with and without Cataracts[1, 2]

Age, Sex, Nutrient	Groups American Normal	American Cataract	Indian Cataract
Age*	53.3 ± 6.9	78.6 ± 2.3	58.2 ± 1.4
Male (female)	2 (4)	7 (2)	5 (7)
Lut/zeax	13.8 ± 0.9	11.8 ± 1.4	25.8 ± 3.5‖≡
β-carotene	ND	ND	ND
Lycopene	ND	ND	ND
Retinol	38.1 ± 4.2	31.3 ± 3.9	50.4 ± 6.3≡
Retinyl ester	25.6 ± 7.1	25.7 ± 4.9	21.7 ± 3.1
α-tocopherol	1573 ± 168	2126 ± 209	2550 ± 203‖
γ-tocopherol	367 ± 64	501 ± 49∓	257 ± 24≡

ND = not detected (<0.1 ng).
[1]Values are means ± SEM.
[2]Analysis of variance comparison procedure was used for statistical analyses of the data. P < 0.05.
* Mean donor age ± SEM.
‖ American normal versus Indian cataract.
≡ American cataract versus Indian cataract.
∓ American normal versus American cataract.
Adapted from Yeum et al., *Invest. Ophthalmol. Vis. Sci.*, 1995. [105]

Table 3
Effect of Aging and Development on Proteolytic Activities

Activity	Source	Development
Intracellular proteolysis [159]	BLEC[1,2]	↓
Ubiquitin-dependent proteolysis in response to stress [124]	Tissue	↓
Neutral proteinase/Proteasome/ High molecular weight protease [160-163]	Tissue	↓
Endopeptidase [123]	BLEC	↓
LAP [113,163]	Tissue	↓
	BLEC	↓
Cathepsins [113]	BLEC	↓
Calpain [164,165]	Tissue	↑
	BLEC	N.D.[3]

[1,2]In cultured cells–aging was simulated by progressive passage of cells in culture. BLEC beef lens epithelial cells; [3]not determined.

III. EPIDEMIOLOGICAL AND CLINICAL STUDIES REGARDING ASSOCIATIONS BETWEEN ANTIOXIDANTS AND CATARACT

Approximately a dozen epidemiological studies examined the associations between cataract and antioxidants. [25,37,126-135] (Please see Chapter 5 for a more thorough discussion of types of studies.) Comparisons are not always straightforward since each of the studies varied in design. Nevertheless, comparisons of the data appear to indicate some agreement with respect to use of nutriture to diminish risk for cataract.

Nine of the studies were retrospective case-control or cross-sectional studies in which levels of cataract patients were compared with levels of individuals with clear lenses. [37,101,126-128,130,131,133,136] Our ability to interpret data from retrospective studies, such as these, is limited by the concurrent assessment of lens status and levels (see Chapter 5). Prior diagnosis of cataract might influence behavior of cases including diet, and it might also bias reporting of usual diet.

Six other studies [25,132,135,137-140] assessed levels and/or supplement use, and then followed individuals with intact lenses for up to eight years. Prospective studies, such as these, are less prone to bias because assessment of exposure is performed before the outcome is present. Some of these studies [25,132,135] did not directly assess lens status, but used cataract extraction or reported diagnosis of cataract as a measure of cataract risk. Extraction may not be a good measure of cataract incidence (development of new cataract), because it incorporates components of both incidence and progression in severity of existing cataract. However, extraction is the result of visually disabling cataract and is the endpoint that we wish to prevent.

Duration of measurement of dietary intake of nutrients may also affect the accuracy of these analyses since cataract develops over many years; one measure may not provide as accurate an assessment of usual intake. Instead, multiple measures over time may offer a better nutritional correlate of cataract.

Hankinson et al. [132] measured intake several times over a four-year period, whereas other studies used only one measure of serum antioxidant status, dietary intake, or supplement use. Jacques et al. [141] measured supplement intake over > 10 years and found different risk ratios for cataract in persons who took vitamin C supplements for different periods of time (see section A below).

In addition to the different study designs noted above, various studies used different lens classification schemes, different definitions of high and low levels of nutrients, and different age groups of subjects. A study (n = 367), which monitored cataract *in vivo* and cataract extraction, but did not find associations between nutriture and cataract, is not described further because the cataract classifications do not match those used on other work. [34]

A. ASCORBATE

As noted above, dietary ascorbate intake is related to eye tissue ascorbate levels. Given potential anticataractogenic and putative procataractogenic roles for ascorbate, the available epidemiological data regarding ascorbate intake and risk for cataract is particularly intriguing.

Vitamin C was considered in approximately ten published studies [37,127,128,130-133,139,141] and observed to be inversely associated with at least one type of cataract in eight of these studies (Fig. 5).

Several studies found correlations between vitamin C supplement use and risk for cataract. In our Nutrition and Vision Project [141], age-adjusted analyses based on 165 women with high vitamin C intake (mean = 294 mg/day) and 136 women with low vitamin C intake (mean = 77 mg/day) indicated that the women who took vitamin C supplements ≥10 years had >70% lower prevalence of early opacities (RR: 0.23; CI: 0.09-0.60) (Fig. 5a) and > 80% lower risk of moderate opacities (RR:0.17; CI: 0.03-0.87) at any site compared with women who did not use vitamin C supplements. [141] Recent reexamination of 600 of the members of the same cohort indicates that comparable data can be anticipated. This corroborated work by Hankinson et al. [132] who noted that women who consumed vitamin C supplements for > 10 years had a 45% reduction in rate of cataract surgery (RR: 0.55; CI: 0.32-0.96) (Fig. 5g). However, after controlling for nine potential confounders including age, diabetes, smoking, and energy intake, they did not observe an association between total vitamin C intake and rate of cataract surgery (see below).

In comparison to the data noted above, Mares-Perlman and coworkers [126] report that past use of supplements containing vitamin C was associated with a reduced prevalence of nuclear cataract (RR: 0.7; CI: 0.5-1.0) (Fig. 5c), but an increased prevalence of cortical cataract (adjusted RR: 1.8; CI: 1.2-2.9) after controlling for age, sex, smoking, and history of heavy alcohol consumption (Fig. 5d).

The inverse relationship is corroborated by data from other studies. Robertson and coworkers [127] compared cases (with cataracts that impaired vision) to age-

and sex-matched controls who were either free of cataract or had minimal opacities that did not impair vision. The prevalence of cataract in consumers of daily vitamin C supplements of >300 mg/day was approximately one-third the prevalence in persons who did not consume vitamin C supplements (RR: 0.30; CI: 0.24-0.77, Fig. 5b).

Elevated dietary ascorbate was also related to benefit with respect to cataract in some studies. Leske and coworkers [128] observed that persons with vitamin C intake in the highest 20% of their population group had a 52% lower prevalence for nuclear cataract (RR: 0.48; CI:0.24-0.99) compared with persons who had intakes among the lowest 20% after controlling for age and sex (Fig. 5c). Weaker inverse associations were noted for other types of cataract (Fig. 5f). Jacques and Chylack observed that among persons with higher vitamin C intakes (>490 mg/day), the prevalence of cataract was 25% of the prevalence among persons with lower intakes (<125 mg/day) (RR: 0.25; CI: 0.06-1.09) (Fig. 5a). [130]

However, Vitale and coworkers observed no differences in cataract prevalence between persons with high (> 261 mg/day) and low (<115 mg/day) vitamin C intakes. [133] The Italian-American Studies group [37] also failed to observe any association between prevalence of cataract and vitamin C intake. In addition, in a large prospective study, comparison of women with high intakes (median = 705 mg/day) to women with low intakes (median = 70 mg/day) failed to reveal any significant correlation with risk for cataract extraction (RR: 0.98; CI: 0.72-1.32). [132]

Attempts to corroborate the above inverse associations between cataract risk and intake using plasma vitamin C levels were generally frustrating. Jacques and Chylack [130] observed that persons with high plasma vitamin C levels (> 90 μM) had less than one-third the prevalence of early cataract as persons with low plasma vitamin C (<40 μM) although this difference was not statistically significant (risk ratio [RR]: 0.29; 95% confidence interval [CI]: 0.06-1.32) after adjustment for age, sex, race and history of diabetes (Fig. 5a). Mohan [131] noted an 87% (RR: 1.87; CI: 1.29-2.69) increased prevalence of mixed cataract (posterior subcapsular and nuclear involvement) for each standard deviation increase in plasma vitamin C levels. Vitale and coworkers [133] observed that persons with plasma levels greater than 80 μM and below 60 μM had similar prevalences of both nuclear (RR: 1.31; CI: 0.61-2.39) and cortical (RR: 1.01; CI: 0.45-2.26) cataract after controlling for age, sex, and diabetes.

Results from one intervention trial have been published and are described below. [142]

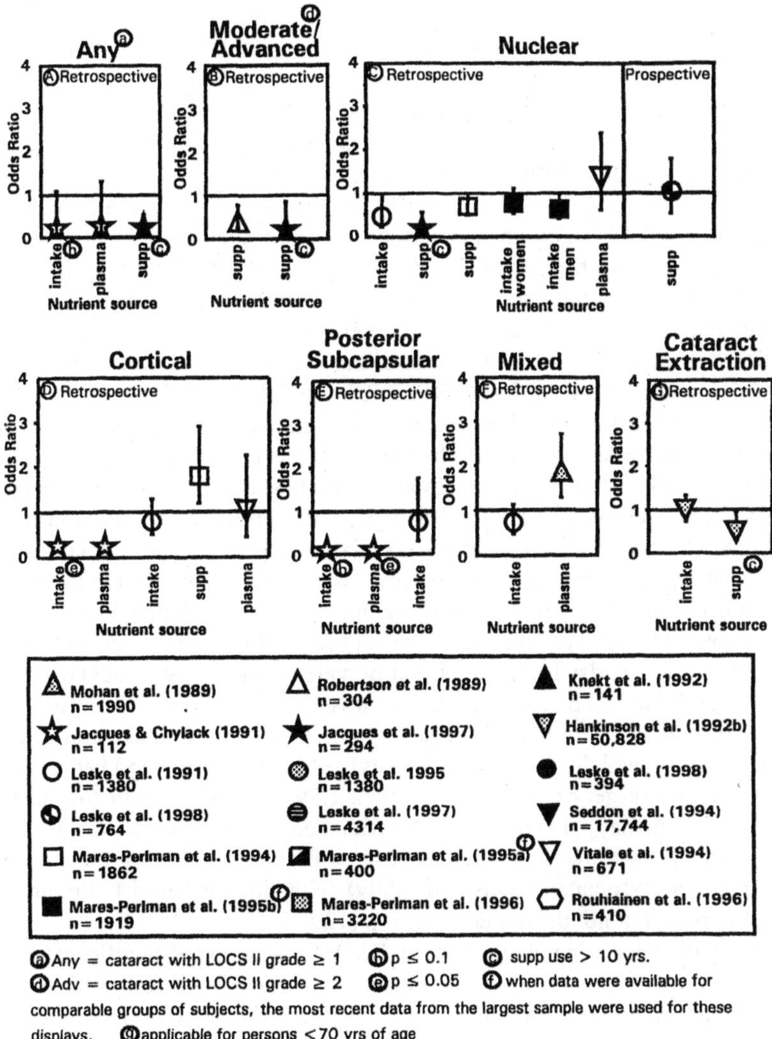

Figure 5. Cataract Risk Ratio, high versus low intake (with or without supplements) or plasma levels of vitamin C. Types of cataract are any, moderate/advanced, nuclear, cortical, posterior subcapsular, mixed, or cataract extraction. Data for retrospective and prospective studies are presented independently. Adapted from Taylor et al., *Vitamin C in Health and Disease*, Marcel Deckker, Inc., New York, 1997.

B. VITAMIN E

Vitamin E, a natural lipid-soluble antioxidant, can inhibit lipid peroxidation [103] and appears to stabilize lens cell membranes. [143] The efficacy of vitamin E as an antioxidant may be affected by ascorbate (see legend to Fig. 3), and also enhances glutathione recycling, perhaps helping to maintain reduced glutathione levels in the lens and aqueous humor. [104]

Consumption of vitamin E supplements was inversely correlated with cataract risk in two studies (Fig. 6). Robertson and coworkers [127] found among age- and sex-matched cases and controls that the prevalence of advanced cataract was 56% lower (RR: 0.44; CI: 0.24-0.77) (Fig. 6b) in persons who consumed vitamin E supplements (>400 I.U./day) than in persons not consuming supplements. Jacques and Chylack (unpublished) observed a 67% (RR: 0.33; CI: 0.12-0.96) reduction in prevalence of cataract for vitamin E supplement users after adjusting for age, sex, race and diabetes. Mares-Perlman and co-workers [126] observed only weak, non-significant associations between vitamin E supplement use and nuclear (RR: 0.9; CI: 0.6-1.5, Fig. 6c) and cortical (RR: 1.2; CI: 0.6-2.3, Fig. 6d) cataract.

The inverse association between vitamin E intake and risk for cataract was corroborated by Leske et al. [128] They observed that after controlling for age and sex, persons with vitamin E intakes among the highest 20% had an approximately 40% lower prevalence of cortical (RR: 0.59; CI: 0.36-0.97, Fig. 6d) and mixed (RR: 0.58; CI: 0.37-0.93, Fig. 6f) cataract relative to persons with intakes among the lowest 20%. Jacques and Chylack observed a nonsignificant inverse association when they related total vitamin E intake (combined dietary and supplemental intake) to cataract prevalence. [130] Persons with vitamin E intake greater than 35.7 mg/day had a 55% lower prevalence of early cataract (RR: 0.45; CI: 0.12-1.79) than did persons with intakes less than 8.4 mg/day. [130] However, Hankinson et al. [132] found no association between vitamin E intake and cataract surgery. Women with high vitamin E intakes (median = 210 mg/day) had a similar rate of cataract surgery (RR: 0.96; CI: 0.72-1.29) as women with low intakes (median = 3.3 mg/day). In partial contrast with their positive correlations between serum α-tocopherol levels and cataract, Mares-Perlman et al. found that dietary vitamin E was associated (nonsignificantly) with diminished risk for nuclear cataract in men, but not in women (Fig. 6c). [129]

Four studies assessing plasma vitamin E levels also reported significant inverse associations with cataract (Fig. 6). Knekt and coworkers [135] followed a cohort of 1419 Finns for 15 years and identified 47 patients admitted to ophthalmological wards for mature cataract. They selected two controls per patient matched for age, sex and municipality. These investigators reported that persons with serum vitamin E concentrations above approximately 20 μM had about one-half the rate of subsequent cataract surgery (RR: 0.53; CI: 0.24-1.1) (Fig. 6g) compared with persons with vitamin E concentrations below this concentration. Vitale and coworkers [133] observed the age-, sex-, and diabetes-adjusted prevalence of nuclear cataract to be about 50% less (RR: 0.52; CI: 0.27-0.99) (Fig. 6c) among persons with plasma vitamin E concentrations greater than 29.7 μM compared to persons with levels below 18.6 μM. A similar comparison showed that the prev-

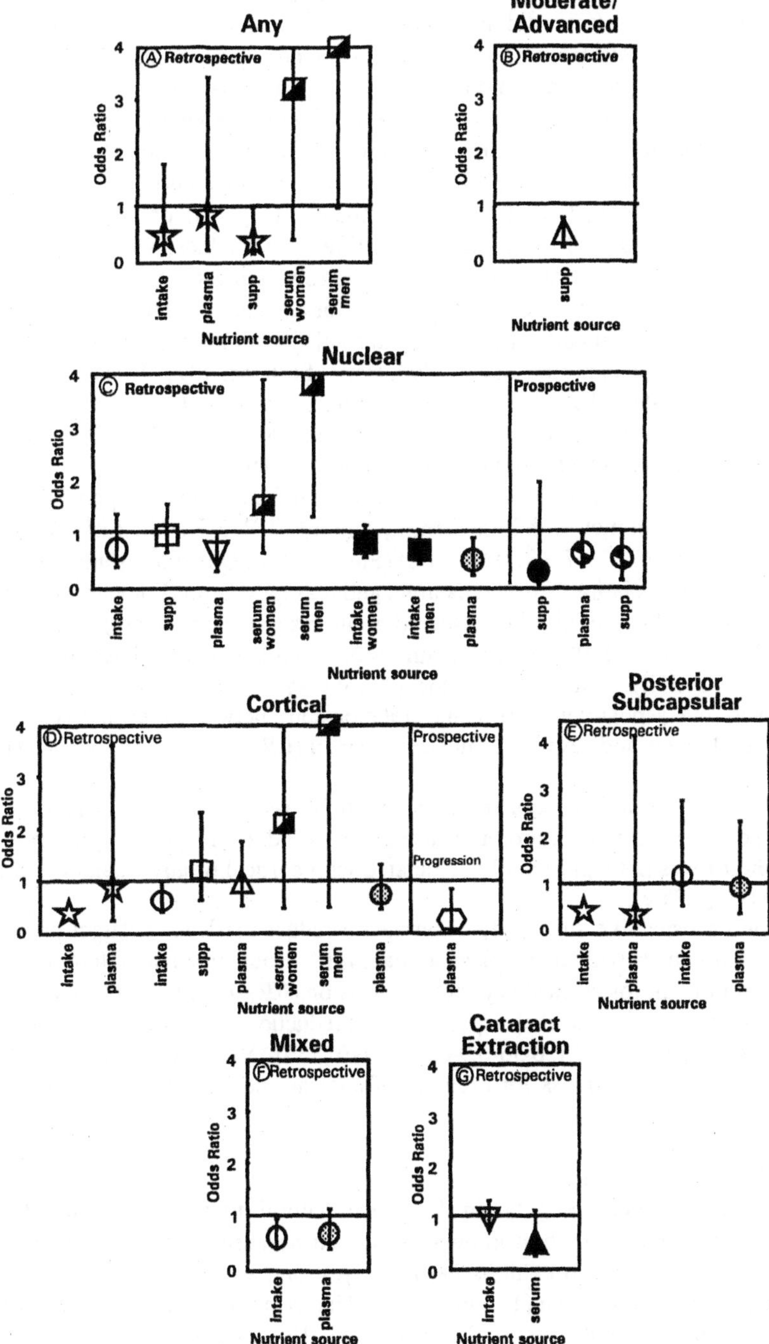

Figure 6. As in Figure 5, but for vitamin E (α-tocopherol). Adapted fromTaylor et al., *Vitamin C in Health and Disease*, Marcel Dekker, Inc., New York, 1997.

alence of cortical cataract did not differ between those with high and low plasma vitamin E levels (RR: 0.96; CI: 0.52-0.1.78) (Fig. 6d). Jacques and Chylack [130] also observed the prevalence of posterior subcapsular cataract to be 67% (RR: 0.33; CI: 0.03-4.13) (Fig. 6e) lower among persons with plasma vitamin E levels above 35 μM relative to persons with levels below 21 μM after adjustment for age, sex, race and diabetes; however, the effect was not statistically significant. Prevalence of any early cataract (RR: 0.83; CI: 0.20-3.40) (Fig. 6a) or cortical cataract (RR: 0.84; CI: 0.20-3.60) (Fig. 6d) did not differ between those with high and low plasma levels. Plasma vitamin E was also inversely associated with prevalence of cataract in a large Italian study after adjusting for age and sex, but the relationship was no longer statistically significant after adjusting for other factors such as education, sunlight exposure and family history of cataract. [37] Leske et al. [101] also demonstrated that individuals with high plasma vitamin E levels had significantly lower prevalence of nuclear cataract (RR: 0.44; CI: 0.21-0.90), but vitamin E was not associated with cataracts at other lens sites.

Mares-Perlman and coworkers noted a significant elevated prevalence of nuclear cataract in men with high serum vitamin E (RR: 3.74; CI: 1.25-11.2) but not in women (RR: 1.47; CI: 0.57-3.82) (Fig. 6c). [70] One other study failed to observe any association between cataract and plasma vitamin E levels. [131]

Mares-Perlman et al. [70] observed an inverse (nonsignificant) relationship (RR: 0.61; CI: 0.32-1.19) between serum γ-tocopherol, which has lower biological vitamin E activity compared to α-tocopherol (Fig. 7b), and severity of nuclear sclerosis, but a positive, significant relationship between elevated serum α-tocopherol levels and severity of nuclear cataract (RR: 2.13; CI: 1.05-4.34) (Fig. 6c).

Whereas serum α-tocopherol appeared to be associated with nonsignificant increases in risk for cortical or any cataract (Figs. 6d, 6a, respectively), serum γ-tocopherol was not significantly associated with cortical or any cataract in these studies (Fig. 7a-c).

Two prospective studies demonstrated a reduced risk for cataract progress among individuals with higher plasma vitamin E. Rouhiainen et al. found a 73% reduction in risk for cortical cataract progression (RR: 0.27; CI: 0.08-0.83) (Fig. 6d) [138], whereas Leske et al. reported a 42% reduction in risk for nuclear cataract progression (RR: 0.58; CI: 0.36-0.94) (Fig. 6c) [139]. Vitamin E supplementation was related to a lower risk for progress of nuclear opacity (RR: 0.43; CI: 0.19-0.99) [139].

C. CAROTENOIDS

The carotenoids, like vitamin E, are also natural lipid-soluble antioxidants. [103] β-carotene is the best known carotenoid because of its importance as a vitamin A precursor. It exhibits particularly strong antioxidant activity at low partial pressures of oxygen (15 torr). [144] This is similar to the ≈20 torr partial pressure of oxygen in the core of the lens. [145] However, it is only one of ~400 naturally occurring carotenoids [146], and other carotenoids may have similar or greater antioxidant potential. [102,103,147,148] In addition to β-carotene, α-carotene, lutein and lycopene are important carotenoid components of the human diet. [149] Carotenoids have been identified in the lens in ≈10 ng/g wet weight concentrations (Table 1). [105,150] There is a dearth of laboratory data which relate carotenoids to cataract formation and there are also no data which relate carotenoid supplement use to risk for cataracts.

Jacques and Chylack [130] were the first to observe that persons with carotene intakes above 18,700 IU/day had the same prevalence of cataract as those with intakes below 5,677 IU/day (RR: 0.91; CI: 0.23-3.78) (Fig. 8a). Hankinson et al. [132] followed this report with a study that reported that the multivariate-adjusted rate of cataract surgery was about 30% lower (RR: 0.73; CI: 0.55-0.97) for women with high carotene intakes (median = 14,558 IU/day) compared with women with low intakes of this nutrient (median = 2,935 IU/day) (Fig. 8e). However, while cataract surgery was inversely associated with total carotene intake, it was not strongly associated with consumption of carotene-rich foods, such as carrots. Rather, cataract surgery was associated with lower intakes of foods such as spinach that are rich in lutein and xanthin carotenoids, rather than ß-carotene. This would appear to be consistent with our observation that the human lens contains lutein and zeaxanthin but no β-carotene. Unfortunately, cataract surgery was not an end point in other studies which considered xanthaphylls. [70,126]

Jacques and Chylack also noted that persons with high plasma total carotenoid concentrations (>3.3 μM) had less than one-fifth the prevalence of cataract compared to persons with low plasma carotenoid levels (<1.7 μM) (RR: 0.18; CI: 0.03-1.03) after adjustment for age, sex, race and diabetes (Fig. 8a). However, they were unable to observe an association between carotene intake and cataract prevalence. [130] Knekt and coworkers [135] reported that among age- and sex-matched cases and controls, persons with serum β-carotene concentrations above approximately 0.1 μM had a 40% reduction in the rate of cataract surgery compared with persons with concentrations below this level (RR: 0.59; CI: 0.26-1.25).

The most recent study that correlated serum carotenoids and severity of nuclear and cortical opacities [70] indicates that higher levels of individual or total carotenoids in the serum were not associated with less severe nuclear or cortical cataract overall, although same sex-related differences in risk were noted (Figs. 8-13). Associations between risk for some forms of cataract and nutriture differed between men and women, for example, nuclear cataract and α-carotene intake (Fig. 9b). [129] Other nutrients for which cataract risk in women vs. men showed opposing relationships to include serum ß-carotene (Fig. 10a and b) and serum lycopene (Fig. 11). A marginally significant trend for lower risk ratio for cortical opacity with increasing serum levels of ß-carotene was observed in men, but not women. Higher serum levels of α-carotene, ß-cryptoxanthin, and lutein were significantly related to lower risk for nuclear sclerosis only in men who smoked. In contrast, higher levels of some carotenoids were often directly associated with elevated risk for nuclear sclerosis and cortical cataract (Figs. 10 and 12), particularly in women.

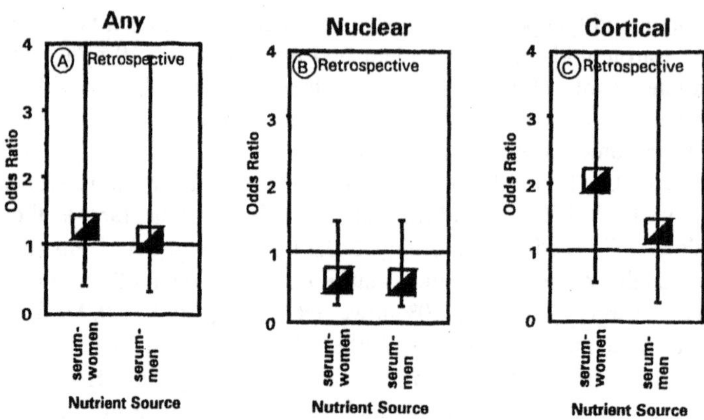

Figure 7. As in Figure 5, but for γ-tocopherol. Adapted from Taylor et al., *Vitamin C in Health and Disease*, Marcel Dekker, Inc., New York, 1997.

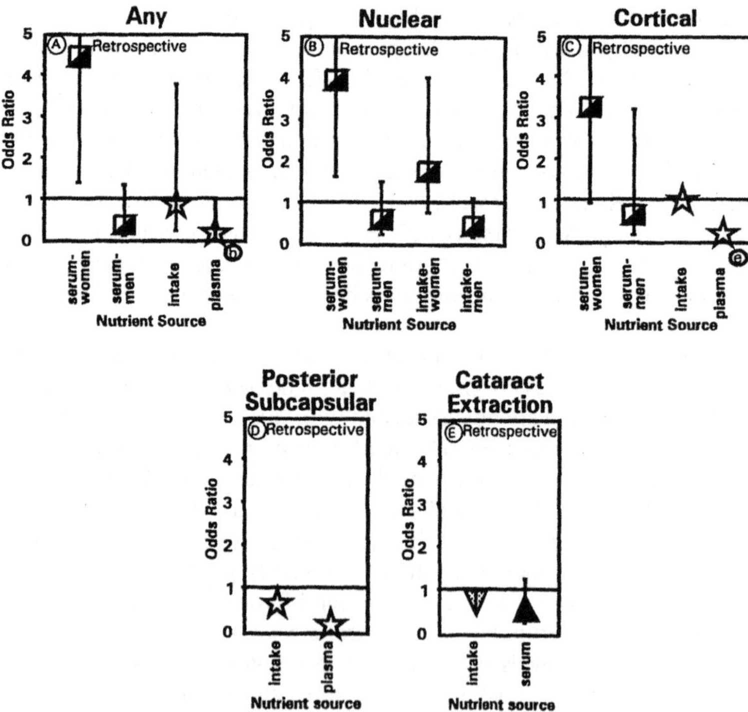

Figure 8. As in Figure 5, but for carotenoids (generally measured as β-carotene). Adapted from Taylor et al., *Vitamin C in Health and Disease*, Marcel Dekker, Inc., New York, 1977.

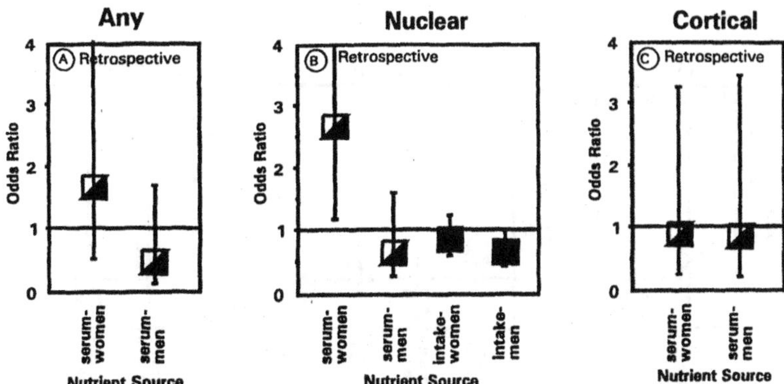

Figure 9. As in Figure 5, but for α-carotene). Adapted from Taylor et al., *Vitamin C in Health and Disease,* Marcel Dekker, Inc., New York, 1977.

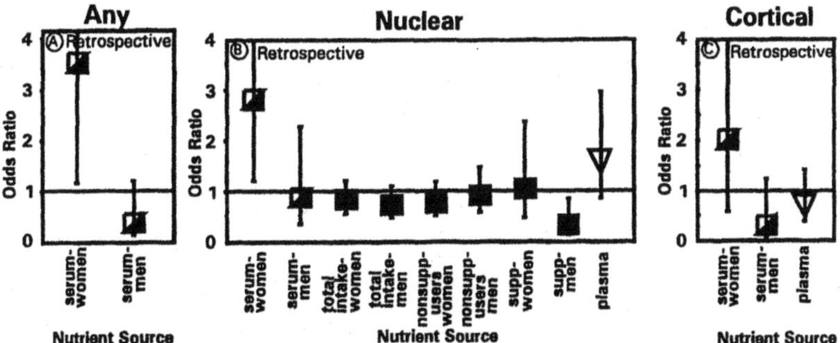

Figure 10. As in Figure 5, but for β-carotene (also see data in Fig. 8). Adapted from Taylor et al., *Vitamin C in Health and Disease,* Marcel Dekker, Inc., New York, 1977.

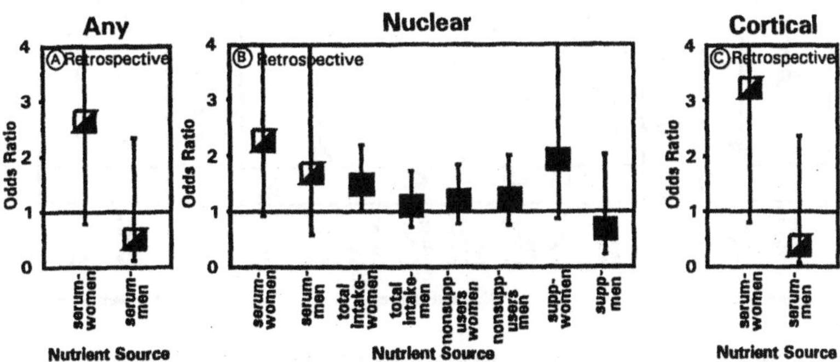

Figure 11. Same as in Figure 5, but for lycopene. Adapted from Taylor et al., *Vitamin C in Health and Disease,* Marcel Dekker, Inc., New York, 1977.

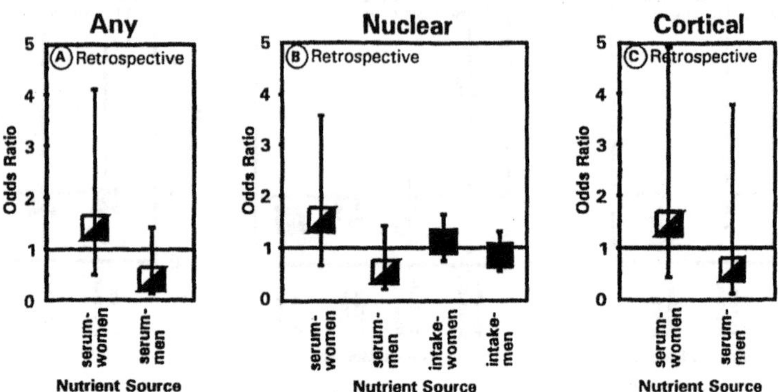

Figure 12. Same as in Figure 5, but for β-cryptoxanthin. Adapted from Taylor et al., *Vitamin C in Health and Disease*, Marcel Dekker, Inc., New York, 1977.

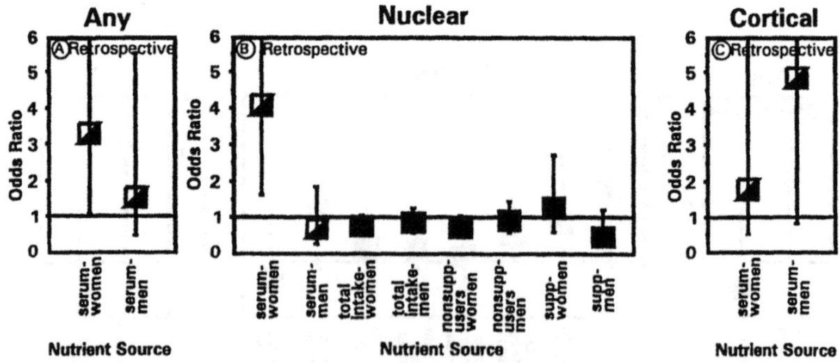

Figure 13. Same as in Figure 5, but for lutein. Adapted from Taylor et al., *Vitamin C in Health and Disease*, Marcel Dekker, Inc., New York, 1977.

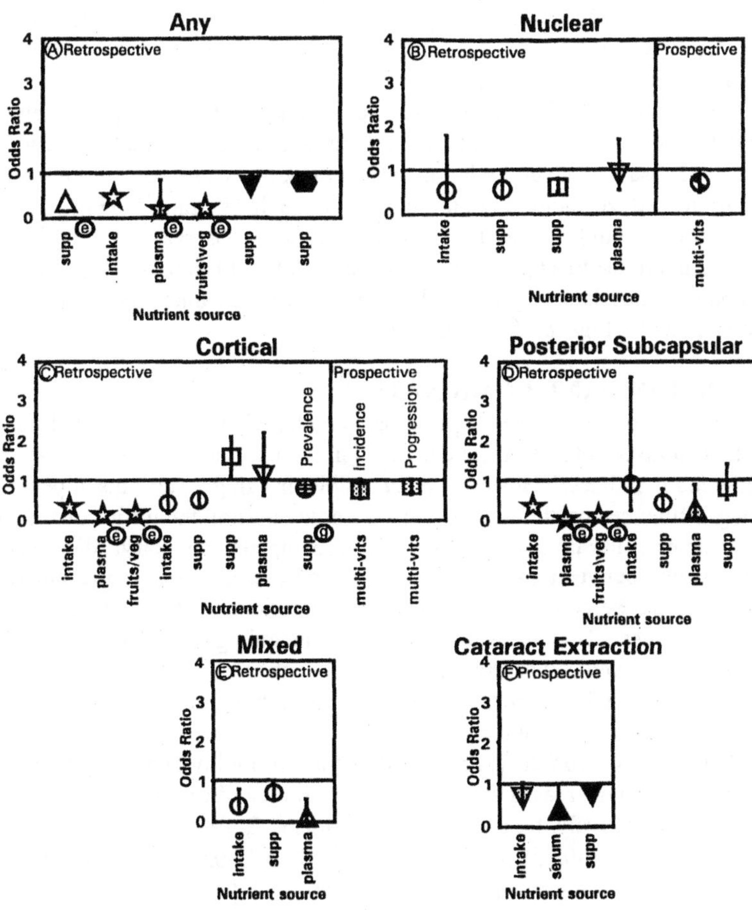

Figure 14. Same as in Figure 5, but for antioxidant nutrient index using multiple antioxidants. Adapted from Taylor et al., *Vitamin C in Health and Disease*, Marcel Dekker, Inc., New York, 1977.

Vitale and colleagues [133] also examined the relationships between plasma β-carotene levels and age-, sex-, and diabetes-adjusted prevalence of cortical and nuclear cataract (Fig. 10b and c). Although the data suggested a weak inverse association between plasma β-carotene and cortical cataract and a weak positive association between this and nuclear cataract, neither association was statistically significant. Persons with plasma β-carotene concentrations above 0.88 μM had a 28% lower prevalence of cortical cataract (RR: 0.72; CI: 0.37-1.42) and a 57% (RR: 1.57; CI: 0.84-2.93) higher prevalence of nuclear cataract compared to persons with levels below 0.33 μM.

Hankinson and coworkers observed correlations between β-carotene intake but not intake of β-carotene-containing foods and risk for cataract extraction. [132] Instead they saw an inverse relation between risk for cataract extraction and intake of lutein and zeaxanthin-containing foods such as spinach (Fig. 14). This observation would appear to be consistent with observations that lutein and zeaxanthin are the most prevalent carotenoids in lens (Table 2). However, Mares-Perlman did not detect significantly altered risk for cataract among consumers of these nutrients (Figs. 8-13). [126,129]

D. ANTIOXIDANT COMBINATIONS

In order to more closely approximate combined effects on cataract risk of the multiple antioxidants which are contained in food, this group was the first to adopt "antioxidant indices." However, it is possible that single nutrients appear to have strong influences on the indices and we now question the utility of the indices. Nevertheless, in an attempt to offer a complete summary, data regarding relationships between antioxidant indices and cataract risk are presented below (Fig. 14). To be consistent with the earlier sections we first describe effects of supplement use. Then the effects of intake, including foods, are summarized.

Robertson and coworkers [127] found no enhanced benefit to persons taking both vitamin E and vitamin C supplements compared with persons who only took either vitamin C or vitamin E.

Leske and coworkers [128] found that use of multivitamin supplements was associated with decreased prevalence for each type of cataract: 60%, 48%, 45%, and 30%, respectively, for posterior subcapsular (RR: 0.40; CI: 0.21-0.77), cortical (RR: 0.52; CI: 0.36-0.72), nuclear (RR: 0.55; CI: 0.33-0.92), and mixed (RR: 0.70; CI: 0.51-0.97) cataracts (Fig. 14b-e). Luthra et al. [136] and Leske et al. [151] reported that supplement consumption was associated with a slight reduction in risk for cortical cataract in a black population (RR: 0.77; CI: 0.61-0.98) in those < 70 years (Fig. 14c).

Multivitamins were also reported to reduce the risk of incident cataracts, as well as progression of existing cataracts in several studies (Fig. 14). Seddon and coworkers [25] observed a reduced risk for incident cataract for users of multivitamins (RR: 0.73; CI: 0.54-0.99). Mares-Perlman et al. [137] reported that mutivitamin users had significant 20% (RR: 0.8; CI: 0.6-1.0) and 30% (RR:0.7; CI: 0.5-1.0) reduction of cortical cataract progression and incidence, respectively (Fig. 14c). Leske et al. reported a 31% reduced risk for progression of nuclear cataract among users of multivitamins (RR: 0.69; CI: 0.48-0.99) [139] (Fig. 14c). Hankinson found no relationship between multivitamin use and risk for cataract extraction. [132].

In these studies it is not clear that synergy between nutrients, with respect to conferring diminished risk for cataract, is indicated.

The first, and perhaps most important, study in terms of revealing the utility of diet indicates that persons who consumed $\geq$ 1.5 servings of fruits and/or vegetables had only ≈20% the risk of developing cataract as those who did not (Fig. 14a). [130] Hankinson and coworkers [132] calculated an antioxidant score based on intakes of carotene, vitamin C, vitamin E and riboflavin and observed a 24% reduction in the adjusted rate of cataract surgery among women with high-antioxidant scores relative to women with low scores (RR: 0.76; CI: 0.57-1.03) (Fig. 14f).

Using a similar index based on combined antioxidant intakes (vitamin C, vitamin E, and carotene, as well as riboflavin), Leske and coworkers [128] found that persons with high scores had 60% lower adjusted prevalence of cortical (RR: 0.42; CI: 0.18-0.97) (Fig. 14c) and mixed (RR: 0.39; CI: 0.19-0.80) (Fig 14e) cataract compared to those who had low scores.

Jacques and Chylack [130] also found that the adjusted prevalence of all types of cataract was 40% (RR: 0.62; CI: 0.12-1.77) and 80% (RR: 0.16; CI: 0.04-0.82) lower for persons with moderate and high-antioxidant index scores (based on combined plasma vitamin C, vitamin E and carotenoid levels), as compared with persons with low scores (Fig. 14a). Mohan and coworkers [131] constructed a somewhat more complex antioxidant scale which included red blood cell levels of glutathione peroxidase, glucose-6-phosphate dehydrogenase and plasma levels of vitamin C and vitamin E. Even though they failed to see any protective associations with any of these individual factors, and even reported a positive association between plasma vitamin C and prevalence of cataract, they found that persons with high- antioxidant index scores had a substantially lower prevalence of cataracts involving the posterior subcapsular region (RR: 0.23; CI: 0.06-0.88) (Fig. 14d) or mixed cataract with posterior subcapsular and nuclear components (RR: 0.12; CI: 0.03-0.56) after multivariate adjustment (Fig. 14e). Knekt and coworkers [135] observed that the rate of cataract surgery for persons with high levels of both serum vitamin E and β-carotene concentrations appeared lower than the rate for persons with either high vitamin E or high β-carotene levels (Fig. 14f). Persons with high serum levels of either had a rate of cataract surgery that was 40% less than persons with low levels of both nutrients (RR: 0.38; CI: 0.15-1.0).

Vitale and coworkers [133] also examined the relationship between antioxidant scores (based on plasma concentrations of vitamin C, vitamin E and β-carotene) and prevalence of cataract, but did not see evidence of any association. The age-, sex-, and diabetes-adjusted risk ratios were close to one for both nuclear (RR: 0.96; CI: 0.54-1.70) and cortical (RR: 1.17; CI: 0.62-2.20) cataract (Fig. 14b and c).

E. INTERVENTION STUDIES

To date only one intervention trial designed to assess the effect of vitamin supplements on cataract risk has been completed. Sperduto and coworkers [142] took advantage of two ongoing, randomized, double-blinded vitamin and cancer trials to assess the impact of vitamin supplements on cataract prevalence. The trials were conducted among almost 4,000 participants aged 45 to 74 years from rural communes in Linxian, China. Participants in one trial received either a multisupplement or placebo. In the second trial, a more complex factorial design was used to evaluate the effects of four different vitamin/mineral combinations: retinol (5000 IU) and zinc (22 mg); riboflavin (3 mg) and niacin (40 mg); vitamin C (120 mg) and molybdenum (30 μg); and vitamin E (30 mg), β-carotene (15 mg), and selenium (50 μg). At the end of the five to six year follow-up, the investigators conducted eye examinations to determine the prevalence of cataract (Fig. 15).

In the first trial there was a significant 43% reduction in the prevalence of nuclear cataract for persons aged 65 to 74 years receiving the multi supplement (RR: 0.57; CI: 0.36-0.90) (Fig. 15a). The second trial demonstrated a significantly reduced prevalence of nuclear cataract in persons receiving the riboflavin/niacin supplement relative to those persons not receiving this supplement (RR: 0.59; CI: 0.45-0.79). The effect was strongest in those aged 65 to 74 years (RR: 0.45; CI: 0.31-0.64). However, the riboflavin/niacin supplement appeared to increase the risk of posterior subcapsular cataract (RR: 2.64; CI: 1.31-5.35) (Fig. 15c). The results further suggested a protective effect of the retinol/zinc supplement (RR: 0.77; CI: 0.58-1.02) and the vitamin C/molybdenum supplement (RR: 0.78; CI: 0.59-1.04) on prevalence of nuclear cataract.

F. CALORIE RESTRICTION AND CONTROL OF BODY MASS INDEX AS A MEANS TO DELAY CATARACT

Restriction of caloric intake extends youth and delays age-related cataract (as well as many other late-life diseases) in these animals (Fig.16).

The decrease in risk for cataract in calorie-restricted Emory mice has some parallels in a recent study which indicates that well-fed male physicians with body mass index below 22 enjoyed less risk for cataract as compared with physicians with body mass indices of >25 [152]. Since cataract is associated with oxidative stress, it might be anticipated that the delay in cataract would be accompanied by elevated ascorbate levels in the protected animals. Nevertheless, in young and old animals, plasma-ascorbate concentrations were lower than in the nonrestricted mice. [77,78,153].

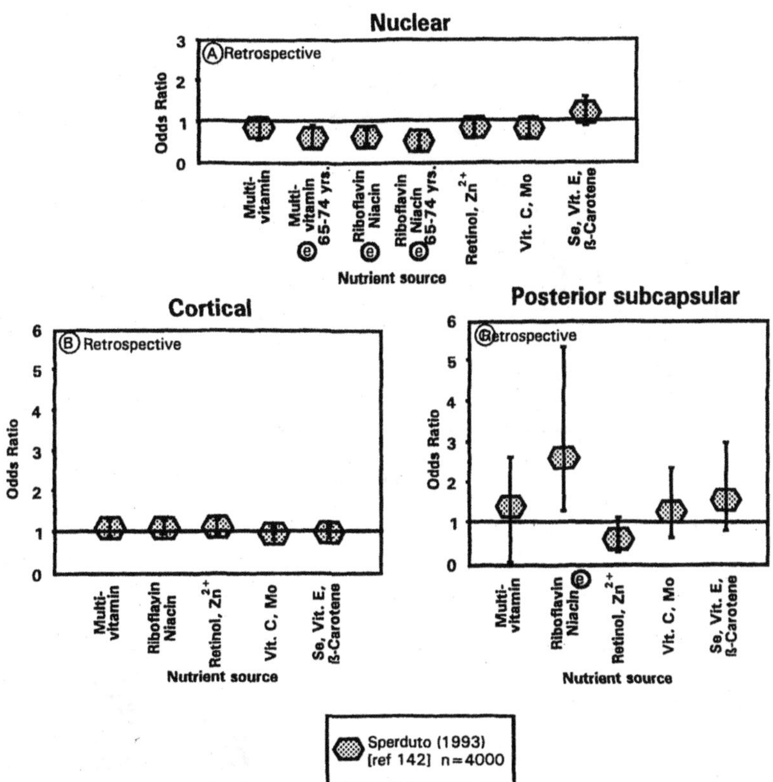

Figure 15. As in Figure 5, but for intervention trials. Adapted from Taylor et al., *Vitamin C in Health and Disease*, Marcel Dekker, Inc., New York, 1977.

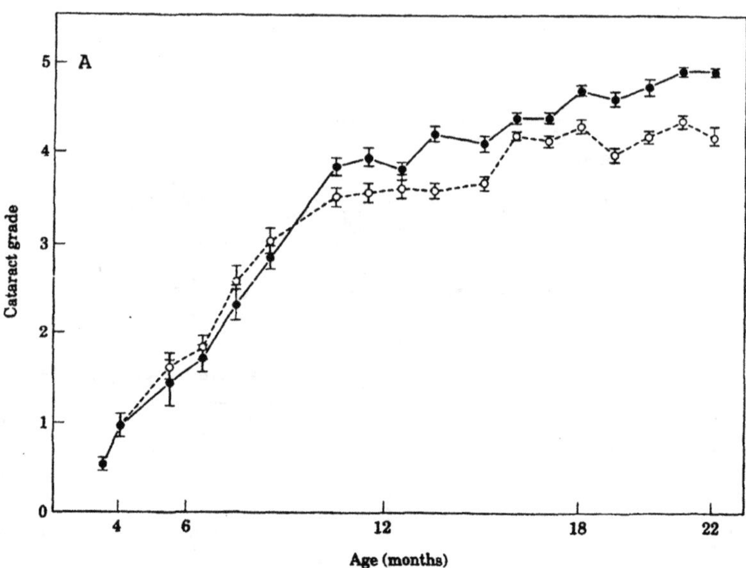

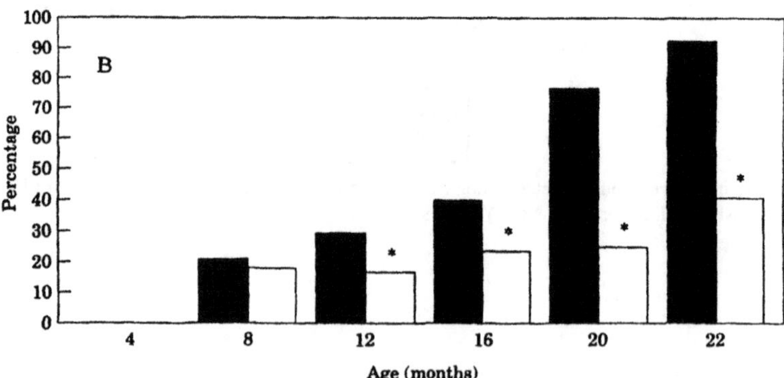

Figure 16
a) Mean cataract grade in calorie restricted and control Emory mice at 3-22 months of age.
• = control mice; ○ = restricted mice; values are means ± SEM. At older ages error bars are approximately equal in size to the symbol for control animals.
b) Percent of lenses with grade 5 cataract. *P , 0.05.
Adapted from Taylor et al., *Exp. Eye Res.*, 61, 1995.

IV. CONCLUSION

Light and oxygen appear to be both a boon and a bane. While necessary for physiological function, when present in excess or in uncontrolled circumstances they appear to be causally related to cataractogenesis. Upon aging, compromised function of the lens is exacerbated by depleted or diminished primary antioxidant reserves, antioxidant enzyme capabilities, and diminished secondary defenses such as proteases. Smoking appears to provide an oxidative challenge and is also associated with an elevated risk of cataract.

The impression created by the literature is that there is some benefit to enhanced antioxidant intake with respect to diminished risk for cataract. Optimal levels of ascorbate would appear to be 250<mg/day; however, more information is essential prior to describing optimal nutriture *vis a vis* cataract. It is difficult to compare the various studies. That the correlations were not always with the same form of cataract may indicate, in addition to the conclusions reached, that the cataracts were graded differently and/or that there are common etiological features of each of the forms of cataract described. Most of the studies noted above utilized case-control designs, and most assessed status only once. Since intake or status measures are highly variable and the effects of diet are likely to be cumulative, studies should be performed on populations for which long-term dietary records are available. It appears that intake studies are preferable to use of plasma measures, if a single measure of status must be chosen. Longitudinal studies and more intervention studies are certainly essential in order to truly establish the value of antioxidants and to determine the extent to which cataract progress is affected by nutriture. More uniform methods of lens evaluation (and earlier detection–see Chapter 13), diet recording, and blood testing, etc., would facilitate conclusions regarding the merits of antioxidants. Optimization of nutriture can be achieved through better diets and supplement use once appropriate levels of specifically beneficial nutrients are defined. In addition to quantifying optimal intake, it is essential to know for how long or when intake of the nutrients would be useful with respect to delaying cataract. It is possible to adjust normal dietary practice to obtain close-to-saturating levels of plasma ascorbate (less than 250 mg/day). [72,132,141,154] Because the bioavailability of ascorbate may decrease with age, slightly higher intakes may be required in the elderly. Thus, the overall impression created by these data suggests that further research in this field will bring significant health benefits.

Poor education and lower socioeconomic status also markedly increase risk for these debilities. [128,131,155,156] These are related to poor nutrition. Since cost-benefit analysis regarding remediation clearly indicates that cataract prevention is preferable (and essential where there is a dearth of surgeons) to surgery, it is not premature to contemplate the value of intervention for populations at risk. The work available, albeit preliminary, indicates that nutrition may provide the least costly and most practicable means to attempt the objectives of delaying cataract.

ACKNOWLEDGMENTS

We acknowledge the assistance of Tom Nowell in the preparation of figures and Paul Jacques for invaluable assistance in evaluating the epidemiological data.

V. REFERENCES

1. **Muller HK,** Buschke W, Vitamin C in linse, kammerwasser und blut normalem und pathologischem linsentstoffwech, *Arch. F. Augenh,* 108, 368-390, 1934.
2. **Taylor A,** Jacques PF, Dorey C K, Oxidation and aging: impact on vision, *J. Toxicol. Indust. Health*, 9, 349-371, 1993.
3. **Bunce GE,** Kinoshita J, Horwitz J, Nutritional factors in cataract, *Ann. Rev. Nutr.,* 10, 233-254, 1990.
4. **Jacques PF,** Chylack LT Jr, Taylor A, Relationships between natural antioxidants and cataract formation, in *Natural Antioxidants Human Health and Disease,* Frei B, Ed, Academic Press, Orlando, FL.
5. **Taylor A,** Vitamin C, in *Nutrition in the Elderly: the Boston Nutritional Status Survey,* Hartz S C, Russell RM, Rosenberg IH, Eds., Smith Gordon Limited, London, UK, 1992, pp. 147-150.
6. **Taylor A,** Cataract: relationships between nutrition and oxidation, *J. Am. Coll. Nutr.*, 12, 138-146, 1993.
7. **Blondin J,** Taylor A, Measures of leucine aminopeptidase can be used to anticipate UV-induced age-related damage to lens proteins: ascorbate can delay this damage, *Mech. Ageing Dev.,* 41, 39-46, 1987.
8. **Blondin J,** Baragi VJ, Schwartz E, Sadowski J, Taylor A, Delay of UV-induced eye lens protein damage in guinea pigs by dietary ascorbate, *Free Radic. Biol. Med.*, 2, 275-281, 1986.
9. **Taylor A,** Jacques PF, Relationships between aging, antioxidant status, and cataract, *Am. J. Clinical Nutr.,* 62, 1439S-1447S, 1995.
10. **Taylor A,** Oxidative stress and antioxidant function in relation to risk for cataract, in *Antioxidants in Disease Mechanisms and Therapeutic Strategies* (A Volume of Advances in Pharmacology Series), Sies H, Ed., Academic Press, San Diego, CA, 1997, pp. 515-536.
11. **Taylor A,** Jacques P, Antioxidant status and risk for cataract, in *Preventive Nutrition: The Guide for Health Professionals*, Bendich A, Deckelbaum RJ, Eds., Humana Press, Totawa, NJ, 1997, pp. 267-283.
12. **Kupfer C,** The conquest of cataract: a global challenge, *Trans. Ophthal. Soc. UK,* 104, 1-10, 1984.
13. **Schwab L,** Cataract blindness in developing nations, *Internat. Ophthalmol. Clinics,* 30, 16-18, 1990.
14. **World Health Organization,** Use of intraocular lenses in cataract surgery in developing countries, *Bull. World Health Organ.,* 69, 657-666, 1991.

15. **Klein BEK,** Klein R, Linton KLP, Prevalence of age-related lens opacities in a population: The Beaver Dam Eye Study, *Ophthalmol.*, 99, 546-552, 1992.

16. **Klein R,** Klein BE, Linton KL, DeMets DL, The Beaver Dam eye study: the relation of age-related maculopathy to smoking, *Am. J. Epidemiol.*, 37, 190-200, 1993.

17. **Leibowitz H,** Krueger D, Maunder C, Milton RC, Mohandas MK, Kahn HA, Nickerson RJ, Pool J, Colton TL, Ganley JP, Loewenstein JI, Dawber TR, The Framingham Eye Study Monograph, *Surv. Ophthalmol.* (suppl), 24, 335-610, 1980.

18. **Chatterjee A,** Milton RC, Thyle S, Prevalence and etiology of cataract in Punjab, *Brit. J. Ophthalmol.*, 66, 35-42, 1982.

19. **Wang G-m,** Spector A, Luo C-q, Tang LQ, Xu LH, Guo WY, Huang YQ, Prevalence of age-related cataract in Ganzi and Shanghai. The Epidemiological Study Group, *Chinese Med. J.,* 103, 945-951, 1990.

20. **Whitfield R,** Schwab L, Ross-Degnan D, Steinkuller P, Swartwood J, Blindness and eye disease in Kenya: ocular status survey results from the Kenya Rural Blindness Prevention Project, *Brit. J. Ophthalmol.*, 74, 333-340, 1990.

21. **Chan CW,** Billson FA, Visual disability and major causes of blindness in NSW: a study of people aged 50 and over attending the Royal Blind Society 1984 to 1989, *Aust. N. Zealand J. Ophthalmol.*, 19, 321-325, 1991.

22. **Dana MR,** Tielsch JM, Enger C, Joyce E, Santoli JM, Taylor HR., Visual impairment in a rural Appalachian community: Prevalence and causes, *JAMA,* 264, 2400-2405, 1990.

23. **Salive ME,** Guralnik J, Christian W, Glynn RJ, Colsher P, Ostfeld AM, Functional blindness and visual impairment in older adults from three communities, *Ophthalmol*ogy, 99, 1840-1847, 1992.

24. **Wormald RPL,** Wright LA, Courtney P, Beaumont B, Haines AP, Visual problems in the elderly population and implications for services, *Br. Med. J.*, 304, 1226-1229, 1992.

25. **Seddon JM,** Christen WG, Manson JE, LaMotte FS, Glynn RJ, Buring JE, Hennekens CH, The use of vitamin supplements and therisk of cataract among US male physicians, *Am. J. Public Health,* 84, 788-792, 1994.

26. **Young RW,** Optometry and the preservation of visual health, *Optom. Vis. Sci.,* 70, 255-262, 1992.

27. **Taylor A,** Tisdell FE, Carpenter FH, Leucine aminopeptidase (bovine lens): synthesis and kinetic properties of ortho, meta, and para substituted leucyl-anilides, *Arch. Biochem. Biophys.,* 210, 90-97, 1981.

28. **Jacques PF,** Taylor A, Micronutrients and age-related cataracts, in *Micronutrients in Health and in Disease Prevention*, Bendich A, Butterworth CE, Eds., Marcel Dekker, New York, 1991, pp. 359-379.

29. **Chylack LT Jr,** Wolfe JK, Singer DM, Leske MC, Bullimore MA, Bailey IL, Friend J, McCarthy D, Wu S, The lens opacities classification system

III, *Arch. Ophthalmol.,* 111, 831-836, 1993.

30. **Chylack LT Jr,** Wolfe JK, Friend J, Singer DM, Wu SY, Leske MC, Nuclear cataract: relative contributions to vision loss of opalescence and brunescence, *Invest. Ophthalmol. Vis. Sci.*, 35, 42632, 1994, abstr.
31. **Wolfe JK,** Chylack LT Jr, Leske MC, Wu SY, LSC Group, Lens nuclear color and visual function, *Invest. Ophthalmol. Vis. Sci.*, 34, 4,2550, 1993. Abstr.
32. **Taylor HR,** West SK, Rosenthal FS, Newland HS, Abbey H, Emmett EA, Effect of ultraviolet radiation on cataract formation, *New Engl. J. Med.,* 319, 1429-1433, *1*988.
33. **Zigman S,** Datiles M, Torczynski E, Sunlight and human cataract, *Invest. Ophthalmol. Vis. Sci.*, 18, 462-467, 1979.
34. **Wong L,** Ho SC, Coggon D, Cruddas AM, Hwang CH, Ho CP, Robertshaw AM, MacDonald DM, Sunlight exposure, antioxidant status, and cataract in Hong Kong fishermen, *J. Epidemiol. Community Health,* 47, 46-49, 1993.
35. **Hirvela H,** Luukinen H, Laatikainen L, Prevalence and risk factors of lens opacities in the elderly in Finland. A population-based study, *Ophthalmol*ogy, 102, 108-117, 1995.
36. **Cruickshanks KJ,** Klein BE, Klein R, Ultraviolet light exposure and lens opacities: The Beaver Dam Eye Study, *Am. J. Public Health*, 82, 1658-1662, 1992.
37. **The Italian-American Cataract Study Group,** Risk factors for age-related cortical, nuclear, and posterior subcapsular cataracts, *Am. J. Epidemiol.*, 133, 541-553, 1991.
38. **Wang G-m,** Spector A, Luo C-q, Tang L-q, Xu L-h, Guo W-Y, Huang Y-q, Prevalence of age-related cataract in Ganzi and Shanghai, *Chinese Med. J.*, 103, 945-951, 1990.
39. **Klein BE,** Cruickshanks KJ, Klein R, Leisure time, sunlight exposure and cataracts. (Review). *Documenta Ophthalmol.*, 88, 295-305, 1994-95.
40. **Javitt JC,** Taylor HR, Cataract and latitude, *Documenta Ophthalmol.*, 88, 307-325, 1995.
41. **Dolin P,** Assessment of the epidemiological evidence that exposure to solar ultraviolet radiation causes cataract, *Documenta Ophthalmol.,* 88, 327-337, 1995.
42. **Zigman S,** Effects of near ultraviolet radiation on the lens and retina, *Documenta Ophthalmol.*, 55, 375-391, 1983.
43. **Brilliant LB,** Grasset NC, Pokhrel RP, Kolstad A, Lepkowski JM, Brilliant GE, Hawks WN, Parajasegaram R, Associations among cataract prevalence, sunlight hours, and altitude in the Himalayas, *Am. J. Epidemiol.,* 118, 250-264, 1983.
44. **Minassian DC,** Baasanhu J, Johnson GJ, Burendei G, The relationship between cataract and climatic droplet keratopathy in Mongolia, *Acta Ophthalmol.*, 72, 490-495, 1994.
45. **Wolff SP,** Cataract and UV radiation, *Documenta Ophthalmol.*, 88, 201-

204, 1995.

46. **Zigman S,** Paxhia T, McDaniel T, Lou MF, Yu N-T, Effect of chronic near-ultraviolet radiation on the gray squirrel lens in vivo, *Inv. Ophthalmol. Vis. Sci.*, 32, 1723-1732, 1991.

47. **Zigler JS,** Goosey JD, Singlet oxygen as a possible factor in human senile nuclear cataract development, *Curr. Eye Res.*, 3, 59-65, 1984.

48. **Varma SD,** Chand O, Sharma YR, Kuck JF, Richards KD, Oxidative stress on lens and cataract formation. Role of light and oxygen, *Curr. Eye Res.*, 3, 35-57, 1984.

49. **Taylor A,** Jahngen-Hodge J, Huang LL, Jacques P, Aging in the eye lens: Roles for proteolysis and nutrition in formation of cataract, *AGE,* 14, 65-71, 1991.

50. **Rao CM,** Qin C, Robison WG Jr, Zigler JS Jr, Effect of smoke condensate on the physiological integrity and morphology of organ cultured rat lenses, *Curr. Eye Res.*, 14, 295-301, 1995.

51. **Shalini VK,** Luthra M, Srinivas L, Rao SH, Basti S, Reddy M, Balasubramanian D, Oxidative damage to the eye lens caused by cigarette smoke and fuel smoke condensates. *Ind. J. Biochem. Biophys.*, 31, 261-266, 1994.

52. **Zigman S,** McDaniel T, Schultz JB, Reddan J, Meydani M, Damage to cultured lens epithelial cells of squirrels and rabbits by UV-A (99.9%) plus UV-B (0.1%) radiation and alpha tocopherol protection, *Mol. Cell Biochem.*, 143, 35-46, 1995.

53. **Smith D,** Palmer V, Kehyias J, Taylor A, Induction of cataracts by X-ray exposure of guinea pig eyes, *Lab Animal*, 22, 34-39, 1993.

54. **Calissendorff BM,** Lonnqvist B, el Azazi M, Cataract development in adult bone marrow transplant recipients, *Acta Ophthalmol. Scandinavica,* 73, 52-154, 1995.

55. **Palmquist BM,** Phillipson B, Barr PO, Nuclear cataract and myopia during hyperbaric oxygen therapy, *Br. J. Ophthalmol.*, 60, 113-117, 1984.

56. **Schocket SS,** Esterson J, Bradford B, Michaelis M, Richards RD, Induction of cataracts in mice by exposure to oxygen, *Israel J. Med.*, 8, 1596-1601, 1972.

57. **Giblin FJ,** Schrimscher L, Chakrapani B, Reddy VN, Exposure of rabbit lens to hyperbaric oxygen in vitro: regional effects on GSH level, *Invest. Ophthalmol. Vis. Sci.*, 29, 1312-1319, 1988.

58. **Giblin FJ,** Padgaonkar VA, Leverenz VR, Lin LR, Lou MF, Unakar NJ, Dickerson JE Jr, Dang L, Reddy VN, Nuclear light scattering, disulfide formation and membrane damage in lenses of older guinea pigs treated with hyperbaric oxygen,. *Exp. Eye Res.*, 60, 219-235, 1995.

59. **Berman ER,** in *Biochemistry of the Eye,* Plenum Press, New York, 1991, pp. 210-308.

60. **Schectman G,** Byrd JC, Gruchow HW, The influence of smoking on vitamin C status in adults, *Am. J. Health,* 79, 158-162, 1989.

61. **Russell-Briefel R,** Bates MW, Kuller LH, The relationship of plasma carotenoids to health and biochemical factors in middle-aged men, *Am.*

J. Epidemiol., 22, 741-749, 1985.

62. **Giraud DW,** Martin HD, Driskell JA, Plasma and dietary vitamin C and E levels of tobacco chewers, smokers, and nonusers, *J. Am. Diet. Assoc.*, 95, 798-800, 1995.
63. **Chow CK**, Thacker RR, Changchit C, Bridges RB, Rehm SR, Humble J, Turbek J, Lower levels of vitamin C and carotenes in plasma of cigarette smokers, *J. Am. Coll. Nutr.*, 5, 305-312, 1986.
64. **Mezzetti A,** Lapenna D, Pierdomenico SD, Calafiore AM, Costantini F, Riario-Sforza G, Imbastaro T, Neri M, Cuccurollo F, Vitamins E, C, and lipid peroxidation in plasma and arterial tissue of smokers and non-smokers, *Atherosclerosis*, 112, 91-99, 1995.
65. **Bolton-Smith C,** Casey CE, Gey KF, Smith SC, Tunstall-Pedoe H, Antioxidant intakes assessed using a food-frequency questionnaire: correlation with biochemical status in smokers and non-smokers, *Br. J. Nutr.*, 65, 337-346, 1991.
66. **Flaye DE,** Sullivan KN, Cullinan TR, Silver JH, Whitelocke RAF, Cataracts and cigarette smoking: the City Eye Study, *Eye*, 3, 379-384, 1989.
67. **West SK,** Munoz B, Emmett EA, Taylor HR, Cigarette smoking and risk of nuclear cataracts, *Arch. Ophthalmol.*, 107, 1166-1169, 1989.
68. **West S**, Does smoke get in your eyes? *JAMA,* 268, 1025-1026, 1992.
69. **Hankinson SE,** Willett WC, Colditz GA, Seddon JM, Rosner B, Speizer FE, Stamper MJ, A prospective study of cigarette smoking and risk of cataract surgery in women, *JAMA,* 268, 994-998, 1992.
70. **Mares-Perlman JA,** Brady WE, Klein BEK, Klein R, Palta M, Bowen P, Stacewicz-Sapuntzakis M, Serum carotenoids and tocopherols and severity of nuclear and cortical opacities, *Invest. Ophthalmol. Vis. Sci.,* 36, 276-88, 1995.
71. **Taylor A,** Davies KJA, Protein oxidation and loss of protease activity may lead to cataract formation in the aged lens, *Free Radic. Biol. Med.,* 3, 371-377, 1987.
72. **Taylor A,** Jacques PF, Nadler D, Morrow F, Sulsky SI, Shepard D, Relationship in humans between ascorbic acid consumption and levels of total and reduced ascorbic acid in lens, aqueous humor, and plasma, *Curr. Eye Res.,* 10, 751-759, 1991.
73. **Taylor A,** Jacques P, Nowell T, Jr, Perrone G, Nadler D, Joswiak B, Vitamin C in human and guinea pig aqueous, lens, and plasma in relation to intake, *Curr. Eye Res.,*16, 857-864, 1997.
74. **Reddy VN,** Glutathione and its function in the lens–an overview, *Exp. Eye Res.*, 150, 771-778, 1990.
75. **Mune M,** Meydani M, Jahngen-Hodge J, Martin A, Smith D, Palmer V, Blumberg JB, Taylor A, Effect of calorie restriction on liver and kidney glutathione in aging Emory mice, *AGE*, 18, 49-49, 1995.
76. **Sastre J,** Meydani M, Martin A, Biddle L, Taylor A, Blumberg J, Effect of glutathione monoethyl ester administration on galactose-induced

cataract in the rat, *Life Chemistry Reports,* 12, 89-95, 1994.

77. **Taylor A,** Jahngen-Hodge J, Smith D, Palmer V, Dallal G, Lipman R, Padhye N, Frei B, Dietary restriction delays cataract and reduces ascorbate levels in Emory mice, *Exp. Eye Res.*, 61, 55-62, 1995.

78. **Taylor A,** Lipman RD, Jahngen-Hodge J, Palmer V, Smith D, Padhye N, Dallal GE, Cyr DE, Laxman E, Shepard D, Morrow F, Solomon R, Perrone G, Asmundsson G, Meydani M, Mune M, Harrison D, Archer J, Dietary calorie restriction in the Emory Mouse: effects on lifespan, eye lens cataract prevalence and progression, levels of ascorbate, glutathione, glucose, and glycohemoglobin, tail collagen breaktime, DNA and RNA oxidation, skin integrity, fecundity and cancer, *Mech. Ageing Dev.*, 79, 33-57, 1995.

79. **Levine M,** New concepts in the biology and biochemistry of ascorbic acid, *New Engl. J. Med.*, 314, 892-902, 1986.

80. **Frei B,** Stocker R, Ames BN, Antioxidant defenses and lipid peroxidation in human blood plasma, *Proc. Nat. Acad. Sci. USA,* 85, 9748-9752, 1988.

81. **Berger J,** Shepard D, Morrow F, Taylor A, Relationship between dietary intake and tissue levels of reduced and total vitamin C in the guinea pig, *J. Nutr.,* 119, 1-7, 1989.

82. **Berger J,** Shepard D, Morrow F, Sadowski J, Haire T, Taylor A, Reduced and total ascorbate in guinea pig eye tissues in response to dietary intake, *Curr. Eye Res.,* 7, 681-686, 1988.

83. **Nakamura B,** Nakamura O, Ufer das vitamin C in der linse und dem Kammerwasser der menschlichen katarakte, *Graefes Arch. Clin. Exp. Ophthalmol.,* 134, 197-200, 1935.

84. **Wilczek M,** Zygulska-Machowa H, Zawartosc witaminy C W. roznych typackzaem, *J. Klin. Oczna*, 38, 477-480, 1968.

85. **Kosegarten DC,** Mayer TJ, Use of guinea pigs as model to study galactose-induced cataract formation, *J. Pharm. Sci.*, 67, 1478-1479, 1978.

86. **Vinson JA,** Possanza CJ, Drack AV, The effect of ascorbic acid on galactose-induced cataracts, *Nutr. Reports Int.*, 33, 665-668, 1986.

87. **Devamanoharan PS,** Henein M, Morris S, Ramachandran S, Richards RD, Varma SD, Prevention of selenite cataract by vitamin C, *Exp. Eye Res.,* 52, 563-568, 1991.

88. **Nishigori H,** Lee JW, Yamauchi Y, Iwatsuru M, The alteration of lipid peroxide in glucocorticoid-induced cataract of developing chick embryos and the effect of ascorbic acid, *Curr. Eye Res.*, 5, 37-40, 1986.

89. **Blondin J,** Baragi VJ, Schwartz E, Sadowski J, Taylor A, Dietary vitamin C delays UV-induced age-related eye lens protein damage, Vitamin C, Ann. NY Acad. Sci., 498, 460-463, 1987.

90. **Garland DD,** Ascorbic acid and the eye, *Am. J. Clin. Nutr.,* 54, 1198S-1202S, 1991.

91. **Naraj RM,** Monnier VM, Isolation and characterization of a blue fluorophore from human eye lens crystallins: in vitro formation from Maillard action with ascorbate and ribose, *Biochim. Biophys. Acta,* 1116,

34-42, 1992.

92. **Bensch KG,** Fleming EE, Lohmann W, The role of ascorbic acid in senile cataract, *Proc. Nat. Acad. Sci. USA,* 82, 7193-7196, 1985.

93. **Vasan S,** Zhang X, Zhang X, Kapurniotu A, Bernhagen J, Teichberg S, Basgen J, Wagle D, Shih D, Terlecky I, Bucala R, Cerami A, Egan J, Ulrich P, An agent cleaving glucose-derived protein crosslinks in vitro and in vivo, *Nature*, 382, 275-278, 1996.

94. **Rathbun WB,** Holleschau AM, Cohen JF, Nagasawa, HT, Prevention of acetaminophen- and naphthalene-induced cataract and glutathione loss by CySSME, *Invest. Ophthalmol. Vis. Sci.,* 37, 923-929, 1996.

95. **Martenssen J,** Steinhertz R, Jain A, Meister A, Glutathione ester prevents buthionine sulfoximine-induced cataracts and lens epithelial cell damage, *Biochemistry*, 86, 8727-8731, 1989.

96. **Rathbun WB,** Killen CE, Holleschau AM, Nagasawa HT, Maintenance of hepatic glutathione homeostasis and prevention of acetaminophen-induced cataract in mice by L-cysteine prodrugs, *Biochem. Pharmacol.*, 51, 1111-1116, 1996.

97. **Vina J,** Perez C, Furukawa T, Palacin M, Vina JR, Effect of oral glutathione on hepatic glutathione levels on rats and mice, *Br. J. Nutr.*, 62, 683-691, 1989.

98. **Clark JI,** Livesey JC, Steele JE, Delay or inhibition of rat lens opacification using pantethine and WR-77913, *Exp. Eye Res.*, 62, 75-84, 1996.

99. **Congdon NG,** Duncan DD, Fisher D, Rieger K, Urist J, Sanchez AM, Vitale S, West SK, Pham T, Cole L, McNaughton C, UV light and lenticular opacities in the Emory Mouse, *Inv. Ophthalmol. Vis. Sci.*, 38, S1020, 1997.

100. **Srivastava S,** Ansari NH, Prevention of sugar induced cataractogenesis in rats by butylated hydroxytoluene, *Diabetes*, 37, 1505-1508, 1988.

101. **Leske MC,** Wu SY, Hyman L, Sperduto R, Underwood B,Chylack LT, Milton, RC, Srivastava S, Ansari N, Biochemical factors in the lens opacities. Case-control study. The Lens Opacities Case-Control Study Group, *Arch. Ophthalmol.*, 113, 1113-1119, 1995.

102. **Schalch W,** Weber P, Vitamins and carotenoids–a promising approach to reducing the risk of coronary heart disease, cancer and eye diseases, *Adv. Exp Med. Biol.*, 366, 335-350, 1994.

103. **Machlin LJ,** Bendich A, Free radical tissue damage: Protective role of antioxidants, *FASEB J.*, 1, 441-445, 1987.

104. **Costagliola C,** Iuliano G, Menzione M, Rinaldi E, Vito P,Auricchio G, Effect of vitamin E on glutathione content in red blood cells, aqueous humor and lens of humans and other species, *Exp. Eye Res.*, 43, 905-914, 1986.

105. **Yeum K-J,** Taylor A, Tang G, Russell RM, Measurement of carotenoids, retinoids, and tocopherols in human lenses, *Invest. Ophthalmol. Vis. Sci.*, 36, 2756-2761, 1995.

106. **Stevens RJ**, Negi, DS, Short, SM, van Kuijk FJGM, Dratz EA, Thomas DW, Vitamin E distribution in ocular tissues following long-term dietary depletion and supplementation as determined by microdissection and gas chromatography-mass spectrometry, *Exp. Eye Res.*, 47, 237-245, 1988.

107. **Creighton MO,** Ross WM, Stewart-DeHaan PJ, Sanwai M, Trevithick JR, Modeling cortical cataractogenesis. VII: Effects of vitamin E treatment on galactose induced cataracts, *Exp.Eye Res.*, 40, 213-222, 1985.

108. **Bhuyan DK,** Podos SM, Machlin LT, Bhagavan HN, Chondhury DN, Soja WS, Bhuyan KC, Antioxidant in therapy of cataract II: Effect of all-roc-alpha-tocopherol (vitamin E) in sugar-induced cataract in rabbits, *Invest. Ophthalmol. Vis. Sci.*, 24, 74, 1983.

109. **Bhuyan KC,** Bhuyan DK, Molecular mechanism of cataractogenesis: III. Toxic metabolites of oxygen as initiators of lipid peroxidation and cataract, *Curr. Eye Res.*, 3, 67-81, 1984.

110. **Hammond BR,** Wooten BR, Snodderly, DM, The density of the human crystalline lens is related to the macular pigment carotenoids, lutein and zeaxanthin, *Optom. Vis. Sci.*, 74, 499-504, 1997.

111. **Fridovich I,** Oxygen: Aspects of its toxicity and elements of defense,*Curr. Eye Res.*, 3, 1-2, 1984.

112. **Giblin FJ,** McReady JP, Reddy VN, The role of glutathione metabolism in detoxification of H_2O_2 in rabbit lens, *Invest. Ophthalmol. Vis. Sci.*, 22, 330-335, 1992.

113. **Eisenhauer DA,** Berger JJ, Peltier CZ, Taylor A, Protease activities in cultured beef lens epithelial cells peak and then decline upon progressive passage, *Exp. Eye Res.*, 46, 579-590, 1988.

114. **Jahngen-Hodge J,** Laxman E, Zuliani A, Taylor A, Evidence for ATP ubiquitin-dependent degradation of proteins in cultured bovine lens epithelial cells, *Exp. Eye Res.*, 52, 341-347, 1991.

115. **Shang F,** Taylor A, Oxidative stress and recovery from oxidative stress are associated with altered ubiquitin conjugatingand proteolytic activities in bovine lens epithelial cells, *Biochem. J.*, 307, 297-303, 1995.

116. **Huang LL,** Jahngen-Hodge J, Taylor A, Bovine lens epithelial cells have a ubiquitin-dependent proteolysis system, *Biochim. Biophys. Acta,* 1175, 181-187, 1993.

117. **Jahngen JH,** Lipman RD, Eisenhauer DA, Jahngen EGE Jr, Taylor A, Aging and cellular maturation cause changes in ubiquitin-eye lens protein conjugates, *Arch. Biochem. Biophys.*, 276, 32-37, 1990.

118. **Jahngen-Hodge J,** Cyr D, Laxman E, Taylor A, Ubiquitin and ubiquitin conjugates in human lens, *Exp. Eye Res.*, 55, 897-902, 1992.

119. **Obin MS**, Nowell T, Taylor A, The photoreceptor G-protein transducin (G_t) is a substrate for ubiquitin-dependent proteolysis, *Biochem. Biophys. Res. Comm.,* 200, 1169-1176, 1994.

120. **Jahngen JH,** Haas AL, Ciechanover A, Blondin J, Eisenhauer D, Taylor A, The eye lens has an active ubiquitin protein conjugation system, *J. Biol. Chem.*, 261, 13760-13767, 1986.

121. **Obin MS,** Jahngen-Hodge J, Nowell T, Taylor A, Ubiquitinylation and ubiquitin-dependent proteolysis invertebrate photoreceptors (rod outer segments): evidence for ubiquitinylationof G_t and rhodopsin, *J. Biol. Chem.*, 271, 14473-14484, 1996.
122. **Jahngen-Hodge J,** Obin MS, Nowell TR Jr, Gong J, Abasi H, Blumberg J, Taylor A, Regulation of ubiquitin conjugating enzymes by glutathione following oxidative stress, *J. Biol. Chem.*, 272, 28218-28226, 1997.
123. **Shang F,** Gong X, Palmer H, Nowell T, Taylor A, Age-related decline in ubiquitin conjugation in responses to oxidative stresses in the lens, *Exp. Eye Res.,* 64, 21-30, 1997.
124. **Shang F,** Gong X, Taylor A, Activity of ubiquitin-dependent pathway in response to oxidative stress: Ubiquitin-activating enzyme is transiently unregulated. *J. Biol. Chem.*, 272, 23086-23093, 1997.
125. **Shang F,** Gong X, Taylor A, Changes in ubiquitin conjugation activities in young and old lenses in response to oxidative stress, *Inv. Opthalmol. Vis. Sci.*, 36, S528, 1995.
126. **Mares-Perlman JA**, Klein BEK, Klein R, Ritter LL, Relationship between lens opacities and vitamin and mineral supplement use, *Ophthalmology*, 101, 315-355, 1994.
127. **Robertson J McD,** Donner AP, Trevithick JR, Vitamin E intake and risk for cataracts in humans, *Ann. NY Acad. Sci.*,570, 372-382, 1989.
128. **Leske MC**, Chylack LT Jr, Wu S, The lens opacities case-control study risk factors for cataract, *Arch. Ophthalmol.*, 109, 244-251, 1991.
129. **Mares-Perlman JA,** Brady WE, Klein BEK, Klein R, Haus GJ, Palta M, Ritter LL, Shoff SM, Diet and nuclear lens opacities, *Am. J. Epidemiol.*, 141, 322-334, 1995b.
130. **Jacques PF**, Chylack LT, Jr, Epidemiologic evidence of a role for the antioxidant vitamins and carotenoids in cataract prevention, *Am. J. Clin. Nutr.*, 53, 352S-355S, 1991.
131. **Mohan M,** Sperduto RD, Angra SK, Milton RC, Mathur RL, Underwood B, Jafery N, Pandya CB, India-US case-control study of age-related cataract, *Arch. Ophthalmol.*, 107, 670-676, 1989.
132. **Hankinson SE,** Stampfer MJ, Seddon JM, Colditz GA, Rosner B, Speizer FE, Willett WC, Intake and cataract extraction in women: a prospective study, *Br. Med. J.*, 305, 335-339, 1992.
133. **Vitale S,** West S, Hallfrisch J, Alston C, Wang F, Moorman C, Muller D, Singh V, Taylor HR, Plasma antioxidants and risk of cortical and nuclear cataract, *Epidemiol.*, 4, 195-203, 1994.
134. **Jacques PF,** Lahav M, Willett WC, Taylor A, Relationship between long-term vitamin C intake and prevalence of cataract and macular degeneration, *Exp. Eye Res.*, 55 (suppl 1), S152, 1992, abstr.
135. **Knekt P,** Heliovaara M, Rissanen A, Aromaa A, Aaran R, Serum antioxidant vitamins and risk of cataract, *Br. Med. J.*, 305, 1392-1394, 1992.
136. **Luthra R**, Wa S-Y, Leske MC, Nemesure B, He Q, BES Group, Lens

opacities and use of nutritional supplements: The Barbados Study, *Invest. Ophthalmol. Vis. Sci.*, 8, S450, 1997.

137. **Mares-Perlman JA,** Brady WE, Klein BEK, Klein R, Palta M, Supplement use and 5-year progression of cortical opacities, *Invest. Ophthalmol. Vis. Sci.*, 37, 137, 1996.

138. **Rouhiainen P**, Rouhiainen H, Salonen TJ, Association between low plasma vitamin E concentration and progression of early cortical lens opacities, *Am. J. Epidemiol.*, 144, 496-500, 1996.

139. **Leske MC**, Chylack LT, Jr, He Q, Wu SY, Schoenfeld E, Friend J, Wolfe J, the LSC Group, Antioxidant vitamins and nuclear opacities– The Longitudinal Study of Cataract, *Ophthalmology*, 105, 831-836, 1998.

140. **Leske MC,** Chylack LT, Jr, He Q, Wu SY, Schoenfeld E, Friend J, Wolfe J, the LSC Group, Risk factors for a nuclear opalescence in a longitudinal study, *Am. J. Epidemiol.*, Jan. 1, 1998 issue.

141. **Jacques PF,** Taylor A, Hankinson SE, Lahav M, Mahnken B, Lee Y, Vaid K, Willett WC, Long-term vitamin C supplement use and prevalence of early age-related lens opacities, *Am. J. Clin. Nutr.*, 66, 911-916, 1997.

142. **Sperduto RD,** Hu T-S, Milton RC, Zhao J, Everett DF, Cheng Q, Blot WJ, Bing L, Taylor PR, Jun-Yao L, Dawsey S, Guo W, The Linxian Cataract Studies: Two nutrition intervention trials, *Arch. Ophthalmol.*, 111, 1246-1253, 1993.

143. **Libondi T**, Menzione M, Auricchio G, In vitro effect of alpha-tocopherol on lysophosatiphatidylcholine-induced lens damage, *Exp. Eye Res.*, 40, 661-666, 1985.

144. **Burton W,** Ingold KU, Beta-carotene: an unusual type of lipid antioxidant, *Science,* 224, 569-573, 1984.

145. **Kwan M,** Niinikoski J, Hunt TK, In vivo measurement of oxygen tension in the cornea, aqueous humor, and the anterior lens of the open eye, *Invest. Ophthalmol. Vis. Sci.*, 11, 108-114, 1972.

146. **Erdman J**, The physiologic chemistry of carotenes in man, *Am. J. Clin. Nutr.,* 7, 101-106, 1988.

147. **Di Mascio P**, Murphy ME, Sies H, Antioxidant defense systems: the role of carotenoids, tocopherols and thiols, *Am. J. Clin. Nutr.,* 53, 194S-200S, 1991.

148. **Krinsky NI**, Deneke SS, Interaction of oxygen and oxy-radicals with carotenoids, *J. Natl. Cancer Inst.*, 69, 205-10, 1982.

149. **Micozzi MS,** Beecher GR, Taylor HR, Khachik F, Carotenoid analyses of selected raw and cooked foods associated with a lower risk for cancer, *J. Natl. Cancer Inst.,* 82, 282-285, 1990.

150. **Daicker B,** Schiedt K, Adnet JJ, Bermond P, Canthaxamin retinopathy. An investigation by light and electron microscopy and physiochemical analyses, *Graefe's Arch. Clin. Exp. Ophthalmol.*, 225, 189-197, 1987.

151. **Leske MC,** Wu SY, Connell AMS, Hyman I, Lens opacities, demographic factors and nutritional supplements in the Barbados Eye Study, *Int. J. Epidemiol.* 26, 1314-1322, 1997.

152. **Glynn RJ,** Christen WG, Manson JAE, Bernheumer J, Hennekens CH,

Body mass index, *Arch. Ophthalmol.*, 113, 1131-1137, 1995.

153. **Taylor A,** Zuliani AM, Hopkins RE, Dallal GE, Treglia P, Kuck JFR, Kuck K, Moderate caloric restriction delays cataract formation in the Emory mouse, *FASEB J.*, 3, 1741-1746, 1989.

154. **Jacob RA,** Otradovec CL, Russell RM, Munro HN, Hartz SC, McGandy RB, Morrow F, Sadowski JA, Vitamin C status and interactions in a healthy elderly population., *Am. J. Clin. Nutr.*,48, 1436-1442, 1988.

155. **Harding JJ,** van Heyningen R, Epidemiology and risk factors for cataract, *Eye*, 1, 537-541, 1987.

156. **McLaren DS**, in *Nutritional Ophthalmology,* 2nd ed., Academic Press, London, 1980.

157. **Hiller R,** Giacometti L, Yuen K, Sunlight and cataract: an epidemiologic investigation, *Am. J. Epidemiol.,*105, 450-459, 1977.

158. **Taylor HR,** West S, Munoz B, Rosenthal FS, Bressler SB, Bressler NM, The long-term effects of visible light on the eye, *Arch. Ophthalmol.,* 110, 99-104, 1992.

159. **Taylor A,** Berger J, Reddan J, Zuliani A, Effects of aging in vitro on intracellular proteolysis in cultured rabbit lens epithelial cells in the presence and absence of serum, *In Vitro Cell. Develop. Biol.,* 27A, 287-292, 1991.

160. **Fleshman KR,** Wagner BJ, Changes during aging in rats lens endopeptidase activity, *Exp. Eye Res.*, 39, 543-551, 1984.

161. **Ray K,** Harris H, Purification of neutral lens endopeptidase: close similarity to a neutral proteinase in pituitary, *Proc. Nat. Acad. Sci. USA,* 82, 7545-7549, 1985.

162. **Murakami K,** Jahngen JH, Lin S, Davies KJA, Taylor A, Lens proteasome shows enhanced rates of degradation of hydroxyl radical modified alpha-crystallin, *Free Radic. Biol. Med.,* 8, 217-222, 1990.

163. **Taylor A,** Brown MJ, Daims MA, Cohen J, Localization of leucine aminopeptidase in hog lenses using immunofluorescence and activity assays, *Invest. Ophthalmol. Vis. Sci.,* 24, 1172-1181, 1983.

164. **Varnum MD,** David LL, Shearer TR, Age-related changes in calpain II and calpastatin in rat lens, *Exp. Eye Res.,* 49, 1053-1065, 1989.

165. **Yoshida H,** Yumoto N, Tsukahara I, Murachi T, The degradation of alpha-crystallin at its carboxyl-terminal portion by calpain in bovine lens, *Invest. Ophthalmol. Vis. Sci.,* 27, 1269-1273, 1986.

166. **Wefers H,** Sies H, The protection by ascorbate and glutathione against microsomal lipid peroxidation is dependent on vitamin E, *FEBS*, 174, 353-357.

167. **Burton GW,** Wronska U, Stone L, Foster DO, Ingold KU, Biokinetics of dietary RRR-alpha-tocopherol in the male guinea pig at three dietary levels of vitamin C and two levels of vitamin E. Evidence that vitamin C does not "spare" vitamin E in vivo, *Lipids,* 25, 199-210, 1990.

168. **Chen S,** A protective role for glutathione-dependent reduction of

dehydroascorbic acid in lens epithelium, *Inv. Ophthalmol. Vis. Sci.,* 36, 1804, 1995.

169. **Sasaki H,** Giblin FJ, Winkler BS, Chakrapani B, Leverenz V, Chu-Johnston CS, Meyer CG, Srilakshmi, JC, Vitamin C elevates red blood cell glutathione in healthy adults, *Am. J. Clin. Nutr.*, 58, 103-105, 1993.

170. **Bohm F,** Edge R, Land EJ, Mcgarvey DJ, Truscott TG, Carotenoids enhance vitamin E antioxidant efficiency, *J. Am. Chem. Soc.*, 119, 621-622, 1997.

171. **Valgimigli L,** Lucarini M, Pedulli GF, Ingold KU, Does beta-carotene really protect vitaminE from oxidation?, *J. Am. Chem. Soc.*, 119, 8095-8096, 1997.

Chapter 5

EVALUATION OF EPIDEMIOLOGIC STUDIES OF NUTRITION AND CATARACT

William G. Christen

I. INTRODUCTION

Basic research studies, including laboratory investigations and studies in animal models, have contributed valuable information regarding a possible connection between nutrition and cataract. In addition to providing mechanisms relating nutrition and cataract, these studies have identified various nutrients that may help to reduce the risk of cataract formation. The relevance of basic research studies to cataract development in humans, however, is unclear because of species differences in the absorption, metabolism, and requirements for various nutrients.[1] Epidemiologic studies in free-living humans provide the most relevant information pertaining to human cataract, but lack the experimenter control, and, therefore, the precision that is possible in basic research studies. An understanding of the relative strengths and limitations of various epidemiologic study designs is essential to a critical evaluation of the published and frequently conflicting reports regarding nutritional determinants of cataract formation.

The purpose of this chapter is to present several basic epidemiologic principles and concepts that are important to consider when evaluating the results of research studies. Consideration will be given initially to possible alternative explanations for observed associations. This will be followed by a brief description of the relative strengths and limitations of several epidemiologic study designs commonly employed in studies of nutrition and cataract. Examples from the research literature will be used to illustrate the specific challenges posed by these design strategies in evaluating alternative explanations for observed associations.

II. ALTERNATIVE EXPLANATIONS FOR ASSOCIATIONS

The goal of epidemiologic research is to determine whether an association exists between an exposure and disease, and whether the relationship is one of cause and effect. While a judgement of causality is based ultimately on a consideration of all available data, with each study contributing only a piece to the puzzle, the process of establishing causality proceeds at several levels. In individual studies, it involves the determination of whether an observed association is valid. That is, does an observed association between a specific measure of nutrition and cataract, for example, reflect the true relationship between this exposure and disease? It is the responsibility of the study investigator (and critical readers of the published literature) to fully consider other explanations for the

0-8493-8565-2/99/$0.00+$.50

findings including whether the results might simply be due to chance? Perhaps there was bias in the way patients were selected for the study, or in the manner in which information was collected. Maybe a third factor, one that is associated with nutritional status and is also a predictor of cataract, is primarily responsible for the association. Questions such as these need to be addressed before the findings in any study can be deemed valid. In short, it is necessary to consider the possibility that the results are due to chance, bias, or confounding.

A. Chance

Chance can never be totally excluded as a possible explanation for a study's findings. Rather, statistical tests and confidence intervals are used to determine the *probability* that the results are due to chance. A discussion of statistical procedures used to evaluate chance can be found elsewhere[2,3,4,5] and is beyond the scope of this chapter. However, a related issue that frequently arises in studies of nutrition and cataract, and deserves a brief mention here, is the issue of multiple comparisons.

In studies of nutritional determinants of disease, the investigator often has the opportunity to examine a large number of possible associations in the data. However, as the number of comparisons in a study increases, so does the likelihood that some statistically significant associations will be found just by chance alone. This can be a particular problem in studies of cataract where investigators are often interested in associations with specific cataract subtypes. While it is certainly plausible that nutritional determinants may be different for the various cataract subtypes, the conduct of multiple comparisons within individual studies increases the risk of chance findings, and probably contributes to the inconsistent results between studies. Investigators and readers of the literature alike need to be aware of this possibility, and take measures to adjust for multiple comparisons where appropriate.

Once chance has been addressed and found to be an unlikely explanation for a study's findings, the investigator can conclude that there is a valid statistical association in the data. But it is still necessary to consider whether the results could be due to bias or confounding.

B. Bias

Bias refers to any consistent difference in the way patients are selected for a study, or in the way data are obtained, reported, or analyzed, that can affect the outcome of the study and lead to a distorted estimate of the "true relationship" between exposure and disease. There are many potential sources of bias in an epidemiologic study but two general types are usually identified: selection bias and information bias.

1. *Selection Bias*

Selection bias occurs when the selection of individuals for inclusion in a study is in some way dependent on the characteristic to be compared. In a study comparing a nutritional measure in persons with and without cataract, selection bias would occur if the probability of being selected for inclusion in the study was related to an individual's nutritional status. Another type of selection bias, commonly referred to as diagnostic bias, would occur if the probability of being identified as a cataract case was linked in some fashion to one's nutritional state.

2. *Information Bias*

Information bias occurs when the methods used to obtain information on exposure or disease differ in a systematic way for the various study groups. Several examples of information bias include interviewer bias, recall bias, and misclassification.

a. Interviewer Bias

Interviewer bias is the selective collection or interpretation of exposure or disease data. Methods used to minimize this source of bias include keeping the interviewer unaware of the subject's exposure or disease status (depending on study type) and to the hypotheses under investigation, and using standardized data collection procedures and instruments.

b. Recall Bias

Recall bias occurs when events are remembered or reported differently by the various study groups. In studies comparing people with and without disease, recall bias is a frequent concern because those with disease tend to recall their exposure history differently, and perhaps more completely, than those without disease.

c. Misclassification

Some degree of misclassification of exposure or disease is unavoidable in any epidemiologic study. Misclassification that is approximately the same for the various study groups is said to be random, or nondifferential, and tends to make the study groups more similar, thereby underestimating any true association between exposure and disease. Misclassification that varies between study groups is called nonrandom, or differential, and is a more serious problem because it can result in either an over- or underestimate of the true association.

In studies of nutritional determinants of disease, misclassification of exposure, especially dietary data, is a particular problem because everyone is exposed to some degree. The strengths and limitations of the various methods used to quantify dietary intake (i.e., dietary recall, food record, diet history, food frequency questionnaire) have been described elsewhere[6] and will not be considered here. Blood-based data, which reflect not only dietary intake but also genetic and lifestyle factors and the intake of other nutrients,[6] are a more direct measure of an individual's nutrient status and are less prone to misclassification. On the other hand, for most nutrients, blood-based data reflect recent intake rather than intake over an extended period. However, regardless of the method used, misclassification will increase if the information obtained is not pertinent to the relevant period of exposure for the disease under study. More specifically, nutritional information collected after a cataract has already developed may not reflect the levels that contributed to the formation of cataract, and will usually lead to further inappropriate classification of study participants. Unfortunately, as with any disease that develops slowly over time, the relevant period of exposure for cataract can be difficult to determine.

d. Loss To Follow-Up

When those that are lost to follow-up are different than those that remain under surveillance in both exposure and disease, serious bias may result.

C. Confounding

If a determinant of disease other than the one under investigation is unevenly distributed between the various study groups, confounding is said to occur. The effect of confounding is to distort the measure of association between exposure and disease because the confounding factor itself produces differences in disease occurrence in the study groups. In studies of nutrition and cataract, confounding is a particular problem because persons who have favorable diets are likely to differ from persons with less-favorable diets on a range of factors that may be related to the risk of developing cataract. The effects of confounding can be at least partially controlled during data analysis, providing adequate information has been collected on other risk factors for disease.

III. EPIDEMIOLOGIC STUDY DESIGNS: STRENGTHS AND LIMITATIONS

Broadly speaking, epidemiologic study designs fall into two categories, descriptive and analytic.[5] *Descriptive* studies are concerned with the distribution of disease in populations or population subgroups and are, therefore, particularly valuable in generating research hypotheses. Examples of descriptive studies include case-reports and case-series, correlational studies, and cross-sectional studies. *Analytic* studies are concerned with testing research hypotheses and are designed to evaluate determinants of disease. A principal distinction between analytic and descriptive studies is the use of a specifically constructed comparison group in the former which enables the testing of research hypotheses. There are two types of analytic studies: observational, including case-control and cohort, and intervention studies or randomized trials. In observational studies, the investigator has no control over exposure status but simply observes who is exposed and who is not, and who gets disease and who does not. In intervention studies, the investigator assigns the exposure and then observes the development of disease over time.

Most of the available epidemiologic data regarding nutrition and cataract have come from cross-sectional, case-control, and cohort studies; thus, the following discussion will focus on these study designs.

A. Cross-sectional Studies

In cross-sectional studies, exposure and disease status for individuals in a well-defined population are determined at one point in time. Therefore, it is often difficult to assess the temporal relationship between exposure and disease. In addition, the investigation of nutritional risk factors is particularly difficult with this study design because current levels of nutritional intake may reflect levels prior to disease development, in which case they may be of etiologic importance, or they may reflect dietary changes made after disease detection.

For example, the relationship of self-reported supplemental vitamin and mineral use and various types of lens opacities was examined in a population-based, cross-sectional analysis of 2,152 persons in the Nutritional Factors in Eye Disease Study.[7] This study had a number of important strengths. Participation rates were high (90% of those eligible) which minimized the importance of selection factors for inclusion in the study and provided confidence that the data were reasonably representative of persons aged 43 to 84 years residing in Beaver Dam, Wisconsin. Lens status was determined with the use of standardized lens photographs and a detailed grading system which minimized the misclassification of cataract. Extensive information on a range of possible risk factors for cataract was collected in a standardized interview conducted at the same time of the eye examination. These data were used to control for confounding during data analysis (analyses were adjusted for the confounding effects of diabetes, annual ambient ultraviolet B exposure, education, smoking, and heavy drinking). Dietary data on food intake and supplement use were collected with the use of a standardized nutritional questionnaire (modified version of a diet history questionnaire developed by the National Cancer Institute) administered during home interviews approximately one month after the eye examination. The use of the standardized questionnaire served to reduce the likelihood of interviewer bias (it is unclear whether the interviewers were kept unaware of the participants' cataract status).

The limitations of the study were due in large part to the cross-sectional design. Because lens status and nutritional status were determined at the same point in time (or approximately so), it was not possible to determine the temporal sequence of events. While the reported nutritional intake may have reflected levels that predated the development of cataract, the reported levels may also have been the result of dietary changes that were made subsequent to the detection of cataract. Participants may have chosen healthier diets and increased the use of antioxidant vitamin supplements following a diagnosis of cataract, in which case cross-sectional data could easily obscure any true protective effect that nutrition might have. Cross-sectional data may also be of limited relevance for the study of diseases that develop slowly over time, such as cataract, in which the relevant exposure period is likely to have occurred many years in the past. The investigators attempted to address this issue by including questions regarding intake ten years prior to the interview, but since comparable data on lens status ten years prior to the study were not available, the temporal sequence of events remained in question. The investigators did find that associations based on reported intake ten years in the past were stronger than associations based on current level of intake but, as they pointed out, this may simply have been the result of recall bias. Persons with cataracts, aware of a possible connection between nutrition and cataract, may have recalled their nutritional history differently than persons without cataract. In essence, other than for characteristics that are unchanging (e.g., gender, blood type, iris color), it is rarely possible to assess the temporal relationship of exposure and disease in cross-sectional studies.

Finally, as with many studies of nutrition and cataract, a large number of comparisons were made in this cross-sectional analysis. Odds ratios and confidence intervals were used to evaluate the role of chance (and to control for confounding), but in view of the multiple comparisons, one should be aware that some of the statistically significant associations observed in this study may have occurred by chance alone.

B. Case-control Studies

In case-control studies, the investigator starts with a group of people with disease (cases) and without disease (controls) and looks backward in time to determine the proportion in each group who had the exposure of interest. Because both exposure and disease have already occurred at the time the study is conducted, case-control studies are particularly vulnerable to bias. For example, selection bias can occur if the decision about who to include in a study as a case or control is in some way related to exposure status. Information bias can occur when those with disease recall their exposure history differently than do those without disease, or when study personnel solicit information or interpret data differently for cases and controls. The case-control design also shares with the cross-sectional design a limited ability to examine the temporal relationship of most exposures and disease, especially when prevalent or existing cases of disease are studied, rather than newly diagnosed cases.

As an example, a wide range of possible risk factors for cataract was examined in a case-control study of 945 cases and 435 controls drawn from a pool of general ophthalmology outpatients examined at one of two clinic sites over a three year period.[8] Medical records of incoming patients were screened for eligibility, and eligible patients were invited to a special study visit for data collection and classification into appropriate study groups. The percentage of eligible case and control patients who agreed to participate was comparatively high and was the same (72.8%) in the two groups, providing a measure of assurance that bias due to nonparticipation was unlikely. Misclassification of case-control status was minimized through the use of a slit-lamp examination and standardized lens classification system to place participants in appropriate study groups. Cases were defined as patients who had age-related nuclear, cortical, or posterior subcapsular opacities in at least one eye that explained a decrease in visual acuity, if any, and controls were defined as patients with no lens opacities and visual acuities of 20/20 or better in both eyes. Specific procedures to minimize bias during data collection were also implemented. Trained study personnel were kept unaware of the specific hypotheses under investigation and of the case-control status of the participant. A standardized protocol was followed in the collection of data on a range of possible risk factors for cataract. Nutritional intake was measured with a standardized food frequency questionnaire. Given these precautionary steps, the possibility of interviewer bias was reduced and any misclassification of nutritional status that might have occurred was likely to be random with respect to case-control status. During data analysis, the investigators examined a number of possible associations and calculated odds ratios and confidence intervals to evaluate the role of chance. The results indicated that several measures of nutritional intake were statistically significantly associated with a decreased risk of one or more subtypes of cataract.

However, before concluding that these results are valid and reflect the true relationship between the nutritional factors and cataract, additional alternative explanations for the findings need to be considered. As before, the critical reader needs to note that the multiple comparisons conducted in this study raise the possibility that some of the statistically significant associations may simply be the result of chance. Recall bias also has to be considered and would have occurred if cases tended to remember or report their dietary history differently from controls. Confounding was decreased by adjusting for the effects of other risk factors for cataract in multivariate analysis. However, as with any observational study, the possibility of uncontrolled confounding remains. Finally, it is also reasonable to consider whether the choice of controls for this study may have introduced some degree of selection bias. Controls should be chosen to represent the population of all individuals who would have been identified and included as cases if they had also developed the disease.[5] In this study, controls were patients with no lens opacities or visual acuity loss who, for the most part, came to the clinic for routine eye examination. If these controls tended to be more health conscious than the larger population of individuals who would have arrived at the clinic had they developed a cataract, then they may also have differed in other ways including, perhaps, having a more favorable diet. Thus, even in the absence of a true relationship between nutrition and cataract, the nutritional status of cases might have appeared inferior to that of the controls, suggesting an association between nutrition and cataract when, in fact, none exists.

C. Cohort Studies

In a cohort, or follow-up study, individuals are categorized according to exposure to a possible risk factor for disease and are followed up over time for the development of new cases of disease. Cohort studies can be either retrospective or prospective. In a retrospective cohort study, both the exposure and disease have already occurred when the study is undertaken whereas in a prospective cohort study, the disease has not yet developed when the study is begun. In both types of cohort study, however, participants are required to be free from the disease under investigation at the time exposure status is defined. Thus, the cohort design has several advantages compared to case-control studies. For one, the temporal relationship between exposure and disease is easier to establish in cohort studies.

Cohort studies are also less susceptible to selection bias and to several types of information bias than are case-control studies. On the other hand, participants may be lost to follow-up in cohort studies which can result in a biased estimate of the association between exposure and disease.

A prospective cohort study design was used to examine the association of reported use of vitamin supplements and risk of cataract among 17,744 participants in the Physicians Health Study who did not report cataract at baseline.[9] Because information on vitamin supplement use was collected at baseline, prior to the diagnosis of cataract, the temporal relationship of supplement use and cataract was not in question in this study. For the same reason, bias resulting from differential reporting of vitamin supplement use according to cataract outcome was not an issue. Loss to follow-up, which is the major threat to validity in cohort studies, was not a problem in this investigation because data regarding the study endpoints was available for over 99% of study participants. Chance was evaluated with rate ratios and confidence intervals. The results indicated a statistically significant decreased risk of cataract for users of multivitamins only. No significant association with risk of cataract was found for two other categories of vitamin supplement use (vitamin C and/or E only, multivitamin and C and/or E). Before concluding that these results are valid, however, other alternative explanations for the findings including several other possible sources of bias and confounding still had to be considered.

Because participants were not examined by study personnel, but instead reported new diagnoses of cataract on annual health questionnaires, the investigators had to address the possibility of misclassification of the cataract endpoint. The investigators indicated that the use of medical record data to confirm the reports of cataract reduced random misclassification of the reported endpoint. Any random misclassification that did occur would have produced an underestimate of the true association between exposure and disease. Nonrandom misclassification was considered unlikely because persons who reviewed the medical records were blinded to the participant's reported vitamin supplement use. In addition, because some cataracts were probably undetected or unreported, the investigators also had to address the possibility of detection bias. The specific concern was that vitamin supplement users may be more health conscious, and therefore have more (or less) medical contacts which would increase (or decrease) the likelihood of having a cataract diagnosed. It was noted that since the participants were physicians, their overall level of medical care was likely to be high, with similar levels for users and nonusers of supplements. Nonetheless, the possibility of some degree of bias due to differential detection of cataract could not be ruled out. Finally, although the investigators adjusted for the effects of a range of possible confounders in data analysis, uncontrolled confounding, resulting from unmeasured confounders or from inadequate control of measured confounders, remained a possibility in this observational study.

IV. FUTURE STUDIES–RANDOMIZED TRIALS

The results of several case-control and cohort studies appear to be compatible with a possible protective role of nutritional factors, particularly vitamins with antioxidant properties, in reducing the risk of cataract. However, an especially important limitation of these observational study designs is uncontrolled confounding. Because diets are self-selected, persons with favorable diets may differ from those with less-favorable diets in important ways, including life-style factors or other dietary practices, that may be predictive of cataract development. While case-control and cohort studies can control for the effects of known confounders, they cannot control for the effects of unknown or unmeasured confounders. Unfortunately, the magnitude of uncontrolled confounding in these observational studies can easily be as large as the small to moderate benefit that might be expected from nutritional factors.

In randomized trials, the exposure status of study participants is under the control of the investigator. When the study population is of a sufficient size, the random assignment of participants to particular exposure or treatment groups tends to assure, on average, the equal distribution of known *and unknown* confounders between the various treatment groups. For this reason, randomized trials provide the most reliable evidence from epidemiologic research.

There have been no completed randomized trials testing possible nutritional determinants of cataract. End-of-trial eye examinations were conducted among a subset of participants in two nutrition intervention trials of cancer in Linxian, China, to assess whether vitamin/mineral supplements affected the *prevalence* of various types of cataract.[10] However, because information on lens status at the beginning of the study was not available, this study was unable to examine the temporal relationship between vitamin treatment and cataract development.

There are several ongoing trials examining nutritional intervention and cataract. The Age Related Eye Disease Study, a 10-year, multicenter randomized trial sponsored by the National Eye Institute, is testing the effects of high dose antioxidants (vitamin C, vitamin E, beta-carotene, and zinc) on the development and progression of AMD and cataract,[1] and should provide the most reliable evidence on this question. The Physicians' Health Study I,[11] testing beta-carotene, and the Physicians' Health Study II, testing beta-carotene, vitamin E, vitamin C, and a multivitamin, both conducted in men, as well as the Women's Health Study,[12] testing vitamin E in women, should also contribute importantly relevant information.

V. SUMMARY

The available epidemiologic data regarding nutritional determinants of cataract have derived principally from cross-sectional, case-control, and prospective cohort studies. While these data are promising and generally appear to support a protective role for nutritional factors in cataract formation, alternative explanations for observed associations frequently are difficult to rule out. In particular, uncontrolled confounding is always a possibility in observational studies, and can easily be as large as the small to moderate benefit that might be expected from nutritional factors. Thus, the most reliable data on which public health recommendations can be based will come primarily from randomized trials.

VI. REFERENCES

1. **Sperduto, R.D.,** Ferris, F.L., and Kurinij N., Do we have a nutritional treatment for age-related cataract or macular degeneration?., *Arch. Ophthalmol.*, 108, 1403, 1990.
2. **Colton, T.,** *Statistics in Medicine*, Little, Brown, Boston, MA, 1974.
3. **Kleinbaum, D.G.,** Kupper, L.L., and Morgenstern, H., *Epidemiologic Research: Principles and Quantitative Methods*, Lifetime Learning Publications, Belmont, CA, 1982.
4. **Rosner, B.,** *Fundamentals of Biostatistics*, PWS-Kent, Boston, MA, 1990.
5. **Hennekens, C.H.,** and Buring, J.E., *Epidemiology in Medicine*, Little, Brown and Company, Boston, MA, 1987.
6. **Willett, W.,** *Nutritional Epidemiology*, Oxford University Press, New York, 1990.
7. **Mares-Perlman, J.A.,** Klein, B.E.K., Klein, R., and Ritter, L.L., Relation between lens opacities and vitamin and mineral supplement use, *Ophthalmology*, 101, 315, 1994.
8. **Leske, M.C.,** Chylack, L.T., Wu, S.-Y., and The Lens Opacities Case-Control Study Group, The lens opacities case-control study: risk factors for cataract, *Arch. Ophthalmol.*, 109, 244, 1991.
9. **Seddon, J.M.,** Christen, W.G., Manson, J.E., Glynn, R.J., LaMotte, F.S., Buring, J.E., and Hennekens, C.H., A prospective cohort study of vitamin supplements and risk of cataract among U.S. male physicians, *Am. J. Pub. Health*, 84, 788, 1994.
10. **Sperduto, R.D.,** Hu, T.-S., Milton, R.C., Zhao, J.-L., Everett, D.F., Cheng, Q.-F., Blot, W.J., Bing, L., Taylor, P.R., Jun-Yao, L., Dawsey, S., Guo, W.-D., The Linxian Cataract Studies: two nutrition intervention trials, *Arch. Ophthalmol.*, 111, 1246, 1993.
11. **Steering Committee of the Physicians' Health Study Research Group,** Final report on the aspirin component of the ongoing Physicians' Health Study, *New Engl. J. Med.*, 321, 129, 1989.
12. **Buring, J.E.,** Hennekens, C.H., The Women's Health Study: summary of the study design, *J. Myocardial Ischemia*, 4, 27, 1992.

Chapter 6

ANIMAL STUDIES ON CATARACT

George Edwin Bunce

I. INTRODUCTION

Howard Schneider, in his opening address of the Centennial Celebration of the Department of Biochemistry, University of Wisconsin at Madison, on August 26, 1983, presented a delightful history of the events that ushered in the paradigm for nutritional studies in the Twentieth Century. [1] The old paradigm was one of chemical analysis of foods as the guide for the design of rations for farm animals and man. The nutritional value of a diet was determined based upon Kjeldahl analysis of nitrogen, an ether extract for fat, total ash content for minerals, total carbohydrates, and water. But experiments feeding single grains (wheat, corn, or oats) to calves revealed that the paradigm was seriously flawed. A young investigator in the Department, E.V. McCollum, recognized that foodstuffs contained vital nutrients not present in isolated and purified macrocomponents. His landmark studies with Marguerite Davis resulting in the recognition of vitamin A also provided the impetus for the new paradigm, namely, that the nutrient value of foodstuffs could be tested by feeding them to small rodents, which could be economically maintained and studied. This, of course, opened the pathway for the discovery of other micronutrients and the recognition of nutritional deficiency diseases.

I open this chapter with these comments for two reasons. One, I so enjoyed the cited article that I wanted to bring it to the attention of others. Two, the material that follows arose from this paradigm (as did much of our current knowledge of nutrition). I shall review those animal studies that have explored the associations between nutrient substances and the development and preservation of function in the mammalian lens.

II. RELATIONS BETWEEN MACRONUTRIENTS AND CATARACT

A. CARBOHYDRATES

The sugar cataract is the most thoroughly studied of all the experimental cataracts. It can be produced in intact animals either by the feeding of diets rich (15-75%) in the monosaccharides xylose, arabinose, or galactose (the galactose containing disaccharide lactose can also be used) [2,3] or by making the animals diabetic following administration of agents such as alloxan or streptozotocin. [4] Monosaccharides enter the lens by diffusion from the aqueous humor. When elevated levels of these sugars are maintained for extended periods of time, the usual metabolic pathways become saturated and the sugars are reduced to the corresponding sugar alcohols by the NADPH-dependent enzyme aldose reductase. Since the sugar alcohol products are neither as readily diffusible nor

0-8493-8565-2/99/$0.00+$.50

rapidly metabolized, they accumulate leading to hypertonicity and osmotic swelling. If the condition is prolonged, progressive degeneration occurs with loss of membrane permeability and disruption of metabolic reactions and ionic balance. Morphologically, the lens progresses through the appearance of vacuoles, cortical cataract and eventually dense nuclear cataract. An extensive literature exists on this subject and a detailed account of this model has been presented. [5]

Prolonged exposure to monosaccharides may also result in nonenzymatic glycosylation and free radical damage in the lens. Reducing sugars can react with lysine or arginine to form a Schiff base that can then rearrange to give an Amadori product. Glycosylated enzymes can show significant loss of function and structural crystallins may undergo crosslinking to yield advanced glycosylation endproducts or AGE's. Van Boekel and Hoenders [6] have examined clear human lenses over an age range of 4 to 81 years and lenses showing senile or diabetic cataract. They found an age-linked increase in glycosylation in (α-crystallins and a two-fold higher increase in age-matched lenses from diabetics. Aldoses can also be a source of free radicals [7] and several investigators have found that antioxidants offer a measure of protection against sugar cataract. Trevithick et al. [8], for example, exposed rat lenses *in vitro* to either normal (5.6 mM) or elevated (56 mM) glucose for 48 hours and observed that the addition of 2.4 uM (α-tocopherol acetate protected the lenses against swelling and deterioration without alteration of sugar uptake or conversion to sorbitol. They also reported that daily injections of 1 g (α-tocopherol/kg body weight prevented cataract in streptozotocin-injected rats. [9] Srivastava and Ansari [10] delayed cataract appearance from 23 to 38 days by supplementing the diet with 0.4% of butylated hydroxytoluene. Yokoyama et al. [11] found that the lenses of scorbutic guinea pigs displayed vacuolation and biochemical abnormalities after exposure to as little as 10% galactose in the drinking water. Pyruvate administered topically in the form of eye drops delayed the onset of cataractous changes and decreased the accumulation of galactitol in rodents. [12]

The sugar cataract, whether initiated by dietary sugars or by diabetic agents, remains probably the most valuable model for studying the biochemical mechanisms of cataractogenesis. Since diabetics have a 3 to 5-fold greater likelihood of developing cataract, it has great clinical value as well.

B. PROTEIN AND AMINO ACIDS

The mammalian lens is packed with structural proteins called crystallins, the density and native conformation of which are crucial to the establishment and preservation of transparency. Intuitively, one might expect that deficits of total protein or individual amino acids would lead to loss of transparency. Curtis et al. [13] described "a white opaqueness of the eye and lens" when various proteins served as sole sources of nitrogen for young growing rats. L-Tryptophan was identified as the first limiting amino acid in these proteins and subsequent studies verified its cataractogenic potential when limiting in the diet of both rats and guinea pigs. [14,15] When L-Trp was held to 0.05 g/100 g diet (35% of the minimum requirement) and all other amino acids were provided in pure form, cataracts were readily visible in 80% of test rats after nine weeks. [16] Elimination of L-Trp from the diet shortened the time to cataract to three weeks. It should be noted that at these severe restrictions, growth of the animals virtually ceased.

The indispensable amino acids show variation in their potential to produce a cataract in rats in response to reduced intake. Hall et al. [17,18] prepared a series of diets that provided three times the minimum requirement of each indispensible amino acid save the one under study which was omitted. Dense nuclear opacities were present after three weeks with omission of either L-Trp, L-Phe, or L-His. Pre-cataractous changes only were noted after three weeks in the absence of L-Leu, L-Ile, L-Val, L-Thr, L-Lys, or L-Met. Omission of L-Arg was without effect.

It is interesting to note that restriction of intake of total protein is more readily tolerated than the imbalances described above. When Hall omitted the entire group of indispensable amino acids, cataract did not appear in the three week test period. [18] McLaren [19] maintained 147 Wistar rats from weaning to advanced maturity on diets that contained either 2 or 4% total protein and saw not a single cataract despite severe limitation of growth. Kauffman and Norton [20] fed 31 weanling pigs diets derived from mixtures of soybean meal and corn and containing either 0, 5, 10, or 12-16% protein. They noted no gross abnormalities of the lens at the conclusion of the study (146 days) and observed that while soft tissues lost nitrogen content, the relative content of lens nitrogen was preserved.

These results show that imbalances of the indispensable amino acids are far more damaging to the lens than restriction of the entire supply. Cataractogenesis in this model may not arise just from interference with protein synthesis alone, but may include some components of metabolic distress arising from the imbalance state. In studies by Bunce et al. [16], the emergence of visible cataract was accompanied by a significant increase in lens wet weight and disappearance of the β-crystallins suggestive of osmotic shifts and/or degradation and changes in protein aggregation patterns. As a model system, however, the tryptophan deficiency cataract is difficult to use because of the extreme debilitation of the subject animals. Protein or amino acid deficiency is probably not an important factor in human cataract except possibly in countries where a low-tryptophan protein such as corn is the prominent staple source of dietary protein but data on this subject are not existent.

III. MICRONUTRIENTS

A. RIBOFLAVIN

The cataractogenic potential of a riboflavin-deficiency state was recognized when this substance was still known as vitamin G. Salmon et al. [21] reported in 1928 that rats fed diets free of "B complex" displayed lens opacities among their many consequences, and Day and Darby [22, 23] established the uniqueness of vitamin G in the prevention of this phenomenon. Riboflavin is the precursor of flavin adenine dinucleotide (FAD) which is the essential cofactor for glutathione reductase. This enzyme plays a vital role in the maintenance of cellular pools of reduced glutathione (GSH). A shift in the intracellular ratio of GSH/GSSG can compromise the peroxide/free radical defense system allowing nonenzymatic oxidation of cellular lipids, proteins, and nucleic acids and changes in this ratio can also exert dramatic effects on lens proteolysis. [24,25,26]

The free radical defense system, however, consists of a complex array of interrelated agents as noted in the previous chapter. It contains multiple mechanisms and redundancy. Some molecules can be renewed while others must be supplied anew in the diet. Enzymes show variable rates of turnover and inductive responsiveness. The nature and size of the oxidant burden is crucial to the damage potential. Viewed from this perspective, it is hardly surprising that studies of dietary riboflavin deficits have exhibited widely divergent results, but the consistent theme has been a confirmation of the cataractogenic potential of this vitamin in the rat [27], pig [28], cat [29], and salmonid fish. [30]

The interactive nature of oxidant burden, riboflavin deficit, and tissue specificity was nicely demonstrated by Srivastava and Beutler. [31,32] When weanling rats were fed an otherwise nutritionally complete but riboflavin-deficient diet for 21 days, erythrocyte glutathione reductase activity fell to 60% of normal as compared with only a 25% decline in the lens. Lens total thiol and reduced GSH showed no change and the lenses were still cataract free after 16 weeks. The same level of riboflavin shortage superimposed upon a 68% galactose diet for 18 days, however, resulted in an increase in cataract from 10% (high galactose alone) to 80%.

The riboflavin-deficiency model offers the opportunity to explore oxidant stress in the lens of intact animals, but its usefulness is lessened by the lengthy periods of time that may be required for endpoint pathology. The addition of heightened, oxidant-burden conditions can shorten this time frame. Riboflavin adequacy could be a problem in human populations subjected to long periods of dietary shortage and oxidant challenge. Children, the elderly, and others enduring prolonged chronic shortages of this vitamin could be at some degree of risk. It is interesting to note that a supplement of riboflavin and niacin together resulted in a significantly reduced prevalence of nuclear cataract, especially in the group aged 65-74 years, in the intervention trial conducted among poorly nourished people in Linxian, China. [33]

B. VITAMINS C AND E

The importance of oxidative stress in the evolution of cataract has generated an intense interest in the role of vitamins E and C in the prevention or delay of this malady. These substances can react directly and non-enzymatically with oxidant molecules, yielding harmless products and thereby terminating propagation of free radical chain reactions. They are also synergistic in that ascorbate and glutathione restore the reduced form of tocopherol. Cataract has not been described as an outcome of an uncomplicated single deficiency of these vitamins in laboratory animals. If a challenge is imposed, however, that can generate a cataract by a mechanism that includes an oxidant stress, then abundant supplies of these vitamins appear to be beneficial.

As an example, Blondin et al. [34] studied the effect of dietary ascorbate on lens damage following postmortem exposure to ultraviolet light. Guinea pigs were fed a semi-purified diet containing either 2 or 50 mg ascorbate/day for 21 weeks. Lens ascorbate concentrations at the end of this period were 3.3 times higher ($P<0.001$) in the high intake group as compared to the low intake group. Lens homogenates were then prepared and subjected to photooxidative stress for up to four hours in the form of UV light. Far fewer high molecular weight aggregates were formed, and there was less enzyme inactivation in the homogenates from the animals fed the extravagant level of ascorbate.

In another study, Bunce and Hess [35] fed a diet utilizing L-amino acids as the sole nitrogen source to female rats during gestation and lactation and varied its content of either L-tryptophan or vitamin E. Nuclear opacities were observed in 42 of 126 pups from 19 dams when L-Trp and vitamin E were both present at suboptimal quantities (75 mg/100g diet and 100 ug/100g diet, respectively). When the diet was low in vitamin E alone, nuclear cataracts were seen in only 7 of 111 progeny from 13 dams. When L-Trp was held at 75 mg/100g diet in the presence of adequate vitamin E, the pups were entirely free of cataract although further limitation of L-Trp (35 mg/100g diet) yielded 75% cataract. Thus the L-Trp requirement to assure normal lens development was dependent upon the dietary level of vitamin E. Presumably oxidative loss of L-Trp was defended by vitamin E.

The literature contains numerous further references to attenuation of cataractogenic injury associated with either *in vitro* or *in vivo* supplements of these vitamins. Many additional specific references can be found in previous reviews on nutrition and cataract by this author. [36,37] Generous supplies of these well-tolerated substances appear to be beneficial in blunting the consequences of oxidant stress in the lens.

C. ZINC, COPPER, MANGANESE AND IRON

The reduction of molecular oxygen to water in the mitochondrion proceeds through the intermediate reduction products, superoxide and hydrogen peroxide. Despite very tight binding of these intermediates to the electron transport chain proteins, a small percentage (perhaps $\approx$5%) escape. The enzymes superoxide dismutase (SOD), glutathione peroxidase (GSHPx), and catalase usually function to remove these metabolites before they inflict damage upon cellular constituents. Cytosolic SOD requires both copper and zinc and its mitochondrial equivalent is manganese-dependent. Catalase requires iron. Selenium, the mineral cofactor for GSHPx, will be discussed separately in the following section.

Cataract has not been among the array of symptoms that arise from nutritional deprivation of zinc, copper, manganese, or iron in warm-blooded animals. It must be said, however, that the vast majority of these studies have been of the short-term variety. The apparent resistance of the mammalian lens to these shortages may result from slow turnover of the parent enzymes and/or adaptive responses. A deficit of zinc has been clearly linked to cataract in fish raised commercially. Ketola observed that cataracts were present in 75-85% of fingerling trout after 16-38 weeks of consuming a "white" fish meal diet. [38] Phytate-rich soybean meal is a major ingredient of commercial salmonid fingerling diets. Increased incorporation of skeletal residues after filleting became popular at that time as a means of enriching these diets with calcium, hence the term "white" fish meal. The combination of phytate and calcium has been demonstrated to greatly reduce the absorption of zinc from the gut. Ketola demonstrated that a supplement of 150 mg zinc/kg diet completely prevented the cataract phenomenon. The reason for the special vulnerability of fish lenses to a dietary zinc deficit has not been established. The author has speculated that it may be related to the occurrence of lens protein phase transitions at ambient cold temperatures.

D. SELENIUM

Following the discovery that selenium is an essential component of GSHPx, it was immediately suspected that cataract might be one outcome of a nutritional deficiency of this element. Lawrence et al. [39] maintained rats on a chromium- and methionine-supplemented Torula yeast diet containing only 20 ppb Se for nine months and continued the employment of this diet in their offspring for an additional six-nine months. Lens concentration of selenium dropped by ten-fold and lens GSHPx activity declined to 15% of controls but the lenses were still free of opacities. Twenty percent of second-generation offspring had opacities (8 of 39 pups) at weaning and the occurrence increased to 40% (4 of 10) in the third-generation. The lenses were described as markedly degenerate and containing a hard opaque nucleus floating in a clear fluid inside the lens capsule. Sprinkler et al. [40] fed a 30% Torula yeast diet containing 18 ppb of selenium but without supplementation of methione and chromium and detected a progressive lens deterioration that culminated in a cataract after 220 days. More recently, Cai [41] found only mild morphological changes in the lens despite significant reductions in lens GSHPx activity and elevations of malondialdehyde, an indicator of oxidative stress. Antioxidant-deprived animals are, however, less able to defend themselves against added oxidant burdens. Langle et al. [42] fed SDZ ICT 322, a compound with prooxidant properties, to rats and detected cataracts after fourteen weeks. The time to cataract was shortened to seven weeks if both selenium and vitamin E were withheld.

Selenium excess, on the other hand, is highly damaging to the lens *in vitro* and cataractogenic in suckling rats or mice. Ostadalova et al. [43] was studying the effect of age on the toxicity of sodium selenite. They administered sodium selenite (20-30 nmoles/g body weight) subcutaneously to 10- to 14-day-old rats and observed little effect on survival but permanent bilateral nuclear cataracts in virtually 100% of animals at 96 hours post injection. When post weaning (21 days or older) rats were injected, selenite was found to be fatal before it yielded cataract. The greater sensitivity of the immature lens may be related to the presence of a supporting vascular bed that atrophies at about 15 days of age and thus reduces delivery of both selenite and oxygen to this tissue.

Selenite interacts directly with glutathione to yield selenodiglutathione. [44] This molecule can then (A) react nonenzymatically with additional molecules of reduced glutathione to yield oxidized glutathione accompanied by regeneration of selenite, (B) react directly with oxygen to form superoxide anion and Se- or S-based free radicals, [45] and (C) can be a substrate for glutathione reductase with consequent reduction of selenite to hydrogen selenide followed by methylation to dimethyl selenide. [46] Production of free radical species simultaneous with a 40% decline in total glutathione [47] damages (among multiple targets) the mechanisms that maintain lens calcium homeostasis. [48] This, in turn, is followed by a 3 to 5-fold elevation of lens calcium, activation of the calcium-dependent proteolytic enzyme calpain II, and fragmentation and aggregation of lens crystallins, the final step that produces the nuclear opacity. [49,50,51] The increased demand for NADPH also stimulates a vigorous increase in activity of the hexose monophosphate shunt and alterations in the concentration of lens free amino acids and glycolytic metabolites. [52]

The selenite model is a highly reproducible and reliable means of generating cataract in living animals in a 3 to 5-day period. It has assisted in the recognition of the role and importance of oxidative stress in lens opacification and in the testing of potential lens-protective agents. It should be noted, however, that excessive exposure to selenite has not been linked to age-related cataract in humans or other animals. The so-called "blind staggers" in selenium-intoxicated herbivores is a neurological rather than a visual defect.

IV. CALORIES

It is fair to say that cataract in humans is principally an age-related phenomenon. Thus any nutritional strategy that prolongs the life span and retards the aging process could be tested for its benefits to the lens. Indeed, caloric restriction has been found to be effective in this regard. Leveille et al. [53] fed female mice diets that delivered either 85 or 50 kcal/week for up to 30 months of age. The calorically restricted diet was enriched with protein, vitamins and minerals so as to insure that caloric deficit was not accompanied by nutrient deficiency. Lens aging was evaluated not by opacification but by measuring the rate of disappearance over time of the water-soluble gamma-crystallin fraction. Mice held to this level of caloric restraint lost this protein at a much slower rate than their ad libitum-fed mates and the difference was consistent and statistically significant. Taylor et al. [54] observed similar results using a rodent model for cataract. Approximately 85% of Emory mice maintained from weaning on a standard diet and allowed to consume their meals ad libitum will spontaneously develop cataract by the age of one year. Reduction of calories alone to 79% of ad libitum levels lowered the incidence of spontaneous cataract to 41%. It is of interest that these caloric-restricted animals did not show markedly altered antioxidant enzyme capabilities and that in some tissues ascorbate levels were significantly decreased.

Masoro and Yu [55] have studied the benefits of caloric restriction upon senescence for over two decades. They have determined that low caloric intakes are generally associated with less lipid peroxidation, and enhanced cytosolic levels of antioxidant molecules and enzymes. Restricted-fed rodents also experienced a significant decline in fasting plasma glucose. As noted previously, oxidant stress and spontaneous glycosylation have been shown to play prominent roles in experimental cataract and in aging in general. Although clinical data from human populations are scanty, it seems plausible to conclude that caloric restraint in humans would also blunt the advance of senescence. This is not likely to be a popular and widely embraced strategy. Nevertheless, given the clear evidence that diabetes enhances cataract (by 3 to 5-fold) as well as diabetic retinopathy and that obesity defined as more than 20% overweight is a major risk factor for maturity-onset diabetes, it is our responsibility to inform the public of these facts and to encourage a healthy lifestyle that includes avoidance of caloric excess.

V. CONCLUSION

Animal studies are a vital component of any investigation of the importance of nutrition to a medical phenomenon. In this chapter I have reviewed the nutrients that have been linked to lens opacification. It seems to be incontrovertible that oxidative stress is a highly significant agent of damage in the aging lens and that glycosylation probably contributes to this pathology. Thus nutritional measures to defend against cataract would be the same as those endorsed to promote longevity, namely optimization of oxidant defenses, minimization of oxidant stress, and avoidance of obesity. In practical terms, this can be achieved by the standard advice of a diet rich in fruits and vegetables, caloric discipline and abstinence from smoking. The moderate use of nutrient supplements such as vitamin E (200 I.U./day) and vitamin C (250 mg/day) may be beneficial.

VI. REFERENCES

1. **Schneider HA.,** Rats, fats, and history, *Perspectives Biol. Med.*, 29, 392-406,1986.
2. **Mitchell HS, Cook GM.,** Galactose cataract in rats, *Arch. Ophthalmol.*, 19, 22-33, 1938.
3. **Meydani M, Martin A, Sastre J, Smith D, Dallal G, Taylor A, Blumberg, J.,** Dose-response characteristics of galactose-induced cataract in the rat, *Ophthalmic Res.*, 26, 368-374, 1994.
4. **Grant WM.,** in *Toxicology of the Eye,* 2nd ed., C. Thomas, Springfield, IL., 1974.
5. **Kinoshita JH.,** Aldose reductase and the diabetic eye, *Am. J. Ophthalmol.*, 102, 685-690, 1986.
6. **Van Boekel MAM, Hoenders HJ**., Glycation of crystallins in lenses from aging and diabetic individuals, *FEBS Lttrs.*, 314, 1-4, 1992.

7. **Hunt JV, Dean RT, Wolff SP.**, Hydroxy radical production and autooxidative glycosylation, *Biochem. J.*, 256,205-212, 1988.
8. **Trevithick JR, Creighton MO, Ross WM, Stewart-DeHaan PJ, Sanwal M.**, Modelling corticol cataractogenesis. 2. In vitro effects on the lens of agents preventing glucose- and sorbitol-induced cataracts, *Can. J. Ophthalmol.*, 16, 32-38, 1981.
9. **Ross WM, Creighton MO, Stewart-DeHaan PJ, Sanwal M, Hirst M, Trevithick JR.**, Modelling cortical cataractogenesis in diabetic rats, *Can. J. Ophthalmol.*, 17, 61- 66, 1982.
10. **Srivastava SK, Ansari NH.**, Prevention of sugar-induced cataractogenesis in rats by butylated hydroxytoluene, *Diabetes,* 37, 1505-1508, 1988.
11. **Yokoyama T, Sasaki H, Giblin FJ, Reddy VN.**, A physiological level of ascorbate inhibits galactose cataract in guinea pigs by decreasing polyol accumulation in the lens epithelium: a dehydroascorbate-linked mechanism, *Exp. Eye Res.*, 58(2), 207-218, 1994.
12. **Henein M, Devamanoharan PS, Ramachandran S, Varma SD.**, Prevention of galactose cataract by pyruvate, *Lens and Eye Tox. Res.*, 9(1), 25-36, 1992.
13. **Curtis PB, Hauge SM, Kraybill HR.**, The nutritive value of certain animal protein concentrates, *J. Nutr.* 5, 503-512, 1932.
14. **MacAvoy JW, van Heyningen R.**, Changes in the cells of the lens bow and epithelium of tryptophan deficient rats, *INSERM Colloq.*, 60,245-250, 1976.
15. VonSallman L,ReidME,GrimesPA,CollinsEM., Tryptophan-deficiency cataract in guinea pigs, *Arch. Ophthalmol.*, 62, 662-672, 1959.
16. **Bunce GE, Hess JL, Fillnow GM.**, Investigation of low tryptophan-induced cataract in weanling rats, *Exp. Eye Res.,* 26, 399-405, 1978.
17. **Hall WK, Bowles LL, Sydenstricker VP, Schmidt HR, Jr.**, Cataracts due to deficiencies of phenylalanine and histidine in the rat. A comparison with other types of cataract, *J. Nutr.*, 36, 277-296, 1948.
18. **Hall WK, Sydenstricker VP, Hock CW, Bowles LL.**, Protein deprivation as a cause of vascularization of the cornea in the rat, *J. Nutr.*, 32, 509-525, 1946.
19. **McLaren DS.**, Growth and water content of the eyeball of the albino rat in protein deficiency, *Br. J. Nutr.*, 12, 254-259, 1958.
20. **Kauffman RG, Norton HW.**, Growth of the porcine eye during insufficiencies of dietary protein, *Growth*, 30, 463-470, 1966.
21. **Salmon WD, Hays RM, Guerrant ND.**, Etiology of dermatitis of experimental pellagra in rats, *J. Infect. Dis.*, 43, 426-441, 1928.
22. **Day PL, Darby WF.**, The inverse relationship between growth and incidence of cataract in rats given graded amounts of vitamin G-containing foods, *J. Nutr.*, 12, 387-394, 1936.
23. **Day PL, Darby WF, Cosgrave KW.**, The arrest of nutritional cataract by the use of riboflavin, *J. Nutr.*, 15, 83-90, 1938.
24. **Shang F, Gong X, Palmer H, Nowell T, Taylor A.**, Age-related decline in ubiquitin conjugation in responses to oxidative stresses in the lens, *Exp. Eye*

Res., 64, 21-30, 1997.

25. **Shang F, Gong X, Taylor A.,** Activity of ubiquitin-dependent pathway in response to oxidative stress: Ubiquitin-activating enzyme (E1) is transiently upregulated, *J. Biol. Chem.*, 272, 23086-23093, 1997.
26. **Jahngen-Hodge J, Obin MS, Nowell TR, Gong J, Abasi H, Blumberg J, Taylor A.,** Regulation of ubiquitin conjugating enzymes by glutathione following oxidative stress, *J. Biol. Chem.*, 272, 28218-28226, 1997.
27. **Shaw JH, Phillips PH.,** The pathology of riboflavin deficiency in the rat, *J. Nutr.*, 22, 345-358, 1941.
28. Miller ER, Johnson RL, Hoefer JA, Luecke RW., The riboflavin requirement of the baby pig, *J. Nutr.*, 52, 405-413, 1954.
29. **Gershoff SN, Andrus SB, Hegsted DM.,** The effect of the carbohydrate and fat content of the diet upon the riboflavin requirement of the cat, *J. Nutr.*, 68, 75-88, 1959.
30. **Halver JE.,** Nutrition of the salmonid fishes. III. Water-soluble vitamin requirements of the chinook salmon, *J. Nutr.*, 62, 225-243, 1957.
31. **Srivastava SK, Beutler E.,** Increased susceptibility of riboflavin-deficient rats to galactose cataract, *Experientia,* 26, 250, 1970.
32. **Srivastava SK, Beutler E.,** Galactose cataract in riboflavin-deficient rats, *Biochem. Med.*, 6, 372-379, 1972.
33. **Sperduto RD, Hu T-S, Milton RC, Zhao J, Everett DF, Cheng Q, Blot WJ, Bing L, Taylor PR, Jun-Yao L, Dawsey S, Guo W.,** The Linxian Cataract Studies: Two nutrition intervention trials, *Arch. Ophthalmol.*, 111, 1246-1253, 1993.
34. **Blondin J, Baragi V, Schwartz E, Sadowski JA, Taylor A.,** Delay of UV-induced eye lens protein damage in guinea pigs by dietary ascorbate, *J. Free Rad. Biol. Med.*, 2, 275-281, 1986.
35. **Bunce GE, Hess, JL.,** Lenticular opacities in young rats as a consequence of maternal diets low in tryptophan and/or vitamin E, *J. Nutr.* 106, 222-229, 1976.
36. **Bunce GE, Kinoshita J, Horwitz J.,** Nutritional factors in cataract, *Annu. Rev. Nutr.*, 10, 233-254, 1990.
37. **Bunce GE.,** Nutrition and eye disease in the elderly, *J. Nutr. Biochem.,* 5, 66-77, 1994.
38. **Ketola HG.,** Influence of dietary zinc on cataracts from rainbow trout, *J. Nutr.*, 109, 965-969, 1979.
39. **Lawrence RA, Sunde RA, Schwartz GL, Hoekstra WG.,** Glutathione peroxidase activity in rat lens and other tissues in relation to dietary selenium intake, *Exp. Eye Res.*, 18, 563-569, 1974.
40. **Sprinkler LH, Harr JR, Newberne PM, Whanger PD, Weswig PH.,** Selenium deficiency lesions in rats fed vitamin E supplemented rations, *Nutr. Rep. Intl.*, 4, 335-340, 1971.
41. **Cai QY.,** Biochemical and morphological changes in the lenses of selenium and/or vitamin E deficient rats, *Biomedical and Environ. Sci.,* 7, 109-115, 1994.

42. **Langle UW, Wolf A, Cordier A.,** Enhancement of SDZ ICT 322-induced cataracts and skin changes in rats following vitamin E- and selenium-deficient diets, *Arch. Toxicol.*, 71, 283-289, 1997.
43. **Ostadalova I, Babicky A, Obenbarger T.,** Cataract induced by administration of a single dose of sodium selenite to suckling rats, *Experientia*, 34, 222-223, 1978.
44. **Tsen CC, Tappel AL.,** Catalytic oxidation of glutathione and other sulfhydryl compounds by selenite, *J. Biol. Chem.*, 233, 1230-1232, 1958.
45. **Seko Y, Saito Y, Kitahara J, Imura N.,** Active oxygen generation by the reaction of selenite with reduced glutathione in vitro, in *Selenium Biology and Medicine*, Wendel A, Ed., Springer-Verlag, New York, NY., 1989, pp.70-73.
46. **Ganther HE.,** Reduction of the selenotrisulfide derivative of glutathione to a persulfide analog by glutathione reductase, *Biochemistry,* 10, 4089-4098, 1971.
47. **Bunce GE, Hess JL.,** Biochemical changes associated with selenite-induced cataract in the rat, *Exp. Eye Res.*, 33, 505-514, 1981.
48. **Wang Z, Bunce GE, Hess JL.,** Selenite and calcium homeostasis in the rat lens: effect on Ca-ATPase and passive calcium transport, *Curr. Eye Res.*, 12, 213-218, 1993.
49. **Bunce GE, Hess JL, Batra R.,** Lens calcium and selenite-induced cataract, *Curr. Eye Res.*, 3, 315-320, 1984.
50. **David LL, Shearer TR.,** Calcium-activated proteolysis in the lens nucleus during selenite cataractogenesis, *Invest. Ophthalmol. Vis. Sci.*, 25,1275-1283, 1984.
51. **Shearer TR, David LL, Anderson RA.,** Selenite cataract: A review, *Curr. Eye Res.*, 6, 289-300, 1987.
52. **Mitton KP, Hess JL, Bunce GE.,** Free amino acids reflect impact of selenite-dependent stress on primary metabolism in rat lens, *Curr. Eye Res.*, 16, 997-1005, 1997.
53. **Leveille PJ, Weindruch R, Walford RL, Bok D, Horwitz J.,** Dietary restriction retards age-related loss of gamma-crystallins in the mouse lens, *Science*, 224, 1247-1249, 1984.
54. **Taylor A, Zuliani AM, Hopkins RE, Dallal GE, Treglia P, Kuck JFR, Kuck K.,** Moderate caloric restriction delays cataract formation in the Emory mouse, *FASEB J.*, 3, 1741-1746, 1989.
55. **Masoro EJ, Shimokawa I, Yu BP.,** Retardation of the aging processes in rats by food restriction, *Ann. N.Y. Acad. Sci.*, 621, 337-352, 1991.

Chapter 7

EVALUATION OF ANTICATARACT REAGENTS

John I. Clark and Toshihiko Hiraoka

I. INTRODUCTION

Demographic and epidemiological studies have established that: 1. lens opacification is the leading cause of blindness and visual loss in the world; 2. cataract is a multifactorial problem associated with heredity, diet, diabetes, smoking and sunlight exposure, all of which have numerous metabolic and nutritional components; 3. age is the most important single factor in cataract incidence and progression [1-16]. Vision impairment in cataract results from opacity or light scattering produced most often by inhomogeneities resulting from formation of large protein aggregates. Aggregation occurs when abnormal molecular interactions favor condensation of cytoplasmic protein within cells. At the earliest stages of opacification, weak non-covalent interactions are important. Covalent bonds and conformational changes are unnecessary. While weak non-covalent interactions between the surfaces of proteins are complex and poorly understood at the molecular level, they provide opportunities for development of simple and safe anticataract agents. The experimental studies of protein aggregation and the epidemiology are consistent in that transparent cell structure involves a variety of common metabolic and nutritional factors that can influence interactions between protein, solvent and membrane constituents of lens cells [17-42]. Development of anticataract therapies requires a method for the characterization of chemical modifications important for lens transparency and vision at the molecular level. The phase diagram for lens cytoplasm has been useful in the identification of chemical and biochemical reagents that act on interactions between lens constituents involved with development and maintenance of cellular transparency [17,23,24,25,27,43,44]. Studies using phase diagrams have demonstrated the potential importance of common cellular metabolites as anticataract agents.

II. PHASE DIAGRAMS AND MOLECULAR INTERACTIONS

Phase diagrams are used in physics, polymer chemistry, materials sciences and biotechnology to describe physical properties of solutions, ceramics and plastics [17,43-46]. A familiar example of a single-component phase diagram describes the physical states of water in terms of temperature and pressure (Figure 1). In thephase diagram for water, the boundary conditions for solid, liquid, and gas are indicated by solid black lines. At normal atmospheric pressure, water undergoes a transition from the liquid to solid at the melting point, 0°C, and from liquid to gas at the boiling point, 100°C. Addition of a second component to water can shift the boundaries for liquid, solid or gas phases to new positions in the phase diagram. The strength of the chemical additives that produce such a shift is commonly measured by the magnitude of the effect on the melting or boiling points of water.

0-8493-8565-2/99/$0.00+$.50

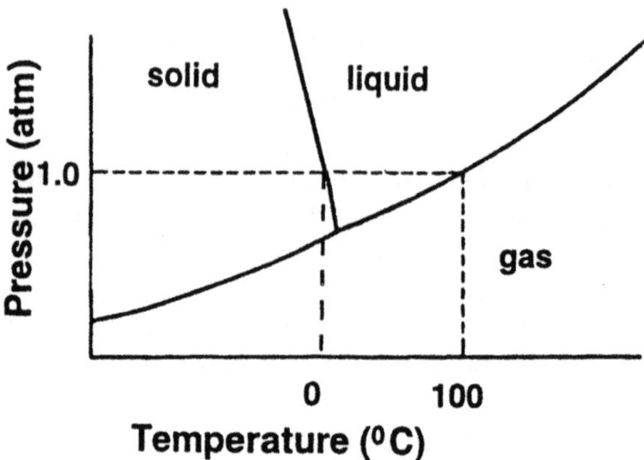

Figure 1. Phase diagram for water. In a phase diagram the conditions ofpressure and temperature for solid, liquid, and gaseous phases of water are separated by solid black lines or phase boundaries. The horizontal dashed line at 1 atmosphere (normal) pressure intersects the solid black phase boundary lines at the points of transition from ice to liquid at 0°C (melting point) and from liquid to steam at 100°C (boiling point). The presence of a second component can shift the phase boundaries and the melting and/or boiling points of water. The use of salt on icy roads is based on the effect of NaCl on the melting point of the solid to liquid transition of water. At atmospheric pressure, NaCl decreases the melting point -3.6 (/mole, and the solid to liquid boundary declines from 0°C to nearly -4°C when 1 M of NaCl is dissolved in water (-). In contrast, the addition of 1 mole of ethyl acetate increases the boiling point of water +2.8(°C/mole) from 100°C to nearly 103°C (-x-). The dotted lines indicate the positions of the new phase boundaries in the presence of NaCl or ethyl acetate. The direction and the magnitude of the effect of numerous additives on the melting and boiling points of water is well documented and tabulated in the *CRC Handbook of Chemistry and Physics* (47).

At the molecular level, transitions between solid, liquid and gas at the melting and boiling points of water are due to the effects of temperature on hydrogen bonds, the primary interactions between water molecules. Addition of salts, carbohydrates or organic solvents can modify the hydrogen bonds between water molecules and change the phase diagram so that transitions occur at temperatures below the melting point for liquid to solid transitions or at temperatures higher than the boiling point for liquid to gas transitions (Figure 1). The effects of chemical additives on interactions between molecular constituents of water are seen in the phase diagram as a change in the melting point and/or boiling points that represent changes in the position of the phase boundaries for water. Even for water, the chemical effects of additives are poorly characterized at the molecular level. Just as phase diagrams can be useful in the identification of chemicals that alter the interactions between water molecules, the phase diagram for lens cytoplasm has been used successfully to identify chemical additives that act on interactions important for transparency and opacity in healthy and diseased lenses [18,23-27].

The phase diagram describes the conditions for transparency and opacity of lens cytoplasm in terms of temperature and protein composition (Figure 2) [45-51]. While the cytoplasm is a complex protein solution, experimental studies found that the phase diagram for lens cytoplasm resembled that of a binary aqueous solution and that the boundary between the conditions for transparent and opaque cytoplasm was formed by the coexistence curve (the solid parabolic line in Figure 2) [43,44, 51]. The transition from transparency to opacity occurred at the phase separation temperature, Tc, which is determined by interactions between the surfaces of lens protein molecules and the surrounding constituents of the complex cytoplasmic environment (45-51). In transparent lens cells, the cytoplasm is a single homogeneous phase in which the predominant structural elements have dimensions that are small relative to the wavelength of visible light (400 to 700 nm) which must be transmitted to the retina.[55,56]. Opaque lens cells contain two separate phases, that coexist as microvolumes of condensed and dilute proteins, having high and low protein concentrations, respectively (see Figure 2B) [43,44]. The structures of the separated coexisting phases are large with respect to the dimensions of the wavelength of visible light (Figure 2B) and can appear in opaque lens cells as droplets, filaments, networks, micelles, crystals or other microscopic structures, depending on the kinetics of the transition and on the chemical nature of the complicated cytoplasmic constituents of the lens. As in the phase diagram for pure water, where the value of the melting point and the freezing point is determined by interactions between constituent water molecules, the value for Tc is determined by interactions between constituent proteins and solvent molecules. The important interactions between the surfaces of cytoplasmic proteins and the surrounding solvent are non-covalent and include hydrogen bonds, van der Waals forces, and electrostatic and hydrophobic interactions. Just as additives alter the melting and freezing points for water, enzymatic and metabolic processes that change the chemical composition of lens cells will alter the Tc and the phase diagram for lens cytoplasm [19,27,28,31]. Endogenous enzymes and metabolites can contribute to lens transparency and protect against lens opacification by modification of protein and solvent components of lens cytoplasm. In theory, the effects of any cytoplasmic modification on transparency should be predictable on the basis of its action on the Tc and the boundaries between transparent and opaque cytoplasm in the phase diagram [19,26,27,51,57]. In our studies, changes in Tc (Figure 2) that were favorable for the transparent single phase were used successfully to identify chemicals for testing as anticataract agents in animal models.

The collective interactions between the protein and solvent constituents of the lens cytoplasm are measured by the phase-separation temperature, Tc, which is defined by the expression:

$$kTc = A\,[E_{ps} - \tfrac{1}{2}(E_{ss} + E_{pp})]$$

where E_{ps} is the attractive energy of interaction between the protein-solvent components. E_{ss} is the attractive energy of interaction between solvent constituents. E_{pp} is the attractive energy of interaction between protein constituents. k is the Boltzmann constant and A is a constant related to the number of interactive sites involved in the transition between transparent and opaque states [19, 24, 57]. We see that the difference between the attractive interactions of like solvent and protein

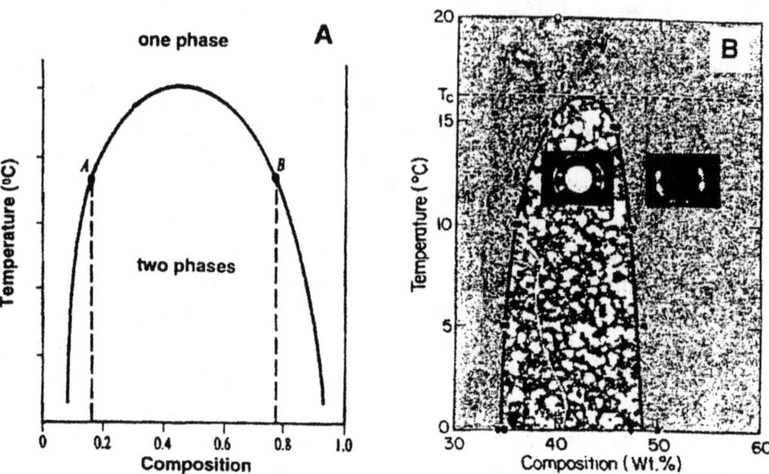

Figure 2. Comparison of a model phase diagram for two-component, binary solutions (A) with phase diagram for lens proteins (B). The composition of each phase is plotted versus temperature. In a binary mixture the boundary line or coexistence curve (solid line) separates the conditions for a single transparent phase from those for opaque coexisting phases. The coexistence curve is determined by plotting the composition of each of the co-existing phases (A & B in Figure 2A) versus the temperature, for temperatures below the phase separation temperature, Tc. When the conditions of temperature and composition are outside the coexistence curve, a single transparent phase is present. The phase diagram can be used to identify conditions favoring a transparent single phase or an opaque two-phase cytoplasm. The phase-separation temperature, Tc, depends on the interactions between molecular constituents. When the phase boundary shifts because of a modification in the interactions between molecular constituents, there is a corresponding shift in Tc. Although the lens cytoplasm consists of a complex solution of proteins, ions and small metabolites, the phase diagram for lens cytoplasm (2B) resembles the phase diagram for a simple binary aqueous solution (2A) [17, 43, 44]. The phase diagram for lens has been determined experimentally using the Tc as a direct measure for the energy of interaction between protein and solvent constituents as described in the equation for Tc (see text). It is important to recognize that a phase separation can be the result of many mechanisms. These mechanisms are exploited in nature to keep normal lens cells in the region of the phase diagram that favors transparent homogenous cytoplasm. The phase diagram allows the characterization of conditions that favor transparency or opacity, without understanding the precise biochemical mechanisms responsible for the microstructure observed in transparent or opaque lens cells. The conditions for phase separation in a lens cell involve multiple interactions, and the process of opacification involves multiple factors. We use the Tc as a direct measure of the collective interactions that are responsible for the multiple factors associated with loss of transparency and cataract formation. Biochemical reagents that modify the protein or solvent constituents of lens cytoplasm to raise or lower Tc are potential cataractogenic or anticataract agents respectively. The inserts in 2B are of an opaque lens on a background showing the microstructure of the opaque phase-separated cytoplasm, and of a transparent lens on a background of transparent homogenous cytoplasm. Wt % is the dry weight percent of lens cytoplasm which is mostly protein.

constituents (E_{ss} + E_{pp}) and the attractive interactions of the protein-solvent constituents, E_{ps} determines the position of the coexistence curve in the phase diagram. Tc is normally well below the physiological temperature of 37°C.

Upward displacement (increased Tc) of the coexistence curve in the phase diagram is favorable for phase separation and protein aggregation. Downward displacement (decreased Tc) of the coexistence curve is favorable for the single transparent phase. During normal lens development in living animals, the Tc decreases as the coexistence curve is displaced downward away from body temperature [58-61]. During cataract formation, abnormal interactions result in an abnormal Tc and an upward displacement of the coexistence curve. While the phase diagram describes the conditions for opacity or transparency, it does not provide specific information on the size and morphology of the cellular microstructures that produce light scattering or on the chemical nature of the interactions responsible for those structures. These may be different in different types of cataracts. In theory, the protective action of chemical reagents can be identified in the absence of detailed chemical and structural information simply by evaluating the effect on interactions measured by Tc [23,24,25,27]. The phase diagram provides a simple method for identification of reagents that are unfavorable or favorable for transparent cell structure.

III. ANIMAL MODELS AND PHASE SEPARATION

In several mammalian models for cataract formation, the Tc has been studied and abnormal phase behavior has been observed as an early indicator of abnormal interactions leading to protein aggregation and lens opacification (Table 1). While the phase diagram allows the characterization of conditions that favor transparency or opacity, the precise biochemical or morphological changes responsible for the transparent or opaque state cannot be evaluated using a phase diagram. The conditions for lens cell transparency involve multiple factors, and the process of cataract formation can involve one or more of these factors as indicated by epidemiological studies. We use Tc as a measure of the collective factors that are responsible for lens transparency and, in the case of cataract, loss of transparency and opacification.

In humans, the relationship between Tc and cataract is more difficult to document because of the variability and the long time constant for formation of mature cataract. Nevertheless, the increased aggregation of proteins and light scattering appear to be similar in humans and in animal models for lens opacification [64-66]. The phase diagrams for solutions of human lens gamma crystallins were found to resemble those of calf gamma crystallins [17,48-51]. Studies are underway to determine the phase diagram for all human lens crystallins and the influence of minor constituents such as cytoskeletal proteins and membranes on Tc. While the composition of the cytoplasm is far from simple, an alteration in one of the numerous protein or solvent components in a lens cell will alter interactions between the molecular constituents as measured by Tc. Our previous studies suggested a connection between lens opacification and abnormal Tc in most, and possibly all, cataracts. Modifications at the molecular level that are favorable for transparency inhibit phase separation and protein aggregation [18, 19, 23, 25, 27, 67].

Table 1

CATEGORY	MODELS
Dietary	Galactose; hyper- and hypoglycemic
Radiation	Gamma and X-ray
Hereditary	Philly; Royal College of Surgeons; Nakano; Emory
Chemical Induced	Selenite; Streptozotocin; Steroid; Alloxan; Cyanate; Calcium
Transgenic/Knockout	HIV protease?; α-crystallin?; SPARC?

Models for cataract formation that are associated with abnormal Tc. Abnormal Tc is a measure of the conditions favorable for cataract in numerous animal models for cataract formation. While the models listed are associated with various categories of cataract, most of the models involved multiple factors, including increased high molecular weight aggregates; post-translational modification of lens proteins; hydration; ion imbalances; and abnormal metabolic levels such as the ratio of reduced to oxidized glutathione. In most animal models Tc is associated with the onset of opacification early in life. In contrast, the Emory mouse forms a cataract late in life (62, 63). All models studied in our laboratory were associated with abnormal Tc. Preliminary studies indicate that abnormal Tc is associated with opacification in transgenic and knockout models for cataract and is currently under investigation.

A study of selected reagents having diverse chemical functionalities, biodistribution and metabolism confirmed the relationship between anticataract activity *in vivo* and effect on Tc *in vitro* (Table 2) [25]. Fourteen reagents were identified in literature reports of their potential to protect against cataract formation in different models under various experimental conditions. The reagents included antioxidants, oxidants, vitamins, chelators, and bioactive peptides. The diverse and chemically different reagents were found to lower Tc over a range from -1° to -248°C and the amount of the decrease was independent of the chemical functionality. In theory, the reagents having the strongest effect on Tc (large negative values) will be the strongest inhibitors of protein aggregation and opacification (see expression for Tc). Antioxidants, oxidants, chelators, thiophosphates, disulfides, sulfhydryl modifiers and cross-linking reagents all decreased Tc which indicated that many chemical factors can contribute to the conditions for transparent lens cell structure.

The selenite model for cataract was selected for our study because of the reproducibility and rapidity of the formation of cataract. The cataract in the selenite model involves nearly all elements of cataract formation in humans, including

Table 2

REAGENT	DTc (°C/mole)	PROTECTION
Glutathione	-248	Good
Glutathione ester	-216	
Pantethine	-212	
L-ascorbate PO_4	-81	Partial
Cystamine-S-PO_4	-75	
Deferoxamine	-139	Minimal
L-ascorbate	-80	
Aminoguanidine	-53	
4-Hydroxy tempo	-44	
WR-77913	-29	
D-penicillamine	-1	

Effects of selected chemical reagents on Tc and opacification. In our studies the reagents tested for a protective effect on lens opacification and on Tc included biochemical metabolites found endogenously, antioxidants, thiophosphates, chelators and a chaotropic agent. The strongest effects on cataract formation *in vivo* were observed with glutathione and pantethine, endogenous biochemicals having the strongest effect on Tc. Ascorbate, tocopherol and other metabolic constituents have a protective action on Tc and on opacification [23,28,31]. It must be noted that some promising endogenous compounds such as cysteine or cystamine derivative, that are effective as anticataract agents can have serious side effects, especially with prolonged use (25,68). The findings suggest that lens cytoplasm contains a variety of endogenous biochemicals that can act collectively to modify interactions between proteins and protect against loss of transparency. These experiments confirmed a correspondence between a large effect on Tc and good protection against cataract formation *in vivo*. Effective inhibitors of lens opacification may be reagents that are multifunctional and act on a variety of interactions between lens cell constituents.

abnormal calcium homeostasis, glutathione metabolism, membrane transport, proteolysis and protein aggregation. A few days after injection of a single 19 (m*M*/kg dose of sodium selenite, a full mature cataract formed in nearly 99% of the injected animals. The rapid formation of the cataract permitted rapid evaluation of the protective effects of each reagent in a reasonable amount of time. Each reagent was injected into the animals as a single dose of 1.5 m*M*/kg, which is rather high. The high concentrations introduced the possibility that numerous complicating factors, including solubility, biodistribution, metabolism and toxicity, could confuse the results. Without knowing the precise levels of eachreagentreaching the lens, there was, nevertheless, a strong correlation between the effects of the reagent on Tc and the effects on cataract formation *in vivo*. The best protection against opacification was provided by reagents having the strongest effect on Tc. The weakest protection correlated with the weakest effect on Tc, with the exception of deferoxamine and ascorbate (Table 2). It should be mentioned that deferoxamine and ascorbate were protective when administered in multiple doses, but not as a single administration used in the protocol for these experiments [34, 69]. The reagents could be administered before or after injection of selenite. This was the first time several anticataract agents had been tested at the same dose in the same animal model for cataract formation. The experimental findings demonstrated that numerous chemical factors may be involved with phase separation in lens cytoplasm and cataract formation in animal models. The studies link endogenous biochemicals with protection against protein aggregation and opacification and suggest that the most effective lead compounds for anticataract agents may be products of common metabolic pathways. In this sense, the results were consistent with epidemiological observations on the potential protective action of common nutrients and metabolites [40,41]. The findings established a correlation between lower Tc and protection against protein aggregation and opacification in living animals.

Of the reagents tested, the thiophosphate, WR-77913, and the disulfide, pantethine, were investigated in more detail. Pantethine is a natural metabolite of pantothenic acid found in all cells and tissues, which may account for its safety at very high doses. Pantethine is an hygroscopic compound comprised of pantoic acid, β-alanine and cystamine, chemical moieties expected to contribute to hydrophilicity. Pantethine is the oxidized, disulfide form of the sulfhydryl, pantetheine, the active component of co-enzyme A which, when phosphorylated, is involved in numerous metabolic pathways, including peptide, membrane, and nucleic acid biosynthesis.

WR-77913 is a radioprotective agent. Comparative studies of the protective effects of WR-77913 and pantethine were conducted in selected rat models for cataract formation (Table 3) [24,26]. The mechanisms of cataract formation included metabolic disorders, free radical formation, oxidation and proteolysis. While there were differences in the primary biological mechanisms of cataract formation, WR-77913 or pantethine were protective in all models. Successful inhibition of opacification required repeated or continuous administration of the anticataract agents except in the radiation or selenite models, where the opacification was initiated by a single exposure to a cataractogenic insult. In contrast, the galactose, streptozocin and Royal College of Surgeons models involved repeated treatments to delay or inhibit the formation of the cataract.

Opacification was delayed by using WR-77913 or pantethine in all models except the selenite model where complete protection was observed. Reversal of opacification was not observed when the WR-77913 or pantethine were administered once the cataract was present. The fact that these protective reagents were effective in several different animal models for cataract was an important finding that demonstrated the potential for development of anticataract agents to treat cataracts of different etiologies.

While all reagents tested could chemically modify lens proteins, the composition of the cytoplasmic solvent can also influence interactions between lens

Table 3

CATARACT MODEL (rat)	PRIMARY MECHANISM OF CATARACT FORMATION	EFFECT OF WR-77913 OR PANTETHINE
Selenite	Abnormal calcium levels and Calpain activation	Protection
Radiation	Free radical	Protection
Streptozotocin	Aldose reductase	Protection
Galactose	Aldose reductase	Protection
Royal College of Surgeons	Hereditary/Oxidation	Protection

Protection against opacification in rat models for cataract using the phosphorothioate, WR-77913, or pantethine. The primary mechanism associated with each cataract model is listed. In all the models, cataract formation is associated with abnormal Tc (see Table 1). When pantethine or WR-77913 were administered prior to or at the earliest stages of cataract formation, the opacification was delayed or inhibited. The observed protective effects of the phosphorothioate, WR-77913 and the disulfide, pantethine, provide experimental support for consideration of the importance of phosphorous and thiol metabolism in protection against cataract formation.

proteins. The expression for the phase-separation temperature, Tc, includes a parameter for interactions with solvent constituents, suggesting that modification of the cytoplasmic solvent alone may have an effect on transparency (see expression for Tc). In separate experiments the composition of the solvent was modified by soaking lenses in D_2O, methanol or selected glycols [70]. The effect on Tc was correlated with the boiling points and heat of vaporization for each solvent which are thermodynamic measures of hydrogen bonds between solvent molecules. These results emphasize that transparent cellular structure can result from the sum of numerous weak, non-covalent interactions. Strong covalent interactions are not required. The magnitude of the energies involved in establishment and maintenance of lens cell transparency can be as small as kT or 0.6 kcal/mole [17], and small changes in the energetics may be sufficient to shift conditions from the opaque to the transparent state. Chemicals that stabilize the weak non-covalent interactions between lens constituents early in the process of cataract formation can be expected to be inhibitors of protein aggregation and protect against lens opacification. The studies confirmed the importance of solvent composition on phase separation, protein aggregation and lens opacification.

IV. TIME COURSE OF CATARACT FORMATION

The difference between the rapid formation of cataract in the selenite model and the slow progression of opacification in humans needs to be considered [65, 66,71]. Light scattering increases continuously with the progressive growth of the size and amount of the scatterers during aging of lens cells. It has been suggested that a small 10% delay in the time constant for the opacification process will have a major impact on blindness and visual impairment in the world [1, 73]. This point emphasizes the kinetics of protein aggregation and opacification rather than the chemical nature of the protein interactions. While the kinetics of protein aggregation and lens opacification are poorly understood, there may be several intermediate stages for intervention during the slow progressive growth of aggregates prior to the irreversible denaturation of lens proteins. Natural mechanisms involving molecular chaperones may act at these intermediate stages [74,75].

Previous experiments on the optimal timing for pantethine effectiveness suggested that the earliest stages of cataract formation are the most responsive to intervention. In the selenite model for cataract, pantethine was administered at selected times after initiation of the cataract induced by injection of sodium selenite [71]. Administration of pantethine, at a concentration of 1.5 m*M*/kg, was effective against opacification *in vivo*, only when administered up to 10 hours following initiation of the cataract by injection of selenite. This is well before large protein aggregates and obvious visible opacity is present. Higher concentrations and/or multiple doses of pantethine may be more effective than a single dose in prolongation of the time for effective administration. Once irreversible covalently bound aggregates are present, chemical reagents that act on non-covalent interactions may be ineffective as inhibitors of protein aggregation and opacification. This result is consistent with the observation that protection against protein aggregation and opacification was not observed in any animal models when anticataract agents were administered after lens opacification was obvious [24-26]. It is important to emphasize that maintenance of the cellular concentrations of metabolites and nutrients like pantethine may contribute to protection against opacification by acting to slow the kinetics of protein aggregation. While this point needs further investigation in animal models and in humans, these experiments suggest that early detection of the opacification process will be important for the development of successful intervention.

V. CHEMICAL MECHANISMS AND PHASE SEPARATION

The epidemiological studies that established relationships between low risk for cataract and common nutrients, including vitamins C, E, A and carotenoids, have emphasized the antioxidant mechanisms of action [2, 6, 8-14, 40, 76]. Antioxidant vitamins participate in a variety of biochemical and physiological pathways that contribute to good health. Given the numerous relationships between oxidation, aging and pathology, it is unsurprising that antioxidants have been studied extensively for their effect on opacification. Experimental studies found that ascorbate, vitamin E and glutathione had protective anticataract action [13, 23, 28, 30, 32-39]. It should be noted that recent studies found that the oxidized, as well as the reduced, forms of metabolites like glutathione and pantethine appear to inhibit protein aggregation and lens opacification [24, 25, 61, 67]. The modification of lens proteins by formation of mixed disulfides may be protective when accompanied by a decrease in the net attraction between lens proteins so that the thermodynamics are unfavorable for phase separations and protein aggregation [19]. While the antioxidant mechanism may explain the protective action of some vitamins and nutrients, oxidants as well as antioxidants can contribute to lens cell transparency. It can be expected that a normal balance between oxidative and anti-oxidative nutrients may be most favorable for maintenance of the balance between the attractive interactions responsible for lens cell transparency as represented in the expression for Tc (see expression for Tc). We emphasize that endogenous metabolites and nutrients are multifunctional, and their physiological activities are not limited to their oxidative/anti-oxidative properties.

The biochemical actions of endogenous metabolites and nutrients found to decrease Tc [17, 18, 31] are under investigation [19,67,70,77]. Pantethine and glutathione are among the most impressive reagents with respect to an effect on Tc. Direct interactions between pantethine or glutathione and crystallins *in vitro* were observed to inhibit the slow, progressive formation of high molecular weight aggregates [67, 75]. Separate studies characterized the chaperone function of α-crystallin, which was enhanced in the presence of pantethine and glutathione [75]. In a chaperone assay, the effect of pantethine was strongest when the aggregating protein was β-crystallin, and the effect of the glutathione was strongest when the aggregating protein was alcohol dehydrogenase. The pantethine appeared to interact with α-crystallin, and the glutathione appeared to interact with the target protein, alcohol dehydrogenase. The constituents of pantethine are pantothenic acid, β-alanine, and cystamine. When tested separately, β-alanine, but not cystamine or pantothenic acid, was found to enhance the action of α-crystallin as a molecular chaperone on the aggregation of β-crystallin [75]. *In vivo*, the effects of pantethine were studied in the selenite model for cataract formation [77]. Degradation of cytoskeletal proteins was one of the first alterations in lens proteins observed during opacification in the selenite and the HIV protease models for lens opacification. When pantethine was administered to prevent opacification, the loss of cytoskeletal proteins was inhibited during the early stages of cataract formation. Since α-crystallins are reported to act on cytoskeletal proteins [78], the protective effects of pantethine and other metabolites may be through an action on the chaperone activity of α-crystallin.

ATP is one of the most important metabolites in lens and is present at concentrations as high as those found in muscle, a much more active tissue [79]. While it is uncertain why the lens has such high concentrations of ATP, oxidative metabolism is important for normal lens development and cellular differentiation. The high concentrations of ATP in lens may be necessary for membrane function, which is especially important in lens cells where extremely high concentrations of protein increase the osmotic activity of the cytoplasm. Recent studies have determined that ATP enhances the chaperone function of human αB-crystallin, similar to other chaperone proteins [80, 81]. In systematic studies cellular transparency was independent of ATP levels, and ATP may participate indirectly in the maintenance of metabolic functions that contribute to balanced cellular homeostasis and lens transparency [82].

These results emphasize the multifunctional nature of natural endogenous metabolites and nutrients in lens cells. The complex chemical nature of anticataract agents makes it difficult to identify a specific mechanism of anticataract action. This complexity justifies the study of pantethine, which is known to be multifunctional, as a model compound for inhibitors of lens opacification. While the endogenous metabolites and nutrients may not involve specific individual targets, the lack of specificity may be important for action on multiple sites that are associated with protein aggregation and opacification in humans. Further studies of natural compounds, including ATP, pantethine, glutathione and ascorbate may demonstrate the effectiveness and safety of multifunctional biochemcials as anticataract agents.

VI. SUMMARY

There are reasons to be optimistic about the potential for development of anticataract therapies that can inhibit or delay protein aggregation during cataract formation. The mechanisms that are responsible for the protective effects of natural compounds like ascorbate, vitamin E, glutathione, and pantethine can be expected to be complex because such biochemical reagents are involved in a variety of physiological and metabolic pathways. It should be recognized that the multifactorial nature of cataract progression may require a multifactorial approach to the development of anticataract therapeutics. Few reagents, if any, would be better than natural endogenous nutrients and metabolites that are both safe and effective. Development of anticataract agents for protection against loss of transparency may involve multiple elements in the cataractogenic process and successful intervention may only require a delay in the progression of protein aggregation and opacification. Additional emphasis on the multifactorial nature of cataract formation needs to be considered in systematic studies of inhibitors of cataract in the aging population. The benefits of a nutritional approach to protection against lens opacification may be related to their potential action on multiple sites that are involved with transparent lens cell structure.

ACKNOWLEDGMENTS

We appreciate the assistance of C. Ganders, T. Cranick, P. Muchowski, and J.M. Clark in preparation and review of this manuscript. Supported by EY04542, from N.E.I.

VII. REFERENCES

1. **Kupfer, C.**, The conquest of cataract: a global challenge, *Trans Ophthalmol Soc UK*, 104, 1-10, 1985.
2. **Hockwin, O.** and Sasaki, K., Eds., *Cataract Pathogenesis: results of epidemiological studies and experimental models*, Dev Ophthalmol, Karger, Basel, 1994, Vol. 26.
3. West, S.K., and Valmadrid, C.T., Epidemiology of risk factors for age related cataract, *Surv Ophthalmol* 39, 323-334, 1995.
4. **Thylefors, B.**, Negrel, A.D., Pararajasegaram, R. and Dadzie K.Y., Global data on blindness, *Bull World Health Org*, 73, 115-121, 1995.
5. **Sperduto, R.D.**, Age related cataracts: Scope of problem and prospects for prevention, *Preventive Med*, 23, 735-739, 1994.
6. **Sperduto, R.D.**, Hu, T.S., Milton, R.C., Zhao, J., Everett, D.F., Cheng, Q., Blot, W.J., Bing, L., Taylor, P.R., Jun-Yao, L., Dawsey, S. and Guo, W., The Linxin cataract studies: two nutrition intervention trials, *Arch Ophthalmol*, 111, 1246-1253, 1993.
7. **Taylor, H.R.** and Sommer, A., Cataract surgery: a global perspective, *Arch Ophthalmol*, 108, 797-798, 1990.
8. **Harding, J.**, Cataract, *Biochemistry, epidemiology and pharmacology*, Chapman and Hall, London, 1991.
9. **Leske, M.C.**, Wu, S.Y., Hyman, L., Sperduto, R., Underwood, B., Chylack, L.T., Milton, R.C., Srivastava, S. and Ansari, N., Biochemical factors in lens opacities: case controlled study. The lens opacities case control study group, *Arch Ophthalmol,* 113, 1113-1119, 1995.
10. **Jacques, P.F.**, Chylack, L.T., Jr. and Taylor, A., Relationships between natural antioxidants and cataract formation, in *Natural antioxidants human health and disease,* Frei, B., Ed., Academic Press, Orlando, Florida, 1994, pp 513-533.
11. **Jacques, P.F.** and Chylack, L.T., Jr., Epidemiologic evidence of a role for the antioxidant vitamins and carotenoids in cataract prevention, *Am J Clin Nutr*, 53, 352S-355S, 1991.
12. **Mares-Perlman, J.A.**, Brady, W.E., Klein, B.E.K., Klein, R., Palta, M., Bowen, P. and Stacewica-Sapuntzakis, M., Serum carotenoids and tocopherols and severity of nuclear and cortical opacities, *Invest Ophthalmol Vis Sci,* 36, 276-288, 1995.
13. **Bunce, G.E.**, Kinoshita, K.J. and Horwitz, J., Nutritional factors in cataract,

Ann Rev Nutr, 10, 233-254, 1990.

14. **Seddon, J.M.**, Christen, W.G., Manson, J.E., LaMotte, F.S., Glynn, R.J., Buring, J.E. and Hennekens, C.H., The use of vitamin supplements and the risk of cataract among US male physicians, *Am J Public Health*, 84, 788-792, 1994.
15. **Minassian, D.C.** and Mehra, V., 3.8 Million blinded by cataract each year: projections for the first epidemiological study of incidence of cataract blindness in India, *Br J Ophthalmol*, 74, 341-343, 1990.
16. **Datiles, M.B.** and Magno, B.V., Cataract: Clinical types, in *Duane's Clinical Ophthalmology*, Tasman, W., Jaeger, E., Eds., Lippincott-Raven, New York, 1996, chap 73.
17. **Clark, J.I.**, Lens cytoplasmic protein solutions: analysis of a biologically occurring aqueous phase separation, *Methods Enzymol*, 228, 525-537, 1994.
18. **Clark, J.I.** and Benedick, G.B., Effects of glycols, aldehydes and acrylamide on phase separation and opacification in the calf lens, *Invest Ophthalmol,* 19, 771-776, 1980.
19. **Pande, J.**, Berland, C., Ogun, O., Melhuish, J. and Benedick, G.B., Suppression of phase separation in solutions of bovine gamma IV crystallin by polar modification of the sulfur containing amino acids, *Proc Natl Acad Sci USA*, 88, 4916-4920, 1991.
20. **Slingsby, C.**, Bateman, O.A. and Simpson, A., Motifs involved in protein-protein interactions, *Mol Biol Rep*, 17, 185-195, 1993.
21. **Tardieu, A.**, Veretout, F., Krop, B., Slingsby, C., Protein interactions in the calf eye lens: interactions between beta crystallins are repulsive whereas in gamma crystallins they are attractive, *Eur Biophys J*, 21, 1-12, 1992.
22. **Veretout,F.**, Delaye, M. and Tardieu, A., Molecular basis of eye lens transparency, *J Mol Biol*, 205, 713-718, 1989.
23. **Eccarius, S.** and Clark, J.I., Effects of aspirin and vitamin E on phase separation in calf lens homogenate, *Ophthalmic Res*, 19, 65-71, 1987.
24. **Clark, J.I.**, Livesey, J.C. and Steele, J.E., Phase separation inhibitors and lens transparency, *Optom Vis Sci*, 70, 873-879, 1993.
25. **Hiraoka, T.**, Clark, J.I., Li, X.Y. and Thurston, G.M., Effect of selected anticataract agents on opacification in the selenite cataract model, *Exp Eye Res*, 62, 11-21, 1996.
26. **Clark, J.I.**, Livesey, J.C. and Steele, J.E., Delay or inhibition of rat lens opacification using pantethine and WR-77913, *Exp Eye Res*, 62, 75-85, 1996.
27. **Clark, J.I.**, Osgood, T.B. and Trask, S.J., Inhibition of phase separation by reagents that prevent X-irradiation cataract in vivo, *Exp Eye Res*, 45, 961-967, 1987.
28. **Hammer, P.** and Benedick, G.B., Effect of naturally occurring cellular constituents on phase separation and opacification in calf lens nuclear homogenates, *Curr Eye Res*, 2, 809-814, 1983.
29. **Kador, P.F.**, Biochemistry of the lens: intermediary metabolism and sugar cataract formation, in *Principles and Practice of Ophthalmology*, Albert, D.M., Jakobiec, F.A., Eds., WB Saunders, Philadelphia, pp 146-167.

30. **Reddy, V.N.**, Glutathione and its function in the lens – an overview, *Exp Eye Res,* 50, 771-778, 1990.
31. **Mitton, K.P.**, Hess, J.L. and Bunce, G.E., Free amino acids reflect the impact of selenite-dependent stress on primary metabolism in rat lens, *Curr Eye Res*, 16, 997-1005, 1997.
32. **Calvin, H.I.**, Zhu, G.P., Wu, J.X., Banerjee, U. and Fu, S.C.J., Progression of mouse buthionine sulfoximine cataracts in vitro is inhibited by thiols or ascorbate, *Exp Eye Res*, 65, 341-347, 1997.
33. **Zigman, S.**, McDaniel, T., Schultz, J.B., Reddan, J. and Meydani, M., Damage to cultured lens epithelial cells of squirrels and rabbits by UV-A (99.9%) plus UV-B (0.1%) radiation and alpha tocopherol protection, *Mol Cell Biochem,* 143, 35-46, 1995.
34. **Devamanoharan, P.S.**, Henein, M., Morris, S., Ramachandran, S., Richards, R.D. and Varma, S.D., Prevention of selenite cataract by vitamin C, *Exp Eye Res,* 52, 563-568, 1991.
35. **Nishigori, H.**, Lee, J.W., Yamauchi, Y. and Iwatsuru, M., The alteration of lipid peroxide in glucocorticoid-induced cataract of developing chick embryos and the effect of ascorbic acid, *Curr Eye Res,* 5, 37-40, 1986.
36. **Garland, D.D.**, Ascorbic acid and the eye, *Am J Clin Nutr,* 54, 1198S-1202S, 1991.
37. Bhuyan, **D.K.** and Bhuyan, K.C., Mechanisms of cataractogenesis III: toxic metabolites of oxygen as initiators of lipid peroxidation and cataract, *Curr Eye Res*, 3, 67-81, 1984.
38. **Robertson, J.M.**, Donner, A.P. and Trevithick, J.R., Vitamin E intake and risk for cataracts in humans, *Ann NY Acad Sci*, 570, 372-382, 1989.
39. **Sasaki, H.**, Giblin, F.J., Winkler, B.S., Chakrapani, B., Leverenz, V. and Shu-Chen, S., A protective role for glutathione-dependent reduction of dehydroascorbic acid in lens epithelium, *Inv Ophthalmol Vis Sci*, 36, 1804-1817, 1995.
40. **Taylor, A.**, Role of nutrients in delaying cataracts, *Ann NY Acad Sci*, 669, 111-124, 1992.
41. **Taylor, A.**, Nutritional and environmental influences on risk for cataract, in *Nutritional and Environmental Influences on the Eye*, Chap 4, (this volume), 1998.
42. **Kilic, F.**, Mitton, K., Dzialoszynski, T., Sanford, S.E. and Trevithick, J.R., Modelling cortical cataractogenesis 14: reduction in lens damage in diabetic rats by a dietary regimen combining vitamins C, E and beta carotene, *Dev Ophthalmol*, 26, 63-71, 1994.
43. **Clark, J.I.** and Benedick, G.B., Phase diagram for cell cytoplasm for the calf lens, *Biochem Biophys Res Comm*, 95, 482-489, 1980.
44. **Delaye, M.A.**, Clark, J.I. and Benedick, G.B., Coexistence curves for phase separation in the calf lens cytoplasm, *Biochem Biophys Res Comm*, 100, 908-914, 1981.
45. **Walter, H.**, Brook, D.E., and Fisher, D., Eds., in *Partitioning in Aqueous Two-phase Systems:Theory, Methods, Uses and Application to Biotechnology*,

Academic Press, Orlando, FL, 1985.
46. **Walter, H.** and Johansson, G., Eds., Aqueous two-phase systems, *Methods Enzymol*, vol. 228, 1994.
47. *CRC Handbook of Chemistry and Physics*, 77th ed., CRC Press, Boca Raton, FL, 1996.
48. **Broide, M.L.**, Berland, C.R., Pande, J., Ogun, O.O. and Benedick, G.B., Binary liquid phase separation of lens protein solutions, *Proc Natl Acad Sci USA*, 88, 5660-5664, 1991.
49. **Berland, C.R.**, Thurston, G.M., Kondo, M., Broide, M.L., Pande, J., Ogun, O. and Benedick, G.B., Solid liquid phase boundaries of lens protein solutions, *Proc Natl Sci USA*, 89, 1214-1218, 1992.
50. **Liu, C.**, Asherie, N., Lomakin, A., Pande, J., Ogun, O. and Benedick, G.B., Phase separation in aqueous solutions of γ-crystallins, *Proc Natl Acad Sci USA*, 93, 377-382, 1996.
51. **Liu, C.**, Lomakin, A., Thurston, G.M., Hayden, D., Pande, A., Pande, J., Ogun, O., Asherie, N. and Benedick, G.B., Phase separation in multicomponent aqueous protein solutions, *J Phys Chem*, 99, 454-461, 1995.
52. **Clout, N.J.**, Slingsby, C. and Wistow, G.J., An eye on crystallins, *Nat Struct, Biol*, 4, 685, 1997.
53. **Kuszak, J.R.**, Peterson, K.L. and Brown, H.G., Electron microscopic observations of the crystalline lens, *Microsc Res Tech*, 33, 441-479, 1996.
54. **Taylor, V.L.**, Al-Ghoul, K.J., Lane, C.W., Davis, V.A., Kuszak, J.R., and Costello, M.J., Morphology of the normal human lens, *Invest Ophthalmol Vis Sci*, 37, 1396-1410, 1996.
55. **Clark, J.I.**, Development and maintenance of lens transparency, in *Principles and Practice of Ophthalmology*, Albert, D.M., Jakobiec, F.A., Eds., WB Saunders, Philadelphia, pp 114-123.
56. **Vaezy, S.**, Clark, J.I. and Clark, J.M., Quantitative analysis of lens cell microstructure in selenite cataract using 2-D Fourier analysis, *Exp Eye Res*, 60, 245-255, 1995
57. **Taratuta, V.G.**, Holschbach, A., Thurston, G.M., Blankschtein, D. and Benedick, G.B., Liquid-liquid phase separation of aqueous lysozyme solutions: effects of pH and salt, *J Phys Chem*, 94, 2140-2144, 1990.
58. **Ishimoto, C.**, Goalwin, P.W., Sun, W., Nishio, I. and Tanaka, T., Cytoplasmic phase separation in formation of galactosemic cataract in lenses of young rats, *Proc Natl Acad Sci USA*, 76, 4414-4416, 1979.
59. **Clark, J.I.**, Giblin, F.J., Reddy, V.N. and Benedick, G.B., Phase separation in X-irradiated lenses of the rabbit, *Invest Ophthalmol*, 22, 186-190, 1982.
60. **Clark, J.I.** and Carper, D.L., Phase separation in lens cytoplasm is genetically linked to cataract formation in the Philly mouse, *Proc Natl Acad Sci USA,* 84, 122-125, 1987.
61. **Clark, J.I.** and Steele, J.E., Phase separation inhibitors, PSI, and prevention of selenite cataract, *Proc Natl Acad Sci USA*, 89, 1720-1724, 1992.
62. **Kuck, J.F.**, Late onset hereditary cataract of the Emory mouse. A model for human senile cataract, *Exp Eye Res,* 50, 659-664, 1990.

63. **Mara, C.V.**, Roh, S., Smith, D., Palmer, V., Path., N. and Taylor, A., Cataract incidence and analysis of lens crystallins in the water-, urea- and SDS-soluble fractions of Emory mice fed a diet restricted by 40% in calories, *Curr Eye Res,* 12, 1081-1091, 1993.
64. **Tanaka, T.** and Benedick, G.B., Observation of protein diffusivity in intact human and bovine lenses with application to cataract, *Invest Ophthalmol*, 14, 449-456, 1975.
65. **Benedick, G.B.**, Chylack, L.T., LiBondi, T., Magnante, P. and Pennett, M., Quantitative detection of the molecular changes associated with early cataractogenesis in the living human lens using quasielastic light scattering, *Curr Eye Res*, 6, 1421-1432, 1987.
66. **Thurston, G.M.**, Hayden, D.L., Burrows, P., Clark, J.I., Taret, V.G., Kandel, J., Courogen, M., Peetermans, J.A., Bowen, M.S., Miller, D., Sullivan, O.M., Storb, R., Stern, H. and Benedick, G.B., Quasielastic light scattering study of the living human lens as a function of age, *Curr Eye Res*, 16, 197-206, 1997.
67. **Friberg, G.**, Pande, J., Ogun, O. and Benedick, G.B., Pantethine inhibits the formation of high Tc protein aggregates in γB solutions, *Curr Eye Res*, 15, 1182-1190, 1996.
68. **Rathbun, W.B.**, Nagasawa, H.T. and Killen, C.E., Prevention of naphthalene-induced cataract and hepatic glutathione loss by the L-cysteine prodrugs, MTCA and PTCA, *Exp Eye Res*, 62, 433-441, 1996.
69. **Wang, Z.**, Hess, J.L. and Bunce, G.E., Deferoxamine effect on selenite-induced cataract formation in rats, *Invest Ophthalmol Vis Sci*, 33, 2511-2519, 1992.
70. **Clark, J.I.**, Phase separation and hydrogen bonding in cells of the ocular lens, *Biopolymers*, 30, 995-999, 1990.
71. **Hiraoka, T.** and Clark, J.I., Inhibition of lens opacification during the early stages of cataract formation, *Invest Ophthalmol Vis Sci*, 36, 2550-2555, 1995.
72. **Libondi, T.**, Mensione, M. and Auricchio, G., *In vitro* effect of alpha-tocopherol on lysophosphatidylcholine-induced lens damage, *Exp Eye Res*, 40, 661-666, 1985.
73. **Benedick, G.B.**, Cataract as a protein condensation disease: The Proctor lecture, *Invest Ophthalmol Vis Sci,* 38, 1911-1921, 1997.
74. **Horwitz, J.**, Alpha crystallin can function as a molecular chaperone, *Proc Natl Acad Sci USA*, 89, 10449-10453, 1992.
75. **Clark, J.I.** and Huang, Q.L., Modulation of chaperone-like activity of bovine α-crystallin, *Proc Natl Acad Sci USA*, 93, 15185-15189, 1996.
76. **Varma, S.D.**, Scientific basis for medical therapy of cataracts by antioxidants, *Am J Clin Nutr*, 53, 335S-345S, 1991.
77. **Matsushima, H.**, David, L.L., Hiraoka, T. and Clark, J.I., Loss of cytoskeletal proteins and lens cell opacification in the selenite cataract model, *Exp Eye Res*, 64, 387-395, 1997.
78. **Wang, K.** and Spector, A., α-crystallin stabilizes actin filaments and prevents cytochalasin-induced depolymerization in a phosphorylation dependent manner, *Eur J Biochem,* 242, 56-66, 1996.

79. **Greiner, J.V.**, Kopp, S.J. and Glonek, T., Distribution of phosphatic metabolites in crystalline lens, *Invest Ophthalmol Vis Sci,* 26, 537-544, 1985.
80. **Muchowski, P.J.** and Clark, J.I., ATP enhanced molecular chaperone functions of the small heat shock protein human αB, *Proc Natl Acad Sci*, 95, 1004-1009, 1998.
81. **Muchowski, P.J.**, Bassuk, J.A., Lubsen, N.H. and Clark, J.I., Human B crystallin, small heat shock protein and molecular chaperone, *J Biol Chem*, 272, 2578-2582, 1997.
82. **Beaulieu, C.F.** and Clark, J.I., ^{31}P-Nuclear magnetic resonance and laser spectroscopic analyses of lens transparency during calcium induced opacification, *Invest Ophthalmol Vis Sci,* 31, 1339-1347, 1990.

Chapter 8

LIGHT AND RISK FOR AGE-RELATED EYE DISEASES

Cathy McCarty and Hugh R. Taylor

I. BACKGROUND

As outlined in Chapters 5 and 6, antioxidants appear to be protective for cataract and age-related maculopathy in both experimental and observational studies. Potential environmental sources of oxidative damage to the lens and retina are cigarette smoke and sunlight exposure. The data related to smoking and risk of age-related eye diseases will be reviewed in the next chapter, while the literature about sunlight and risk of age-related eye disease will be reviewed in this chapter.

The visible spectrum of light comprises red, orange, yellow, green, blue, indigo and violet, while the ultraviolet spectrum is classified according to wave length (Figure 1). UV-C is short wave radiation, below 290 nm, that is generally only encountered in special situations such as arc welding or germicidal sterilising lamps. Because the cornea absorbs nearly all radiation below 280 nm (Figure 2), protective eyewear is essential for occupational settings with exposure to UV-C. UV-B, 290-320 nm, causes sunburn. At 320 nm (UV-B), more than half of the radiation is transmitted through the cornea to the lens (Figure 2). UV-A (near UV) is long wave radiation in the range 320 to 400 nm that is partially absorbed by the ozone layer. It produces suntanning and photosensitivity reactions and is associated with skin cancer. At 380 nm, approximately 3% of the radiation is absorbed by the retina, while 78% is absorbed by the lens. The irradiance of UV-C, UV-B and UVA-A, respectively, in watts per square metre is 6.4, 21.1, and 85.7, but will vary with the exact distance of the earth from the sun at a particular time.

The amount of UV reaching the ocular structures is affected by the environment. Over 90% of UV can penetrate clouds and 95% of incident UV penetrates water, 50% down to 2 metres. Fresh snow reflects 80% of UV and sand reflects 25% of UV. Previous research in a group of Chesapeake Bay watermen has shown that personal protection behaviours, such as the use of a brimmed hat and sunglasses, can have an 18-fold difference in ocular UV-B exposure [1-5], while ambient levels of UV-B vary only 4-fold by latitude [6]. Recently, this research has been replicated for other job categories in the Salisbury Eye Evaluation Project [7]. Ocular ambient exposure ratios for UV-B, the proportion of ambient UV-B that reaches the eye, were found to be affected by season of the year (highest in the winter) and were reduced by 34% by the use of hats. They did not vary by job category. Ocular ambient exposure ratios for visible light displayed a seasonal effect similar to UV-B, but were not significantly affected by the use of hats.

0-8493-8565-2/99/$0.00+$.50

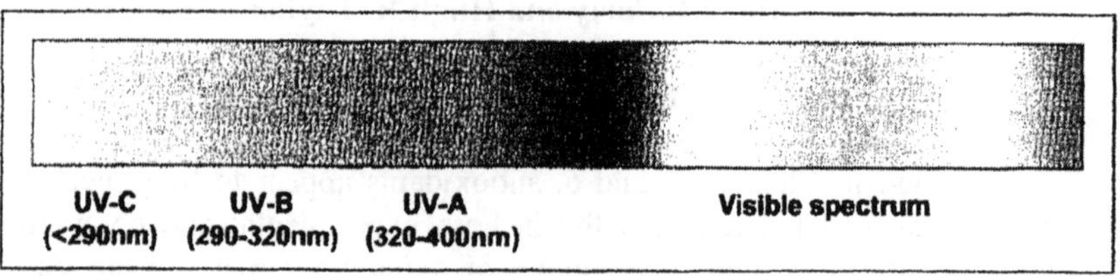

Figure 1. Ultraviolet and visible light spectra.

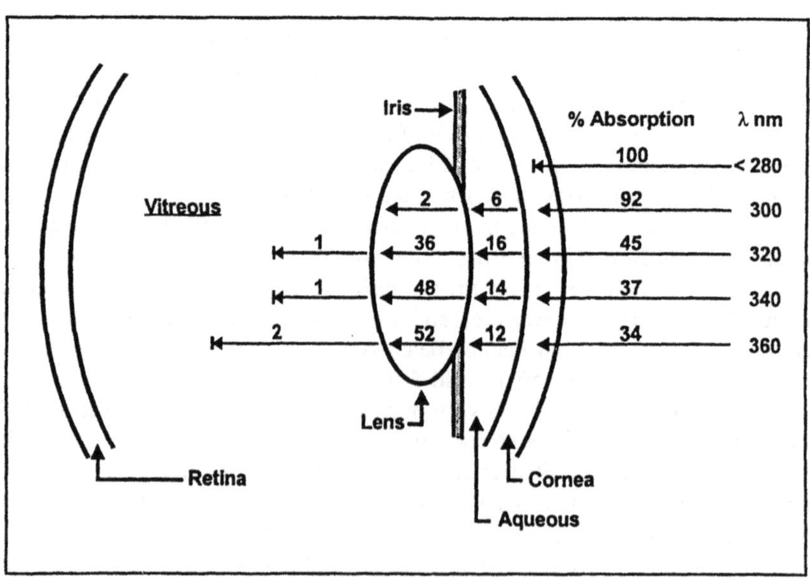

Figure 2. Percent of ambient UV absorbed by the ocular media [8].

Ultraviolet radiation, specifically UV-B in the range 290 to 320 nm, has been implicated in the development of age-related cataract. Experimental evidence has shown that the lens absorbs radiation in the UV-B range (Figure 2), but epidemiological evidence to prove a causal association between UV-B and cataract has not been entirely consistent. Three recent reviews of UV-B and cataract have concluded that the epidemiologic evidence is convincing for a causal relationship between UV-B and cataract [6,9,10], while another investigator rejects the UV-B hypothesis entirely [11]. Much of the disparity in conclusions has resulted from inadequate assessment of exposures and/or outcomes. Systematic misclassification of exposures or outcomes in study subjects tends to bias studies towards nonsignificant results (see Chapter 7 regarding study design).

Studies in which personal ocular UV-B exposure has not been assessed are subject to the ecologic fallacy. The ecologic fallacy occurs when it is assumed that everyone in the population (or a certain subgroup, such as workers) has the same level of exposure and thus the same risk of disease. Ecological studies are good for hypothesis generation, but not for hypothesis testing. Caution must be exercised when making conclusions about individual risk on the basis of data collected on groups.

A review of the epidemiologic evidence to establish an association between an exposure such as UV-B and an outcome such as cataract must consider the epidemiologic criteria for causality. These criteria are 1) consistency of results, 2) strength of the association (odds ratio or relative risk), 3) dose-response (often assessed with a test for trend), 4) temporality, 5) biological plausibility and 6) specificity [12]. The epidemiologic evidence related to sunlight and the age-related eye diseases cataract, age-related macular degeneration and pterygium will be summarised using these epidemiologic criteria for causality.

Equally important to assessment of causality and aetiology is the relative contribution of a statistically significant risk factor to the prevalence and incidence of a given health outcome in the population. When possible, population attributable risks (PAR) have been calculated for published studies with the formula $PAR=p(RR-1)/p(RR-1)+1$ where p is the proportion of people in the population with the risk factor (sunlight exposure) and RR is the relative risk or odds ratio (Tables 1 to 3). The interpretation of the population attributable risk is the percentage of the outcome in the population studied that is due to the risk factor. Larger values of PAR indicate that a greater proportion of the outcome is caused by the risk factor.

Table 1
Summary of Epidemiologic Studies of UV-B and Cataract

Study & type	Study cohort	Exposure measure	Outcome measure	Effect size (CL)	Dose resp.	PAR
Anduze [43] case study	200 West Indians	occupation location	cataract surgery	N/A	N/A	N/A
Chatterjee [13] ecological	1269 Punjab Indians	occupation location	senile or aphakic	n.s.	no	0%
Brilliant [21] ecological	873 Nepalese	sunlight hours, latitude, skyline	senile cataract	OR=3.8 (N/A) for 12 hrs sunlight	yes	N/A
Taylor [22] ecological	350 Australian Aborigines	latitude, sunlight hours	any cataract	OR=1.3 to 4.2 (N/A)	yes	N/A
Hollows [23] ecological	64,307 Aborigines 41,254 Non-Aborigines	latitude	any cataract	OR=1.53 to 3.0 (N/A)	yes	N/A
Javitt [44] ecological	U.S. Medi-care data	latitude	cataract surgery	3% increase for each 1° latitude	N/A	N/A
Wojno [45] case control	66 Wisconsin patients	use of spectacles	cortical nuclear PSC	OR=1.41 OR=1.90 OR=2.25 (N/A)	N/A	9% 18% 24%
Collman [27] case control	274 North Carolinians	lifetime sunlight exposure	cortical nuclear PSC	n.s. n.s. n.s.	N/A	0% 0% 0%
Dolezal [14] case control	320 Iowans	lifetime sunlight exposure	senile nuclear	n.s. OR=1.73 (1.03,2.9)	N/A	0% 6%
Bochow [28] case control	336 Maryland residents	lifetime personal ocular UV exposure	PSC	β=1.45 (.41, 2.5)	N/A	N/A

Study & type	Study cohort	Exposure measure	Outcome measure	Effect size (CL)	Dose resp.	PAR
Mohan [15] case control	1990 New Delhi patients	cloud cover, altitude	cortical nuclear PSC	OR=1.28 OR=1.28 OR=1.28 (1.1,1.47)	N/A	N/A
Leske [46] case control	1380 Massachusetts patients	time in sun, use of hats and sunglasses	cortical nuclear PSC mixed	n.s. OR=0.61 (.37,.99) n.s. OR=1.44 (1.1,1.94)	N/A	0% 0% 0% 8%
Rosmini [24] case control	1477 Italian patients	sunlight exposure index	cortical nuclear mixed	OR=2.26 (1.14,4.5) n.s. n.s.	yes	6% 0% 0%
Hiller [25] cohort	U.S. adults	sunshine hours	any cataract	F>10.0	yes	N/A
Hiller [26] cohort	U.S. adults	average daily UV-B counts	cortical nuclear PSC	RR=3.6 (N/A) n.s. n.s.	yes	52% 0% 0%
Taylor [18] cohort	838 Maryland watermen	lifetime personal ocular UV-B exposure	cortical nuclear	OR=1.6 (1.01,2.6) n.s.	yes	N/A 0%
Cruickshanks [19] cohort	4926 Wisconsin adults	lifetime personal sunlight exposure	cortical nuclear PSC	OR=1.4 for men (1.02,1.8) n.s. n.s.	N/A	12% 0% 0%
Wong [29] cohort	367 Hong Kong fishermen	lifetime sunlight exposure	cortical nuclear PSC	increased risk, but n.s.	N/A	N/A
Hirvela [47] cohort	500 elderly Finnish	outdoor occupation	cortical nuclear	RR=0.90 to 1.38 (N/A) n.s.	N/A	0-38 0%
Burton [48] cohort	797 adults in 2 villages of northern Pakistan	relative ambient UV and occupation location	any cataract	p<0.01 for outdoor workers	N/A	N/A
Taylor [20] cohort	3271 Melbourne adults	lifetime personal ocular UV-B exposure	cortical nuclear PSC	OR=1.38 (1.07,1.8) n.s. n.s.	yes	8.7% 0% 0%

Table 2
Summary of Epidemiologic Studies of Sunlight and AMD

Study & type	Study cohort	Exposure measure	Outcome measure	Effect size	Dose resp.	PAR
Hyman [49] case control	228 cases in Baltimore	residential and recreational exposure to sunlight	photo AMD with vision loss	n.s.	N/A	0%
Eye Disease C/C Study [50] case control	U.S. multi-centre trial with 421 cases	lifetime sunlight exposure	photo AMD with visual acuity <6/6	n.s.	n.s.	0%
Darzins [51] case control	409 cases from Australia	lifetime ocular sun exposure, tanning ability	photo AMD	n.s.	N/A	0%
West, Taylor [52,53] cohort	838 Maryland watermen	lifetime personal ocular blue light exposure	photo AMD	OR=1.35 (1.0,1.81) for geo atrophy	N/A	N/A
West, Taylor [52,53]	838 Maryland watermen	lifetime personal ocular UV exposure	photo AMD	n.s.	N/A	0%
Cruickshanks [54] cohort	4926 Wisconsin adults	lifetime amount of time spent outdoors	photo AMD	OR=1.44 (1.01,2.0) to 2.26 (1.06,4.8)	yes	13% to 20%

Table 3
Summary of Epidemiologic Studies of Sunlight and Pterygium

Study & type	**Study cohort**	**Exposure measure**	**Outcome measure**	**Effect size**	**Dose resp.**	**PAR**
Detels [60] ecological	Canada, India, Thailand, Taiwan	latitude, radiation, occupation (sawmills)	corneal flashlight exam	n.s.	N/A	0%
Moran [56] ecological	>100,000 Australian Aborigines and non-Aborigines	UV zone	clinical slitlamp exam	2.5x increased risk zone 5 (n. Aust) vs zone 1 (s. Aust) in Aborigines	yes	43%
Mack-enzie [57] case control	278 Brisbane hospital patients	occupational UV exposure	pterygium treatment	OR=14.1 (2.8,70.6) for ≥50% time outdoors aged 0-5	yes	30%
Taylor [61] cohort	350 Australian Aborigines	occupation and residence	clinical slitlamp exam	p=.006 for outdoor workers	N/A	N/A
Taylor [58] cohort	838 Maryland watermen	lifetime personal ocular UV-B exposure	clinical slitlamp exam	OR=6.36 (1.77,5.31) for upper quartile	yes	34%

The PAR allows for the assessment of the potential public health implication of statistically significant risk factors.

Sunlight/UV is a rather unique risk factor because there is nearly universal exposure to the risk factor in the population. Therefore, the population attributable risk of sunlight for age-related eye disease, if the association is true in the community, is potentially very high even if the odds ratio or relative risk is low.

II. EPIDEMIOLOGIC EVIDENCE RELATED TO CATARACT

A. CONSISTENCY

The key findings of the epidemiologic studies about sunlight and cataract are summarized in Table 1. They are listed in order from the "weakest" study design, a case study, to the "strongest" epidemiologic study design, a cohort study (see Chapter 7 regarding study design). Across the different study designs, the results are quite consistent in revealing a significant association between exposure and outcome. The only study in which a positive association between sunlight exposure and cataract was not demonstrated was an ecological study conducted in India that had no individual measures of exposure [13].

The best epidemiologic data are derived from cohort studies because this study design can address the issue of temporality and is less subject to recall bias by the participants. In all of the eight cohort studies from five continents, cataract was found to be associated with sunlight exposure, specifically UV-B.

Data specific to the type of cataract are preferable because the three types of cataract (cortical, nuclear, posterior subcapsular - PSC) may have different aetiologies. Generally, UV-B has been shown to be associated only with cortical cataract, although there are a few exceptions. In two case-control studies, nuclear cataract was found to be associated with sunlight [14,15]. One potential explanation for these findings only in case-control studies is survivor bias. Data from Beaver Dam Eye Study (a cohort study) reveal that nuclear cataract is a predictor of subsequent mortality [16]; thus, the people with nuclear cataract who survive long enough to participate in a case-control study may differ from the general population in many aspects, such as their lifetime exposure to sunlight. This positive association between nuclear cataract and subsequent mortality has also been demonstrated in the Chesapeake Bay Watermen Study, a cohort study [17].

PSC cataract was shown to be associated with sunlight in several of the case control studies, but in none of the cohort studies. This may be due in part to the rarity of PSC cataract in the cohort studies and inadequate statistical power. Case-control studies are better than cohort studies for the study of rare outcomes.

It is important to collect information about personal exposure because personal behaviours have been shown to have an 18-fold impact on the ocular dose of UV-B [1-5]. By collecting detailed personal information about both exposure and outcome, the ecological fallacy is less likely to occur and the results are more likely to be valid. Personal ocular UV-B exposure was assessed in the Chesapeake Bay Watermen Study [18], the Beaver Dam Eye Study [19], and the Melbourne Visual Impairment Project [20]. In all three of these cohort studies, personal ocular UV-B exposure was found to be associated with cortical cataract.

B. STRENGTH

The strength of the relationship between UV-B and cataract is demonstrated by the size of the odds ratios, which are as large as a 4-fold increased risk in cataract with high sunlight hours [21]. Anywhere from 6% to 38% of cortical cataract is potentially caused by sunlight exposure, the highest estimate of risk associated with outdoor occupation.

C. DOSE RESPONSE

Dose response was assessed in nine studies [13,18,20-26] and was demonstrated in all but one of them [13]. It does not appear that there is a ceiling effect of UV-B exposure, but rather a continuous relationship.

D. TEMPORALITY

To establish temporality, it is necessary to determine that a given risk factor exposure (such as UV-B) has occurred before the health event. Cohort studies are the best type of epidemiologic study to establish temporal events. Case control studies can lead to spurious results because people sometimes change their health behaviours after being diagnosed with disease. Therefore, assessment of concurrent behaviours and health outcomes can be misleading. This may be especially relevant with respect to cataract studies as people with cataract may tend to avoid sunlight exposure due to photophobia.

Seven of the studies included measurements of lifetime sunlight exposure, thus allowing assessment of temporality [14,18-20,27-29]. In all but one of these studies [29], lifetime sunlight exposure, specifically UV-B, was found to be significantly associated with the prevalence of cataract.

E. BIOLOGICAL PLAUSIBILITY

Research in laboratory animals and with cadaver lenses has shown that UV-B is absorbed by the lens and that cataract can be induced by the introduction of UV-B radiation [30-33].

Theoretically, the inferior and nasal portion of the lens are more exposed to sunlight because of the lack of shading effect of the nose, eyelids and eyebrows [34-36], and because of peripheral light focussing by the anterior eye [37]. Therefore, if UV-B is related to cataract development, cortical opacities should be more frequent in the inferior-nasal quadrant of the lens. In the three studies where location of opacity has been investigated, cortical opacities were more common in the inferior-nasal region, providing further biological support of the UV-B hypothesis [38-40].

Increased ambient temperature has also been shown to be associated with senile cataract [41,42]. Both temperature and UV-B levels vary by latitude; therefore, any potential confounding or effect modification is difficult to ascertain.

F. SPECIFICITY

In reality, no epidemiologic relationship is ever completely specific. This lack of specificity has been the ongoing argument by cigarette companies that cigarettes do not cause lung cancer. Everyone who smokes cigarettes will not develop lung cancer. Likewise, people develop lung cancer who have never smoked cigarettes. Despite lack of specificity, it is possible to have sufficient evidence from epidemiologic studies to support a causal relationship between an exposure and a health outcome.

In terms of specificity of the exposure, the Chesapeake Bay Watermen Study researchers showed that the relationship between ultraviolet radiation and cortical cataract was specific to UV-B and not related to UV-A or visible light [18].

G. SUMMARY

The association between UV-B and age-related cortical cataract is consistent, strong, exhibits a dose-response relationship, has the correct temporal relationship, and is biologically plausible and specific; thus, it meets the epidemiologic criteria for causality. Furthermore, as much as half of the cortical cataract in the population, as summarised by the PAR, may be due to ocular UV-B exposure [26].

III. EPIDEMIOLOGIC EVIDENCE RELATED TO AMD

A. CONSISTENCY

There have been five studies that included assessments of sunlight and AMD (Table 2). None of the three case-control studies [49-51] found a significant relationship between sunlight and AMD, but each of the cohort studies [52-54] showed an increased risk of AMD with higher lifetime exposures to sunlight. Although these are inconsistencies between the study findings, the consistent results of the cohort studies, which are the stronger epidemiologic study type and less prone to bias, suggest that the potential sunlight/AMD relationship cannot be dismissed. Further data are needed.

B. STRENGTH

In the two cohort studies where a significant relationship was shown, the odds ratios were 1.3 and 1.4. They are not extraordinarily large odds ratios, but remember that potentially everyone in the population is exposed to sunlight in their lifetime. In the Beaver Dam Eye Study [54], investigators found that between 13% and 20% of AMD in the population could be explained by excess sunlight exposure.

C. DOSE-RESPONSE

A potential dose response effect has been evaluated in only two of the reported studies [50,54]. The tests for trend were not significant in the case-control study [50] and were significant in the cohort study [54]. Again, the available data are equivocal, but do not remove the possibility of a causal relationship between sunlight and AMD.

D. TEMPORALITY

In four of the five studies [50-54], data on lifetime sunlight exposure were collected. Again, only the two cohort studies [52-54] found a significant relationship between lifetime sunlight exposure and AMD. The case-control study that did not assess lifetime sunlight exposure history may be particularly subject to bias in the current behaviours of the cases. People with AMD may not have as much current sunlight exposure because of mobility problems due to their visual impairment.

E. BIOLOGICAL PLAUSIBILITY

It has been suggested that AMD may be the result of repeated oxidative insults and the outer retina is susceptible to damage by solar radiation, particularly blue light [55]. As shown in Figure 2, nearly all of the ultraviolet radiation is absorbed by the other ocular structures before reaching the retina.

Investigators from the Chesapeake Bay Watermen Study revealed that recent sunlight exposure (the previous 20 years) was strongly related to geographic atrophy, suggesting that the normal mechanisms of retinal photo-oxidative repair may decrease with age. Therefore, the elderly may be susceptible to damage from sunlight doses that were "safe" when they were young.

The role of cigarette smoking in the aetiology of AMD will be reviewed in Chapter 9.

F. SPECIFICITY

Although the relationship between sunlight and AMD is not specific, a potential causal effect of sunlight on the aetiology of AMD cannot be dismissed based solely on this criterion.

G. SUMMARY

More data are needed to determine whether sunlight is causally related to AMD. It certainly seems that the ultraviolet spectrum is not related to AMD and that future research should be directed at visible light, particularly blue light. Prospective data with lifetime ocular sunlight exposure information are necessary.

IV. EPIDEMIOLOGIC EVIDENCE RELATED TO PTERYGIUM

Pterygium is a fairly major public health problem; 10% of males and 4.4% of females aged 40-59 were found to be affected in a study conducted in Australia [56]. Limited data are available on putative risk factors for pterygium.

A. CONSISTENCY

There have been five studies into the potential effect of sunlight on pterygium (Table 3). Four of the five studies found that ultraviolet light was related to an increased risk of pterygium. The only study where sunlight was not found to be related to pterygium was an ecological study where individual exposure was not assessed.

B. STRENGTH

In the five studies where sunlight was shown to be associated with pterygium, the relationship was very strong, ranging from a 2.5-fold increased risk in Australian Aborigines [56] to an odds ratio of 14 in Brisbane hospital patients [57]. Due to the high odds ratios and the nearly universal exposure of the population to sunlight, the population attributable risks were quite high. They suggest that 30-43% of pterygium is caused by excess sunlight exposure (Table 3).

C. DOSE-RESPONSE

A dose-response effect was found in all of the three studies [56-58] in which the results of this examination were reported.

D. TEMPORALITY

Only one study included the assessment of lifetime ocular UV-B exposure [58]. In that cohort study of Maryland watermen, men in the upper quartile of lifetime ocular UV-B exposure were more than six times as likely to have pterygium as men in the lowest quartile of lifetime ocular UV-B exposure.

E. BIOLOGICAL PLAUSIBILITY

Coroneo et al. have summarised the biological rationale for a causal relationship between UV and pterygium [37,59]. They suggest that peripheral focussing of light on the nasal aspect of the limbus by the anterior eye supports this relationship. This would also explain the fact that pterygium occurs most commonly on the nasal side of the cornea.

F. SPECIFICITY

As mentioned previously, it is nearly impossible to have a completely specific relationship between exposures and outcomes in epidemiologic studies, but this does not preclude the determination of causality from epidemiologic research.

In only one study, the Chesapeake Bay Watermen Study, was the relationship between pterygium and other light spectra investigated [58]. These investigators found that not only was pterygium significantly related to UV-B, but also to UV-A and visible light. Therefore, pterygium may be caused by broad band sunlight rather than just the UV-B.

G. SUMMARY

The association between UV-B and pterygium meets the epidemiologic criteria for causality, and more than one-third of the pterygium in the population may be due to ocular UV-B exposure.

V. SUNLIGHT AND OTHER OCULAR DISEASES

The role of solar UV radiation in the development of climatic droplet keratopathy, ocular melanoma, pinguecela and carcinoma in situ was reviewed recently by a WHO task group [8]. They concluded that there is limited or insufficient evidence to link UVR exposure with climatic droplet keratopathy, pingueculae and cancers of the anterior ocular structures.

VI. CONCLUSION

In conclusion, the epidemiologic data support a role for sunlight in the development of cataract and pterygium, and possibly AMD, but more data are needed. Age is the strongest predictor of any of these diseases, but is not modifiable. Therefore, sunlight has the potential to be one of the major modifiable risk factors for cataract, AMD and pterygium. It is therefore prudent to recommend that people protect their eyes from the sun, both visible light and UV-B, through the avoidance of the midday sun and the use of brimmed hats and sunglasses.

VII. REFERENCES

1. **Rosenthal FS**, Safran M, Taylor HR. The ocular dose of ultraviolet radiation from sunlight exposure, *Photochem Photobiol,* 42,163-71,1985.
2. **Rosenthal FS**, Bakalian AE, Taylor HR. The effect of prescription eyewear on ocular exposure to ultraviolet radiation, *Am J Public Health,* 76,1216-20,1986.
3. **Rosenthal FS**, Bakalian AE, Lou CQ, Taylor HR. The effect of sunglasses on ocular exposure to ultraviolet radiation, *Am J Public Health,* 78,72-4,1988.
4. **Rosenthal FS**, Phoon C, Bakalian AE, Taylor HR. The ocular dose of ultraviolet radiation to outdoor workers, *Invest Ophthalmol Vis Sci,* 29,649-56,1988.
5. **Rosenthal FS**, West SK, Munoz B, Emmett EA, Strickland PT, Taylor HR. Ocular and facial skin exposure to ultraviolet radiation in sunlight: a personal exposure model with application to a worker population, *Health Phys,* 61,77-86,1991.
6. **McCarty C**, Taylor H. Recent developments in vision research: Light damage in cataract, *Invest Ophthalmol Vis Sci,* 37,1720-3,1996.
7. **Duncan DD**, Munoz B, Bandeen-Roche K, West SK, Salisbury Eye Evaluation Team. Visible and ultraviolet-B ocular-ambient exposure ratios for a general population, *Invest Ophthalmol Vis Sci,* 38,1003-11,1997.
8. **Programme for the Prevention of Blindness**. WHO, Ed., *The Effects of Solar UV Radiation on the Eye*, 1994.

9. **West SK**, Valmadrid CT. Epidemiology of risk factors for age-related cataract, *Surv Ophthalmol,* 39,323-34,1995.
10. **Dolin PJ**. Assessment of epidemiological evidence that exposure to solar ultraviolet radiation causes cataract, *Doc Ophthalmol*, 88,327-37,1994.
11. **Harding JJ**. The untenability of the sunlight hypothesis of cataractogenesis, *Doc Ophthalmol,* 88,345-9,1994.
12. **Mausner, JS**, Kramer, S, in *Epidemiology. An Introductory Text.* W.B. Saunders Company, Philadelphia, 1985.
13. **Chatterjee A**, Milton RC, Thyle S. Prevalence and aetiology of cataract in Punjab, *Br J Ophthalmol,* 66,35-42,1982.
14. **Dolezal JM**, Perkins ES, Wallace RB. Sunlight, skin sensitivity, and senile cataract, *Am J Epidemiol,* 129,559-68,1989.
15. **Mohan M**, Sperduto RD, Angra SK, Milton RC, Mathur RL, Underwood BA, Jaffery N, Pandya CB, Chhabra VK, Vajpayee RB. India-US case-control study of age-related cataracts. India-US Case-Control Study Group, *Arch Ophthalmol,* 107,670-6,1989.
16. **Klein R**, Klein BE, Moss SE. Age-related eye disease and survival. The Beaver Dam Eye Study, *Arch Ophthalmol,* 113,333-9,1995.
17. **Vitale S**, West S, Munoz B, et al. Watermen Study II: mortality and baseline incidence of nuclear opacity. [Abstract] *Invest Ophthalmol Vis Sci,* 33,1152,1992.
18. **Taylor HR**, West SK, Rosenthal FS, Munoz B, Newland HS, Abbey H, Emmett EA. Effect of ultraviolet radiation on cataract formation, *N Engl J Med,* 319,1429-33,1988.
19. **Cruickshanks KJ**, Klein BE, Klein R. Ultraviolet light exposure and lens opacities: the Beaver Dam Eye Study, *Am J Public Health,* 82,1658-62,1992.
20. **McCarty CA**, Taylor HR. Risk factors for age-related cataract in Australia, *Exp Eye Res*, 67, S158, 1998.
21. **Brilliant LB**, Grasset NC, Pokhrel RP, Kolstad A, Lepkowski JM, Brilliant GE, Hawks WN, Pararajasegaram R. Associations among cataract prevalence, sunlight hours, and altitude in the Himalayas, *Am J Epidemiol,* 118,250-64,1983.
22. **Taylor HR**. The environment and the lens, *Br J Ophthalmol,* 64,303-10,1980.
23. **Hollows F**, Moran D. Cataract–the ultraviolet risk factor, *Lancet,* 2, 249-50,1981.
24. **Rosmini F**, Stazi MA, Milton RC, Sperduto RD, Pasquini P, Maraini G. A dose-response effect between a sunlight index and age-related cataracts. Italian-American Cataract Study Group, *Ann Epidemiol,* 4,266-70,1994.
25. **Hiller R**, Giacometti L, Yuen K. Sunlight and cataract: an epidemiologic investigation, *Am J Epidemiol,* 105,450-9,1977.
26. **Hiller R**, Sperduto RD, Ederer F. Epidemiologic associations with nuclear, cortical, and posterior subcapsular cataracts, *Am J Epidemiol,* 124,916-25,1986.

27. **Collman GW**, Shore DL, Shy CM, Checkoway H, Luria AS. Sunlight and other risk factors for cataracts: an epidemiologic study, *Am J Public Health,* 78,1459-62,1988.
28. **Bochow TW**, West SK, Azar A, Munoz B, Sommer A, Taylor HR. Ultraviolet light exposure and risk of posterior subcapsular cataracts, *Arch Ophthalmol,* 107,369-72,1989.
29. **Wong L**, Ho SC, Coggan D, Cruddas AM, Hwang CH, Ho CP, Robertshaw AM, MacDonald DM. Sunlight exposure, antioxidant status, and cataract in Hong Kong fisherman, *J Epidemiol Comm Health,* 47,46-9,1993.
30. **Lerman S**. Human ultraviolet radiation cataracts, *Ophthalmic Res,* 12,303-14,1980.
31. **Zigman S**, Datiles M, Torczynski E. Sunlight and human cataracts, *Invest Ophthalmol Vis Sci,* 18,462-7,1979.
32. **Andley UP**, Weber JG. Ultraviolet action spectra for photobiological effects in cultured human lens epithelial cells, *Photochem Photobiol,* 62,840-6,1995.
33. **Merriam JC**. The concentration of light in the human lens, *Trans Am Ophthalmol Soc,* 94,803-918,1996.
34. **Sliney DH**. Epidemiological studies of sunlight and cataract: the critical factor of ultraviolet exposure geometry, *Ophthalmic Epidemiol,* 1,107-19,1994.
35. **Sliney DH**. UV radiation ocular exposure dosimetry, *Photochem Photobiol B,* 31,69-77,1995.
36. **Sliney DH**. Ocular exposure to environmental light and ultraviolet–the impact of lid opening and sky conditions, *Dev Ophthalmol,* 27,63-75,1997.
37. **Coroneo MT**, Muller-Stolzenburg NW, Ho A. Peripheral light focusing by the anterior eye and the ophthalmohelioses, *Ophthalmic Surg,* 22,705-11,1991.
38. **Klein BEK**, Klein R, Linton KL. Prevalence of age-related lens opacities in a population. The Beaver Dam Eye Study, *Ophthalmology,* 99,546-52,1992.
39. **Schein OD**, West S, Munoz B, Vitale S, Maguire M, Taylor HR, Bressler NM. Cortical lenticular opacification: distribution and location in a longitudinal study, *Invest Ophthalmol Vis Sci,* 35,363-6,1994.
40. **Graziosi P**, Rosmini F, Bonacini M, Ferrigno L, Sperduto RD, Milton RC, Maraini G. Location and severity of cortical opacities in different regions of the lens in age-related cataract, *Invest Ophthalmol Vis Sci,* 37,1698-703,1996.
41. **Miranda MN**. Environmental temperature and senile cataract, *Trans Am Ophthalmol Soc,* 78,255-64,1980.
42. **Sliney DH**. Physical factors in cataractogenesis: ambient ultraviolet radiation and temperature, *Invest Ophthalmol Vis Sci,* 27,781-90,1986.
43. **Anduze AL**. Ultraviolet radiation and cataract development in the U.S. Virgin Islands, *J Cataract Refract Surg,* 19,298-300,1993.

44. **Javitt JC**, Taylor HR. Cataract and latitude, *Doc Ophthalmol,* 88,307-25,1994.
45. **Wojno T**, Singer D, Schultz RO. Ultraviolet light, cataracts, and spectacle wear, *Ann Ophthalmol,* 15,729-32,1983.
46. **Leske MC**, Chylack LT, Jr., Wu SY. The Lens Opacities Case-Control Study. Risk factors for cataract, *Arch Ophthalmol,* 109,244-51,1991.
47. **Hirvela H**, Luukinen H, Laatikainen L. Prevalence and risk factors of lens opacities in the elderly in Finland. A population-based study, *Ophthalmology,* 102,108-17,1995.
48. **Burton M**, Fergusson E, Hart A, Knight K, Lary D, Liu C. The prevalence of cataract in two villages of northern Pakistan with different levels of ultraviolet radiation, *Eye,* 11,95-101,1997.
49. **Hyman LG**, Lilienfeld AM, Ferris FL, 3rd, Fine SL. Senile macular degeneration: a case-control study, *Am J Epidemiol,* 118,213-27,1983.
50. **The Eye Disease Case-Control Study Group**. Risk factors for neovascular age-related macular degeneration, *Arch Ophthalmol,* 110,1701-8,1992.
51. **Darzins P**, Mitchell P, Heller RF. Sun exposure and age-related macular degeneration. An Australian case-control study, *Ophthalmology,* 104,770-6,1997.
52. **West SK**, Rosenthal FS, Bressler NM, Bressler SB, Munoz B, Fine SL, Taylor HR. Exposure to sunlight and other risk factors for age-related macular degeneration, *Arch Ophthalmol*, 107,875-9,1989.
53. **Taylor HR**, Munoz B, West S, Bressler NM, Bressler SB, Rosenthal FS. Visible light and risk of age-related macular degeneration, *Trans Am Ophthalmol Soc,* 88,163-73,1990.
54. **Cruickshanks KJ**, Klein R, Klein BEK. Sunlight and age-related macular degeneration. The Beaver Dam Eye Study, *Arch Ophthalmol,* 111,514-518,1993.
55. **Sliney DH**, Mueller HA, Ham WT. Retinal sensitivity to damage from short wavelength light, *Nature,* 260,153-5,1976.
56. **Moran DJ**, Hollows FC. Pterygium and ultraviolet radiation: a positive correlation, *Br J Ophthalmol,* 68,343-6,1984.
57. **Mackenzie FD**, First LW, Battistutta D, Green A. Risk analysis in the development of pterygia, *Ophthalmology,* 99,1056-61,1992.
58. **Taylor HR**, West SK, Rosenthal FS, Munoz B, Newland HS, Emmett EA. Corneal changes associated with chronic UV irradiation, *Arch Ophthalmol,* 107,1481-4,1989.
59. **Coroneo MT**. Pterygium as an early indicator of ultraviolet radiation: a hypothesis, *Br J Ophthalmol,* 77,734-9,1993.
60. **Detels R**, Dhir SP. Pterygium: a geographical study, *Arch Ophthalmol,* 78,485-91,1967.
61. **Taylor HR**. Aetiology of climatic droplet keratopathy and pterygium, *Br J Ophthalmol,* 64,154-63,1997.

Chapter 9

SMOKING AND THE RISK OF EYE DISEASES

Sheila K. West

I. SMOKING: HISTORY AND MAGNITUDE OF THE PROBLEM

Before Europe "found" the New World, the use of tobacco was common in the Americas. Reports of smoking were brought to Europe by early explorers, including Christopher Columbus, who wrote of the use of a Y-shaped pipe called a tabaca by the residents of the Caribbean. In a cosmic trade for infectious diseases unknown in the New World, these explorers brought tobacco leaves to Europe, and the use spread. Tobacco belongs to the genus *Nicotiana*, named for Jean Nicot, French ambassador to Portugal who introduced it to France. Cigarette smoking became common among Europeans after French and British soldiers adopted the habit from Turkish soldiers during the Crimean War. The automatic cigarette making machine was perfected in Durham, North Carolina, in 1883, and large-scale production became possible.

Even in older times, the use of tobacco had its detractors, although for reasons other than health. King James I disliked the smell of this "sot-weed" and forbade its use in England, with no success. Now one of the leading tobacco growing states in the U.S., Virginia at one time discouraged tobacco growing because farmers neglected food crops in favor of the "high cash value" crop. In fact, bundles of tobacco leaves were used as currency in Virginia, Maryland, and the Carolinas. Early settlers in New England passed laws to prohibit smoking because it was a non-productive pastime, again with little impact.

By the early 1960s the health hazards of cigarette smoking were apparent. In 1964, the Surgeon General of the United States, backed by an expert committee of 11 scientists, issued a report that the use of tobacco was a major health hazard and a cause of lung cancer, chronic bronchitis, emphysema, and heart diseases.[1] In a gesture of public concern, the cigarette companies responded by writing the Cigarette Advertising Code, which banned health claims from cigarette advertising and suggested reducing the amount of advertising aimed at young persons. An empty gesture indeed, as cigarettes were never primarily marketed as a health aid, and the economic value of attracting the populace to smoking at a young age was, and is, considerable. Thus, from the languid gaze of a sultry movie star pouting her lips behind a curling wisp of cigarette smoke to the frenetic "cool" of Joe Camel with his omnipresent dark glasses and hip music, the promotion of smoking to the public has been sophisticated and relentless.

In attempts to educate the public and stem the rising rates of smoking, the United States Government passed a law in 1965 requiring a health warning on every pack of cigarettes sold in the U.S. In 1970, another law was passed that banned cigarette advertising on radio and television. Currently, all 50 states in the U.S. prohibit tobacco sales to minors, and, in 1997, the Food and Drug Administration (FDA) established 18 as the minimum age to legally purchase tobacco products.[2] Recently, the FDA officially declared cigarettes "addicting," a fact

0-8493-8565-2/99/$0.00+$.50

which came as no surprise to the more than 48 million current smokers and to the public health workers employed in smoking-cessation programs.

The legislative approach seems to have had little impact on smoking. Approximately 24 billion packages of cigarettes are purchased annually in the United States, which is second only to China in tonnage of tobacco grown. Smoking is increasing among adolescents[3] and 88% of current smokers started by the age of 18.[4] Tobacco retailers still sell products to minors, and even enforcement of the law has questionable effects on the access of adolescents to tobacco products.[5] In the United States, it is estimated that every day approximately 3,000 children begin smoking.[6]

II. HEALTH EFFECTS

The health effects resulting from long-term smoking are legion; rare is the study of chronic disease that doesn't reveal some association with smoking. Five major categories lead the list of smoking-related diseases: heart disease and stroke, lung and other cancers, and chronic obstructive pulmonary disease. To this list, some would add age-related eye diseases, and the rest of this chapter will review the data linking smoking and chronic eye diseases.

A myriad of chemicals are contained in tobacco smoke, which is really an aerosol of particulates. Toxic chemicals include nicotine, benzo(a)pyrene, beta-naphthalamine, nickel, cadmium, arsenic, and lead. Gases identified in cigarette smoke include carbon monoxide, methanol, acetone, hydrogen cyanide, ammonia, benzene, formaldehyde, and nitrosamines. Such a toxic cocktail contains a number of ingredients that could harm the lens, retina, and other ocular structures. However, the thousands of chemicals contained in tobacco smoke make it difficult to identify the single agent or combination of agents responsible for the adverse health effects. For example, in the cancer literature, many of the chemicals in tobacco smoke are known to be tumor initiators, tumor promoters, or complete carcinogens. Moreover, other chemicals can have synergistic effects with smoking, thus enhancing the risk of adverse health outcomes. As an example, there is a multiplicative interaction of alcohol use and smoking for the risk of oral cancer.

The mechanisms by which tobacco smoking causes adverse health effects have not been definitively described, and little data are available on the mechanisms for ocular damage. In general, nicotine causes vasoconstriction and other hemodynamic effects, as well as stimulation of nicotinic receptors with probable activation of central nervous system neurohumoral pathways; carbon monoxide causes hypoxia leading to compensatory polycythemia; and smoking is associated with hypercoagulability. The pathology seen with smoking includes direct, smoking-related, pulmonary changes of loss of cilia, increased goblet cells, inflammation, mucous plugging, and loss of alveoli and small arteries. Smoking is associated with accelerated atherosclerosis, endothelial cell damage, and increased activity of enzymes that break down elastin and other connective tissue.

In considering the effects of smoking, and particularly nicotine, two aspects of the pharmacology must be kept in mind. The complex dose-response characteristics make some effects difficult to judge.[7] For example, in low doses, nicotine may produce one set of effects and in high doses the complete opposite effect. Second, tolerance to at least some of the effects of smoking does occur, and often rapidly. Thus, acute exposures may not be relevant models for understanding long-term effects.

Most of the studies of the effect of smoking on ocular function have evaluated the acute effects on blood flow in animal and human models. Autoregulation of the choroidal and ophthalmic artery circulation does occur, which may ameliorate the more pronounced effects of smoking on vasculature. For example, while acute effects of smoking include increased systolic and diastolic blood pressure and heart rate, little change was seen on ocular pulse amplitude.[8]

In another study of the acute effects of smoking on retinal blood flow, smoking caused a significant reduction in retinal blood flow in both normal and diabetic volunteers.[9] Oxygen reactivity, a marker for vascular autoregulation, was reduced significantly in the normal group and eliminated in the diabetic volunteers. These data suggest that smoking, at least acute doses, does reduce retinal blood flow and the ability of the retinal vessels to respond to hypoxia. In another small study, 2-4 mg of nicotine in a gum base were administered to glaucoma and normal subjects, and responses of the ophthalmic artery flow velocity studied. The peak systolic-flow velocity and mean envelope-flow velocity were increased, while finger blood flow was significantly decreased after nicotine administration.[10] These studies used different techniques to study blood flow, and in different types of vasculature, but suggest that small vessel blood flow is reduced.

Because of the hemodynamic effects of smoking, it is reasonable to postulate an effect of smoking on diabetic eye disease. In addition to a possible vasoconstrictive effect, smoking has been shown to increase the level of carboxyhemoglobin, which reduces the oxygen-carrying capacity of the blood. Together, these effects may decrease the delivery of oxygen to the retina and may play a role in the progression of diabetic retinopathy.

III. DIABETIC RETINOPATHY

The most comprehensive evaluation of the risk factors for diabetic retinopathy is part of the Wisconsin Epidemiological Study of Diabetic Retinopathy (WESDR), where a population-based cohort of insulin-dependent and non-insulin-dependent diabetics have been followed for up to 10 years.[11] The incidence and progression of retinopathy were evaluated based on fundus photography and strict criteria for presence of multiple signs of diabetic retinopathy. In the ten-year follow up, neither smoking status nor dose of cigarettes smoked was related to risk of retinopathy or progression. Other studies have also found that cigarette smoking was not related to retinal changes, either longitudinally[12] or cross-sectionally.[13] However, some studies have found cigarette smoking to be related to non-clinically significant evidence of diabetic retinopathy such as small microaneurysms[13] or background retinopathy stages 2 and 3.[12]

IV. AGE-RELATED CATARACT

Despite the possibility of surgical intervention, cataract remains the leading cause of blindness in the world today.[14] Even in technologically advanced countries like the United States, cataract is a leading cause of visual impairment, especially among African Americans. Despite the availability of surgery, the costs are not inconsiderable, making the identification of factors that induce or drive the progression of cataract a research priority (see Chapter 4). Epidemiological research on risk factors for cataract has identified several factors that may be amenable to intervention, of which smoking is one of the most important.[15] Cataract is the result of opacification of the crystalline lens, sufficient to cause visual symptoms. There are at least three types of age-related cataract, with different risk factors associated with each type.

Several mechanisms have been proposed for the lens damage among smokers. One hypothesis maintains that smoking causes additional oxidative stress by lowering circulating anti-oxidants.[16] Smokers do appear to have lower serum values for some anti-oxidants compared to non-smokers.[17] Whether this is related to decreased dietary intake, interference with absorption, or another mechanism is unclear. In a prospective study of 50,828 nurses for risk of cataract extraction associated with anti-oxidant status, an interaction was reported between smoking and anti-oxidants status.[18] Smoking negated the protective effect of anti-oxidant status for risk of cataract extraction, although the interaction term in the model was not significant. Cataract extraction is an imperfect surrogate for measuring the degree of lens opacification, as several socioeconomic factors are associated with obtaining surgery for cataract and with smoking; so this interaction needs further replication.

Smoking may also result in systemic absorption of compounds capable of chronic accumulation and causing oxidative damage to lens proteins.[19] Harding has proposed that higher levels of cadmium and lead from smoking may lead to lens damage.[20] Significant accumulation of cadmium in both the blood and lens of smokers has been reported.[21] Harding further postulates that exposure to thiocyanate from smoking may also cause lens damage through carbamylation of enzymes, lens proteins, and crystallins; smokers do have elevated levels of cyanide and thiocyanate in blood, although lens levels have not been measured.

Epidemiological studies do support an association between smoking and lens opacities. Smoking and lens opacities have been associated in at least eleven studies, with diverse populations, using different study designs, and different lens opacity grading systems, where such methodologies were used at all (see Table 1).[22-32] The consistency of the association with estimated relative risks between 2 and 3, and the consistency of the association with opacity type, add credence to the validity of the finding. A cross-sectional study of 838 Chesapeake Bay fishermen was the first to link nuclear opacities with smoking,[22] and in studies where lens opacity type has been evaluated, most have confirmed that link.[26-32] The data have shown a dose-response relationship, with the increasing odds of nuclear opacity associated with increasing pack-years of smoking. Prospective studies have linked current smoking with the risk of developing new nuclear opacities or surgery for nuclear opacities[28,29,32] and the progression of existing nuclear opacities.[31] Three studies have linked Posterior Subcapsular (PSC) opacities with smoking,[28-30] but others have not found any relationship with opacities other than nuclear.[22,26,27,32]

The value of stopping smoking is less clear. There have been no randomized studies on the effect of smoking cessation and possible changes in the risk of cataract, although other smoking-related diseases do show a reversion to the risk of non-smokers the longer the time since quitting. In one cross-sectional and one prospective study, past smokers who quit over ten years ago had a risk of nuclear opacity, and progression of nuclear opacity, similar to those who never smoked.[22,31]

The attributable risk of nuclear cataract due to smoking is about 20%;[31] this appears to be one risk factor for cataractogenesis that can be altered through public health measures.

V. AGE-RELATED MACULAR DEGENERATION

Age-related macular degeneration (AMD) is an umbrella designation for a disorder that has multiple different forms, ranging from the appearance of drusen, to growth of new blood vessels into the macula. These different forms may well have different etiologies. The advanced forms of AMD, choroidal neovascularization or exudative disease and geographic atrophy, are the primary reasons for vision loss with this disease. Although less common than cataract, the impact of AMD in the elderly population is becoming greater because there is no known treatment that will reverse vision loss. A major imperative exists for determining the pathogenesis of this disease and identifying factors that can be altered to reduce the risk of AMD.

Because the degeneration occurs in the macular region where visible light is focused, an oxidative damage model for the development of AMD has been proposed. Furthermore, since smoking appears to increase the oxidative stress, and to reduce the level of plasma anti-oxidants, smoking is proposed as a risk factor for AMD. In addition to depressing ascorbate and carotenoid blood levels, cigarette smoking may also cause a reduction in macular pigment density (pigment containing retinal carotenoids).[33] Other researchers who favor a vascular abnormality origin for the development of AMD also find justification for smoking as a risk factor on the basis of the effects on vasculature described above.

Two problems plague the study of the relationship of smoking to AMD in epidemiological studies. The first is that advanced AMD is a disease of the very old; about 7% of persons age 75 and older in the white population have AMD.[34] However, the life expectancy of smokers is much less than that of non-smokers. At age 70, an estimated 78% of male non-smokers are still alive as compared to 57% of smokers (86% and 75% respectively for women).[35] The paucity of smokers who survive to develop AMD results in diminished power to detect the association in all but the largest studies. Furthermore, if there is selective loss of smokers with advanced AMD, the association will be correspondingly biased.

One method to circumvent this conundrum is to study the association of

Table 1
Summary of Cigarette Smoking and Cataract

Lead Author	Population	Design	Cataract Assessment	Association[1]
West[22] (1989)	838 fishermen	Cross-sectional	Photographs for nuclear, cortical, PSC	Nuclear Cataract: 40% ↑ risk with 40 Pack Years. Quitting > 10 yrs ago assoc. with ↓ risk
Clayton[23] (1982)	931 surgery cases 325 controls	Case-control	Cases presenting for surgery (no type specific)	Heavy smoking 2X more common in cases
Klein[24] (1985)	1370 diabetics	Cross-sectional	Clinical exam for nuclear, PSC	Current smoking assoc. with cataract
Harding[25] (1988)	300 surgery cases 609 controls	Case-control	Cases presenting for surgery (type not specified)	Heavy smoking assoc. with cataract (OR = 2.0)
Flaye[26] (1989)	1029 volunteers	Cross-sectional	Clinical exam for nuclear, cortical, PSC	Leske[27] (1991)
Leske[27] (1991)	945 clinic cases 435 controls	Case-control	Photographs for nuclear, cortical, PSC	OR = 1.68 for current smoking and risk of nuclear cataract

Table 1 (continued)

Christen[28] (1992)	22,071 male physicians	Prospective	Self-report plus medical record and loss of vision	RR = 2.1 for current smokers of > 20 cig/day. For nuclear, RR = 2.24; For PSC, RR = 3.17. Past smokers, no risk of NS but ↑ risk of PSC
Hankinson[29] (1992)	50,828 female nurses	Prospective	Cataract extraction	For all cataract, RR = 1.58 for 65-pack years, RR = 2.59 for PSC, 1.79 for nuclear
Klein[30] (1993)	4926 population-based sample	Cross-sectional	Photographs for nuclear, cortical, PSC	For nuclear, OR = 1.09 for 10-pack years For PSC, OR = 1.06 for 10 pack years (only for men)
West[31] (1995)	442 fishermen	Prospective	Photographs for nuclear	RR for progression of nuclear = 2.4 for current smokers
Hiller[32] (1997)	660 partaking in Framingham Eye Study with no lens opacities	Prospective	Clinical exam for nuclear, cortical, PSC	RR = 2.37 for incidence of nuclear among heavy smokers

smoking with early AMD, or precursor lesions. However, there is no agreement on the constituents of early AMD, and signs such as hyperpigmentation, confluent drusen, or very large drusen appear to have their own, distinct risk factors. Moreover, some signs are common, such as drusen, or unstable, such that they become virtually non-informative as to who will eventually develop severe AMD. It is not clear, then, that risk factors for these entities are really adding to the knowledge of risk factors for advanced AMD.

Against this backdrop of uncertainty, it is not surprising that there is some uncertainty in the association of smoking with AMD. In six cross-sectional studies, findings included smoking not related to AMD, protective for early AMD, associated only with exudative AMD, or associated with all forms of AMD.[36-41] In the Framingham Eye study, the investigators relied on clinical assessment of AMD coupled with a visual acuity criterion, and the analyses were not controlled for other risk factors except age and gender.[38] No association with smoking and AMD was observed. In a survey of 500 Finnish residents, AMD was determined based on fundus photographs.[41] No association with either early or advanced AMD was observed, although there was a suggestion of increased risk in advanced AMD. In the Chesapeake Bay fishermen study, early AMD (primarily large drusen cases) was assessed on the basis of photographs.[37] In a multiple logistic regression model, smoking appeared to be protective against early AMD, although no dose-response relationship was observed. The fishermen were heavy smokers, and most, 80%, were smokers at some point. It is possible that differential survival bias may have produced this result,[42] although others have found no evidence that early AMD is associated with mortality.[43]

Other cross-sectional studies have found evidence for an association. In the Beaver Dam Eye Study, Blue Mountain Eye Study, and Rotterdam Study, AMD was characterized in a population using photographic documentation, and divided into early and advanced AMD. In Beaver Dam, early AMD was not associated with smoking status, pack years smoked, or passive smoking. However, exudative AMD was related to current smoking, with odds in females and males of 2.50 and 3.29, respectively.[36] Similarly, the Rotterdam study found a strong, increased risk of exudative AMD with current smoking, with an odds of 6.6; former smokers had an increased odds of 3.2, and those who quit more than 20 years previously had no increased risk.[39] In both studies, no association was seen between geographicatrophy and smoking. In the Blue Mountain Eye study, current smoking was associated with exudative AMD and geographic atrophy. Smoking was also related to early AMD, with odds of 1.75.[40]

Four case-control studies have equally conflicting results, although two suffer from inadequate sample sizes. In a study of 421 cases of exudative AMD and 615 controls, cases were more likely to smoke compared to controls.[44] Both former smokers and current smokers had increased risk of exudative AMD, with odds of 1.5 and 2.2, respectively. Two small, underpowered, case-control studies found no significant association between smoking and AMD.[45,46] A larger case-control study found an increased odds of AMD in male, but not in female smokers.[47]

Two prospective studies, one in male physicians and one in female nurses, have examined the issue of smoking and development of AMD.[48,49] In both studies, AMD was determined on the basis of self report of incident cases and validated by medical records from eye care providers. AMD was defined as characteristic signs of AMD (drusen, confluence, etc.) with vision loss to 20/30 or worse, and exudative AMD. In both studies, the incidence of AMD was related to current smoking of at least 20 cigarettes per day, with a relative risk of 2.5 in men, and 2.4 in women. Past smokers had a slightly lower, but still elevated risk compared to those who never smoked. In both studies, the incidence rate for exudative disease was higher in smokers, and both studies demonstrated a dose-response relationship. These prospective data provide strong evidence for an association between smoking and advanced AMD.

The strongest and most consistent relationship to emerge from all these studies is the association of current smoking with exudative AMD, with little evidence for an association with early AMD. The lack of association with early AMD may be due to several factors. First, the characterization of specific clinical signs as "early AMD" may be incorrect, or at least not very precise, for population studies. Thus, misclassification has biased the results towards the null. Further work on improving the specificity of classifying early AMD is probably warranted. There is also the possibility that smoking is a risk factor for progression of AMD to the severe, exudative form, but not related to incidence of early forms. Thus, an association with early lesions would be unlikely, as few will progress. The prospective studies did not address this issue, because their definition of AMD in essence excluded early AMD. The definition of "incidence" in these studies included progression to advanced AMD. Current, ongoing, prospective studies will no doubt address these questions in the future.

VI. OTHER EYE DISEASES

The mechanism by which smoking might cause glaucoma is not at all clear, although the effect on connective tissue, on vasculature, and the nervous system can all be invoked. A case-control study in 1987 found a significant association between glaucoma and current smoking, after adjusting for other risk factors.[50] The association was not observed when comparing glaucoma "suspects" to controls. Three cross-sectional studies found no evidence of an association between smoking and glaucoma.[51-53] While methods of diagnoses of glaucoma or ocular hypertension were different, none of the studies found any evidence to suggest an association. In two studies, the number of cases of glaucoma were relatively small, but the cases and controls were population-based and not subject to detection or selection biases. The larger study in Barbados of 302 glaucoma cases in a population of 4,314 blacks found no association as well.

A prospective study of 647 persons with ocular hypertension was carried out to determine factors associated with progression of visual field loss.[54] Smoking at baseline was not associated with progression in the 68 persons who developed a visual field defect. Clearly, there has not been the wealth of data on smoking and glaucoma that characterizes the science in the other age-related eye diseases.

However, at present there is little reason to presume there is an association worth pursuing.

There has been some work suggesting smoking is a risk factor for the development of Grave's disease, possibly enhancing the severity of the cases that develop endocrine ophthalmopathy (outer signs associated with excessive thyroid-related hormone concentration). Hypoxia, causing stimulation of fibroblasts, is one possible explanation for this association.[55-57]

VII. SUMMARY

Smoking appears to be strongly related to two main causes of visual loss in the world today, cataract and exudative age-related macular degeneration. Dose-response relationships have been demonstrated, and the evidence supports the value of quitting smoking to reduce the risk. The fact that cigarette smoking is associated with so many age-related diseases, such as cardiovascular disease and cancer, raises the question of why there is a lack of specificity in smoking-related illnesses. The myriad of chemicals in cigarette smoke is one explanation, and these may have different, and interactive, effects on various organ systems. It is reasonable to expect that multiple effects from the particulates and gases in smoke could result in multiple pathology.

Another possibility worth further exploration is that smoking interacts with other risk factors, notably genetic factors, to produce a characteristic pathologic response in certain individuals. This line of reasoning provides a framework to explain why not all smokers develop lung cancer, or age-related macular degeneration. Fruitful research should delve into mechanisms of the interaction between factors that put persons at high risk of disease.

The resemblance between smoking changes and premature senescence is also of interest. Cataracts, cardiovascular disease, aging dermatological changes, and immunological changes are all features of the aging process. Perhaps the effect of smoking is more uniform than otherwise thought, by acting to accelerate the aging process at the cellular level, allowing other, individual factors to dictate the form the aging process will take in a person.

Regardless of the mechanism by which smoking causes pathology, there is no question of the toll it exacts. In the United States in 1993, tobacco use was responsible for more than 420,000 deaths annually, and at younger ages.[58] Most smokers want to quit, but are tobacco dependent, having been addicted since childhood. The challenge for the future is not just settling with the tobacco industry for payments to reimburse society for the cost of health care services (costs that the tobacco industry can pass on by raising prices). Rather, an industry which has made immense profits from lying to the American public and addicting its children must be held accountable for instigating measures that will result in decreasing smoking, especially smoking among adolescents.

VIII. REFERENCES

1. **Report of the Surgeon General,** The health consequences of smoking, Washington D.C. US Public Health Service, Department of Health Education and Welfare,1964.
2. **Food and Drug Administration,** Regulations restricting the sale and distribution of cigarettes and smokeless tobacco to protect children and adolescents. Final rule. Fed Regist 61(168), 44396-5318, 1996.
3. **Johnston, L.D., O'Malley, P.M. and Bachman, J.G.,** National survey results on drug use from the monitoring the future study, 1975-1995. Vol 1. Secondary school students. Rockville, MD. National Institute on Drug Abuse, NIH pub No 96-4139, 1996.
4. **Department of Health and Human Services,** Preventing tobacco use among young people. A report of the Surgeon General. Washington D.C. Government Printing Office, 1994.
5. **Rigotti, N.A., DiFranza, J.R., Chang, Y.C., Tisdale, T., Kemp, B. and Singer, D.E.,** The effect of enforcing tobacco sales laws on adolescents' access to tobacco and smoking behavior, *New Eng. J. Med.*, 337, 1044-1051, 1997.
6. **Koop, C.E. and Kessler, D.,** Final report of the Advisory Committee on Tobacco Policy and Public Health, July 1997.
7. **Benowitz, N.L.,** Pharmacologic aspects of cigarette smoking and nicotine addiction, *New Eng. J. Med.*, 319, 1318-1330, 1988.
8. **Schmidt, K.G., Mittag, T.W., Pavlovic, S. and Hessemer, V.,** Influence of physical exercise and nifedipine on ocular pulse amplitude, *Graefes Arch. Clin. Exp. Ophthalmol.* 234, 527-32, 1996.
9. **Morgado, P.B., Chen, H.C., Patel, V., Hebert, L. and Kohner, E.M.,** The acute effect of smoking on retinal blood flow in subjects with and without diabetes, *Ophthalmology,* 101, 1220-1226, 1994.
10. **Rojanapongpun, P. and Drance, S.M.,** The effects of nicotine on the blood flow of the ophthalmic artery and the finger circulation, *Graefes Arch. Clin. Exp. Ophthalmol.,* 231, 371-374, 1993.
11. **Moss, S.E., Klein, R., and Klein, B.E.,** Cigarette smoking and ten year progression of diabetic retinopathy, *Ophthalmology*, 103, 1438-1442, 1996.
12. **Marshall, G., Garg, S.K., Jackson, W.E., Holmes, D.L. and Chase, H.P.,** Factors influencing the onset and progression of diabetic retinopathy in subjects with insulin dependent diabetes mellitus, *Ophthalmology*, 100, 1133-1139, 1993.
13. **Sparrow, J.M., McLeod, B.K., Smith, T.D., Birch, M.K. and Rosenthal, A.R.,** The prevalence of diabetic retinopathy and maculopathy and their risk factors in the non-insulin treated diabetic patients of an English town, *Eye*, 7, 158-163, 1993.
14. **Thylefors, B.,** The World Health Organization's programme for the prevention of blindness, *Int. Ophthalmol.*, 14, 211-219, 1990.
15. **West, S.K. and Valmadrid, C.T.,** Epidemiology of risk factors for Age

Related Cataract, *Surv. Ophthalmol.*, 39, 323-334, 1995.

16. **Taylor, A., Jacques, P.F. and Epstein, E.M.,** Relations among aging, antioxidant status, and cataract, *Am. J. Clin. Nutr.*, 62, 1439s-1447s, 1995.
17. **Kallmer, A.B., Hartman, D. and Hornig, D.,** On the requirements of ascorbic acid in man. Steady state turnover and body pool in smokers, *Am. J. Clin. Nutr.*, 34, 1347-1355, 1981.
18. **Hankinson, S.E., Stampfer, M.J., Seddon, J.M., Colditz, G.A., Rosner, B., Speizer, F.E. and Willett, W.C.,** Nutrient intake and cataract extraction in women: a prospective study, *Brit. Med. J.,* 35, 335-339, 1992.
19. **Shalina, V.K., Luthra, M., Srinivas, L., Rao, S.H., Basti, S. and Reddy, M.,** Oxidative damage to the eye lens caused by cigarette smoke and fuel smoke condensates, *Indian J. Biochem. Biophys.*, 31, 261-266, 1994.
20. **Harding, J.,** Cataract: biochemistry, epidemiology, and pharmacology, Chapman and Hall, London, England, 1991. p. 199.
21. **Ramakrishnan, S., Sulochana, K.N., Selvaraj, T., Abdul Rahim, A., Lakshmi, M. and Arunagiri, K.,** Smoking of beedies and cataract: cadmium and vitamin C in the lens and blood, *Br. J. Ophthalmol.*, 79, 202-206, 1995.
22. **West, S.K., Munoz, B., Emmett, E.A. and Taylor, H.R.,** Cigarette smoking and risk of nuclear cataracts, *Arch. Ophthalmol.*, 107, 1166-1169, 1989.
23. **Clayton, R.M., Cuthbert, J., Duffy, J., Seth, J., Phillips, C.I., Barthalmew, R.S. and Reid, J.,** Some risk factors associated with cataract in S.E. Scotland: a pilot study, *Trans. Ophthalmol. Soc. UK,* 102, 331-336, 1982.
24. **Klein, B.K., Klein, R. and Moss, S.E.,** Prevalence of cataract in a population based study of persons with diabetes mellitus, *Ophthalmology*, 92, 1191-1196, 1985.
25. **Harding, J. and van Heyningen, R.,** Drugs, including alcohol, that act as risk factors for cataract, and possible protection against cataract by aspirin-like analgesics and cyclopenthiazide, *Br. J. Ophthalmol.*, 72, 809-814, 1988.
26. **Flaye, D.E., Sullivan, K.N., Cullinan, T.R., Silver, J.H. and Whitelock, R.,** Cataracts and cigarette smoking. The City Eye Study, *Eye*, 3, 379-384, 1989.
27. **Leske, M.C., Chylack, L.T. and Wu, S.Y.,** The lens opacity case control study group. The lens opacity Case Control Study: Risk factors for cataract, *Arch. Ophthalmol.*, 109, 244-251,1991.
28. **Christen, W.G., Manson, J.F., Seddon, J.M., Glynn, R.J., Buring, J.E., Rosner, B. and Hennekens, C.H.,** A prospective study of cigarette smoking and risk of cataract in men, *JAMA,* 268, 989-993, 1992.
29. **Hankinson, S.E., Willett, W.C., Colditz, G.A., Seddon, J.M., Rosner, B., Speizer, F.E. and Stampfer, M.J.,** A prospective study of cigarette smoking and risk of cataract surgery in women, *JAMA,* 268, 994-998, 1992.
30. **Klein, B.K., Klein, R., Linton, K.P. and Franke, T.,** Cigarette smoking and lens opacities: the Beaver Dam Eye Study, *Am. J. Prev. Med.*, 9, 27-30, 1993.
31. **West, S.K., Munoz, B., Schein, O.D., Vitale, S., Maguire, M., Taylor, H.R. and Bressler, N.M.,** Cigarette smoking and risk for progression of nuclear opacities. *Arch. Ophthalmol.*, 113, 1377-1380, 1995.
32. **Hiller, R., Sperduto, R.D., Podgor, M.J., Wilson, P., Ferris, F.L., Colton,**

T., D'Agostino, R.B., Roseman, M.J., Stockman, M.E. and Milton, R.C., Cigarette smoking and the risk of development of lens opacities. The Framingham studies, *Arch. Ophthalmol.*, 115, 1113-1118, 1997.

33. **Hammond, B.R., Wooten, B.R. and Snodderly, D.M.,** Cigarette smoking and retinal carotenoids: implications for age related macular degeneration, *Vision Res.*, 36, 3003-3009, 1996.
34. **Klein, R., Klein, B.K. and Linton, K.P.,** Prevalence of age related maculopathy in the Beaver Dam Eye Study, *Ophthalmology,* 99, 933-943, 1992.
35. **Barendregt, J.J., Bonneux, L. and Van der Maas, P.J.,** The Health care costs of smoking, *New Eng. J. Med.*, 337, 1052-1057, 1997.
36. **Klein, R., Klei: B.E., Linton, K.P. and DeMets, D.,** The Beaver Dam Eye Study. The relation of age related maculopathy to smoking, *Am. J. Epidemiol.*, 137, 190-200, 1993.
37. **West, S.K., Rosenthal, F., Bressler, N.M., Bressler, S.B., Munoz, B., Fine, S.L. and Taylor, H.R.,** Exposure to Sunlight and other risk factors for age related macular degeneration, *Arch Ophthalmol.,* 107, 875-879, 1989.
38. **Kahn, H.A., Leibowitz, H.M., Ganley, J.P., Kini, M.M., Colton, T., Nickerson, R.S. and Dawber, T.R.,** The Framingham Eye Study: association of ophthalmic pathology with single variables previously measured in the Framingham Heart Study, *Am. J. Epidemiol.*, 106, 33-41, 1977.
39. **Vingerling, J.R., Hofman, A., Grobbee, D.E. and de Jong, P.T.,** Age related macular degeneration and smoking. The Rotterdam Study, *Arch. Ophthalmol.*, 114, 1193-1196, 1996.
40. **Smith, W., Mitchell, P. and Leeder, S.R.,** Smoking and age related maculopathy. The Blue Mountain Eye Study, *Arch. Ophthalmol.,* 114, 1518-1523, 1996.
41. **Hirvela, H., Luukinen, H., Laara, E. and Laatikainen, L.,** Risk factors of age related maculopathy in a population of 70 years of age or older, *Ophthalmology*, 103, 871-877, 1996.
42. **Riggs, J.E.,** Smoking and Alzheimer's diesease: protective effect or differential survival bias?, *Lancet,* 342, 793-794, 1993.
43. **Klein, R., Klein, B.E. and Moss, S.E.,** Age related eye disease and survival. The Beaver Dam Eye Study, *Arch. Ophthalmol.,* 113, 333-339, 1995.
44. **Eye Disease Case Control Study Group,** Risk factors for neovascular age related macular degeneration, *Arch. Ophthalmol.,* 110, 1701-1708, 1992.
45. **Maltzman, B.A., Mulvihill, M.N. and Greenbaum, A.,** Senile macular degeneration and risk factors, a case control study, *Ann. Ophthalmol.*, 11, 1197-1201, 1979.
46. **Blumenkranz, M.S., Russell, S.E., Robey, M.G., Kott-Blumenkranz, R. and Penneys, N.,** Risk factors in age related maculopathy complicated by choroidal neovascularization, *Ophthalmology,* 93, 552-557, 1986.
47. **Hymen, L.G., Lilienfeld, A.M., Ferris, F.L. and Fine, S.L.,** Senile macular degeneration. A case-control study, *Am. J. Epidemiol.*, 118, 213-227, 1983.
48. **Seddon, J.M., Willett, W.C., Speizer, F.E. and Hankinson, S.E.,** A

prospective study of cigarette smoking and age related macular degeneration in women, *JAMA,* 276, 1141-1146, 1996.

49. **Christen, W.G., Glynn, R.G., Manson, J.E., Ajani, U.A. and Buring, J.E.,** A prospective study of cigarette smoking and risk of age related macular degeneration in men, *JAMA,* 276, 1147-1151, 1996.
50. **Wilson, M.R., Hertzmark, E., Walker, A.M., Childs-Shaw, K. and Epstein, D.L.,** A case control study of risk factors in open angle glaucoma, *Arch. Ophthalmol.,* 105, 1066-1071, 1987.
51. **Ponte, F., Guiffre, G., Giammanco, R. and Dardanoni, G.,** Risk factors of ocular hypertension and glaucoma, The Casteldaccia Eye Study, *Doc. Ophthahlmol.,* 85, 203-210, 1994.
52. **Klein, B.E., Klein, R. and Ritter, L.L.,** Relationship of drinking alcohol and smoking to prevalence of open-angle glaucoma. The Beaver Dam Eye Study, *Ophthalmology,* 100, 1609-1613, 1993.
53. **Leske, M.C., Connell, A.S., Wu, S., Hyman, L.G. and Schachat, A.P.,** Risk factors for open angle glaucoma. The Barbados Eye Study, *Arch. Ophthalmol.,* 113, 918-924, 1995.
54. **Quigley, H.A., Enger, C., Katz, J., Sommer, A., Scott, R. and Gilbert, D.,** Risk factors for the development of glaucomatous visual field loss in ocular hypertension, *Arch. Ophthalmol.,* 112, 644-649, 1994.
55. **Prummel, M.F. and Wiersinga, W.M.,** Smoking and risk of Grave's disease, *JAMA,* 269, 479-82, 1993.
56. **Winsa, B., Mandahl, A. and Karlsson, F.A.,** Graves disease, endocrine ophthalmology and smoking, *Acta Endocrinol.,* 128, 156-60, 1993.
57. **Metcalfe, R.A. and Weetman, A.P.,** Stimulation of extraocular muscle fibroblasts by cytokines and hypoxia. Possible role in thyroid associated ophthalmopathy, *Clin Endocrinol.,* 40, 67-72, 1994.
58. **Centers for Disease Control and Prevention,** Cigarette smoking attributable mortality and years of potential life lost: United States, 1990, *Morb. Mortal Wkly. Rep.,* 42, 645-649, 1993.

Chapter 10

GRADING OF AGE-RELATED MACULOPATHY AND AGE-RELATED MACULAR DEGENERATION

Moshe Lahav

I. INTRODUCTION

Degeneration is an acquired tissue change which is secondary to a variety of physical or environmental influences. Age-related macular degeneration (AMD) is defined as macular changes associated with aging. Degenerative changes in the macula include drusen, pigmentation, atrophy and choroidal neovascularization with exudation and bleeding. These changes in the macula may lead to the cicatrical form of age-related macular degeneration, which is manifested by the formation of a fibrovascular scar. A typical appearance of early AMD includes small yellow bodies or crystals called drusen (rocks in German), which are seen in the macula and have been associated with the degeneration related to aging, hence the old name of Senile Macular Degeneration. Additional changes include pigmentation, areas of pigment epithelial atrophy known as atrophic or dry AMD, and choroidal neovascularization with leakage also known as wet AMD.

Dystrophy is a tissue change which is related to familial tendency or heredity. A prime example is found in corneal dystrophy where abnormal metabolic products accumulate and cause decreased vision. Drusen of the macular region or elsewhere in the ocular fundus can be seen as a manifestation of a dystrophy in younger individuals. These form various patterns such as Giant Dominant Hereditary Drusen or Doyne Honeycomb Retinal Dystrophy. [1] Recently, specific gene loci have been related to some of the phenotypes, such as Malattia Leventinese which is manifested as dominant Radial Drusen [2] and in Stargardt's disease. [3]

Age-related drusen tend to be clustered in families. [4-11] Recently a more frequent association of AMD with defects in the Stargardt's gene has been identified. [3] Therefore, in these instances the term Age-related Maculopathy (ARM) is more suitable than age-related macular degeneration, and Drusen Associated Maculopathy (DAM) conveys an even more accurate description.

II. CLINICAL PATHOLOGICAL CORRELATION

A. CLINICAL DESCRIPTION

The presence of drusen is considered to be an indicator of ARM and AMD. It is customary to differentiate clinically between hard and soft drusen. Hard drusen are small yellow-white deposits 50-200µm in diameter with well-defined margins seen as shiny crystals. Soft drusen are larger or yellowish excrescence with indistinct margins. These may coalesce or undergo absorption leaving atrophic areas behind. Pigmentary changes such as clumping or hyper- and hypopigmentation are seen as well. In some cases, leaky choriocapillaries may lead to retinal pigment epithelial (RPE) detachment thus converting the degeneration from "Dry" to "Wet". A full blown neovascular sprout from the choroid may

0-8493-8565-2/99/$0.00+$.50

invade the basement membrane (BM) into the subretinal space and leak, exude or bleed and cause exudative maculopathy.

B. HISTOPATHOLOGY

Drusen is an ophthalmoscopic diagnosis of yellow spots in the retinal pigment epithelial basement membrane (RPE-BM) complex. The deposits may have either of the following characteristics: (1) intra-RPE deposits, (2) pre-RPE-BM deposits which are amorphous with wide-spaced collagen, (3) intra- RPE-BM excrescence, (4) sub-RPE-BM deposits of curvilinear phospholipids which are more likely to be products of metabolic error, (5) intra-Bruch's membrane, pre- and inter-choriocapillaries deposits of amorphous granular material and which increase in quantity with aging. [12,13] The material external to the basement membrane of the RPE on top of Bruch's membrane is composed of a curvilinear phospholipids deposit which is diffused throughout the macular region. Focal thickenings, which are manifested as poorly delineated, rather large 250-500 μm promontories, appear as soft drusen. These soft drusen are not stationary; they may coalesce or disappear leaving RPE atrophic areas behind. They can be associated with RPE clumping or phagocytosis of pigment granules from disintegrating cells leading to hyperpigmentation. Calcium deposits may be present after absorption of the soft drusen.

C. CONSIDERATIONS REGARDING CORRELATIONS BETWEEN PATHOLOGY AND RETINA DISEASE

To study the natural history of age-related macular degeneration where the etiology is unknown, several assumptions have to be made. These include

1. Age-related changes such as the various deposits and fragmentation of collagen can be due to a slow repair process related to cellular aging. Various physical insults such as ultraviolet radiation, nutritional factors, such as a low amount of antioxidant protection or vascular ischemia, can also be contributing factors.

2. It has to be determined whether drusen, either hard or soft, are part of the aging process or are the result of a hereditary defect which is manifested later in life.

3. Since the drusen are easily identifiable markers it is easier to quantify and follow drusen associated in maculopathy (DAM), keeping in mind that other forms of AMD exist as well.

4. One should try and separate the hard drusen, which is more likely to be associated with the aging process, from the soft drusen, which indicated diffuse RPE changes and may be more likely to be associated with a genetic abnormality.

III. REVIEW OF GRADING SYSTEMS FOR MACULAR DEGENERATION

A. INITIAL ATTEMPTS

The early reports on the natural history and prognosis of macular degeneration did not utilize a quantitative method to follow up the development of the disease. These studies noted the presence of drusen and determined how many of the eyes with drusen developed choroidal neovascular membranes or atrophic changes which are the vision-reducing events in many cases. AMD was defined as RPE changes, increased pigmentation, hard and soft drusen, exudation, and geographic atrophy. [4] Attempts to classify AMD into subgroups by the number and appearance of drusen resulted in a simple classification system [14] and included the following criteria:

1. Five or more large drusen within the center of the fovea.
2. More than 20 small or intermediate drusen.
3. One or more areas of demarcated atrophy at least 1mm in size.
4. Focal hypo or hyperpigmentation 0.5 mm cumulative in size.
5. Exudative changes.

To study the natural history, progress and treatment of AMD, it is essential to have a reproducible, universally accepted grading system, preferably one that can be quantitative with respect to the various elements of maculopathy. Clinically, the most important feature is visual acuity. However, for grading purposes, description of the various morphologic indicators of degeneration is widely used.

It is generally agreed that drusen are one marker which can be easily recognized. The drusen may vary in size, number, distribution, demarcation and degree of confluence. The earlier attempts to quantitate AMD recognized small (<100 μm diameter) medium (100-200 μm diameter) and large (≥200 μm diameter) drusen. The distribution of drusen was graded into three groups: within 1500 μm of foveal center, within 3000 μm the foveal center, and beyond 3000 μm from the foveal center. The drusen was recognized as well or poorly demarcated. Confluence of drusen was graded into subgroups as none ≤ 3 drusen, more than 3 drusen within an area of less than 1000 μm in diameter. A large area of confluent drusen occupies >1000 μm. Other changes such as pigmentation or the presence of neovascular membrane were also noted. [16]

B. DIGITAL TECHNIQUES

Since the correlation between graders varied greatly, an attempt was made to computerize the recognition and analysis of the drusen-containing area. [15,16] Using such techniques, the macula area, which is occupied by drusen, and changes in the pattern of drusen can be determined longitudinally over time. In this system the observer has to determine the type of drusen. Other changes such as pigmentation, vascularization or atrophy have to be edited manually. The great advantage of such a system is that it records a surface area. Since soft drusen is a disseminated disease of the macula (with the areas that are more prominent seen as soft drusen), surface area measurements would appear to be more precise than simply estimating or counting the number of drusen (Fig. 1). This system was applied in one study which found reproducibility of sequential reading to be 6.1% and that of photoduplicates 2.3%. [15] With this technique it was possible to demonstrate that eyes with smaller drusen areas have mostly hard drusen, as well as to show an increase in drusen area over time. The authors also showed that eyes with larger drusen areas have soft drusen and an overall decrease in drusen area over time, thus demonstrating that drusen undergo dynamic formation and resorption over time. [16]

C. OTHER ATTEMPTS TO GRADE MACULAR CHANGES

In other systems the development of exudative or atrophic changes were assigned special grades in addition to the number of hard or soft drusen. In these studies atrophic areas were graded as smaller than, and equal or larger than a 700 μm standard. Grade 4 or 4 plus have grade 3 large confluent drusen. Grades 4,3, or plus grade 2 have small drusen ≥20 within 1500 μm of the foveal center. Grades 4,3,2 plus have 15 small drusen within 1500 μm or 10 small drusen between 1500-3000 μm. Risk factors for development of choroidal neovascularation were found to be: the presence of large and confluent drusen, soft drusen, and focal hyperpigmentation within 1500 μm of the foveal center. [17-18]. These systems are hard to reproduce and, therefore, a more standardized technique had to be developed to achieve a universal reproducible classification.

D. RECENT CLASSIFICATION METHODS

The grading system becomes slightly more complex but more arbitrary in a transition from qualitative to quantitative methods. These attempts to develop a grading method led to the most elaborate system available today, that of the Wisconsin Age-related Maculopathy Study. [19] The grading is the basis of a recently published international classification system. [20] This system reviews stereoscopic standardized photographic pairs centered on the disc and macula, also known as field 1 and 2 of the modified Airlie House classification system for diabetic retinopathy. The viewing light is standardized at 6200K (bluer than sun light). Magnification is X3 for the fundus camera and X5 for the Donaldson stereoscopic viewers (total of X15). To define the subfields in the macula, standardized grids of three circles 400, 1500 and 3000 μm, respectively, with two diagonally crossed lines are used (Fig. 2). Three sets of open circles are used to define the size of the drusen and the area involved (Fig. 3). The system takes into account the characteristics of drusen, other lesions of AMD and other associated abnormalities.

1. Drusen

Grading characteristics are size, predominant type, area and degree of confluence. Circle one used to measure size and equals $C_0 = 63$ μm; $C_1 = 125$ μm; $C_2 = 250$ μm (Fig. 3).

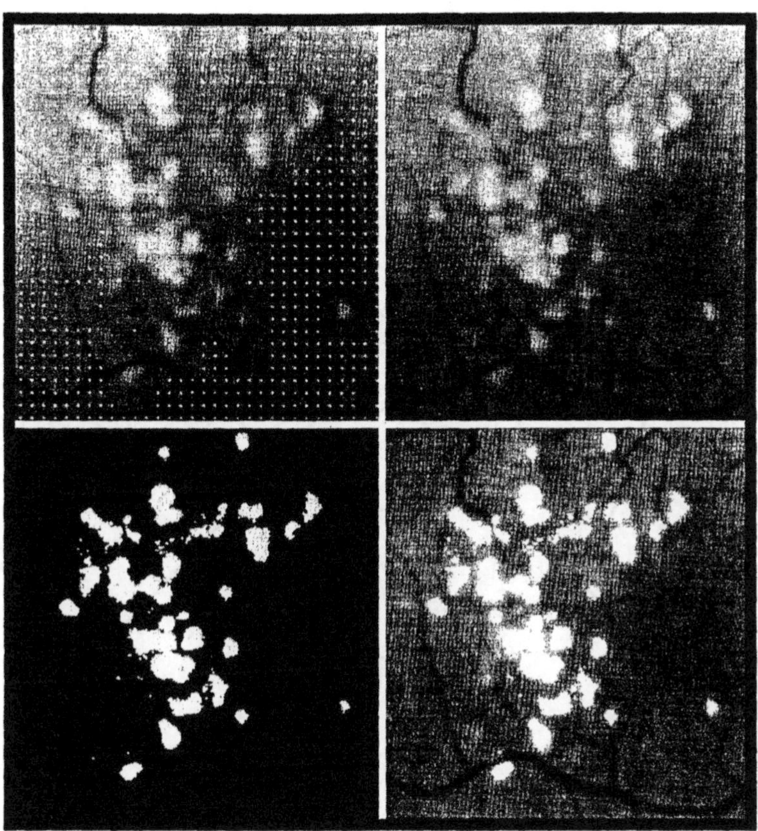

Fig. 1. Drusen detection from fundus photographs. Top right–digitized image. Top left–black dots represent areas that might contain drusen. Bottom left–the foveal processed image output indicating drusen as white and background as black. The area occupied by drusen in this image is 7.1%. Bottom right–the detected drusen superimposed on the original image (reprinted courtesy of *Ophthalmology* from Peli E. and Lahav M. Drusen measurement from fundus photographs using computer image analysis, *Ophthalmology* 93: 1575-1580, 1986.)

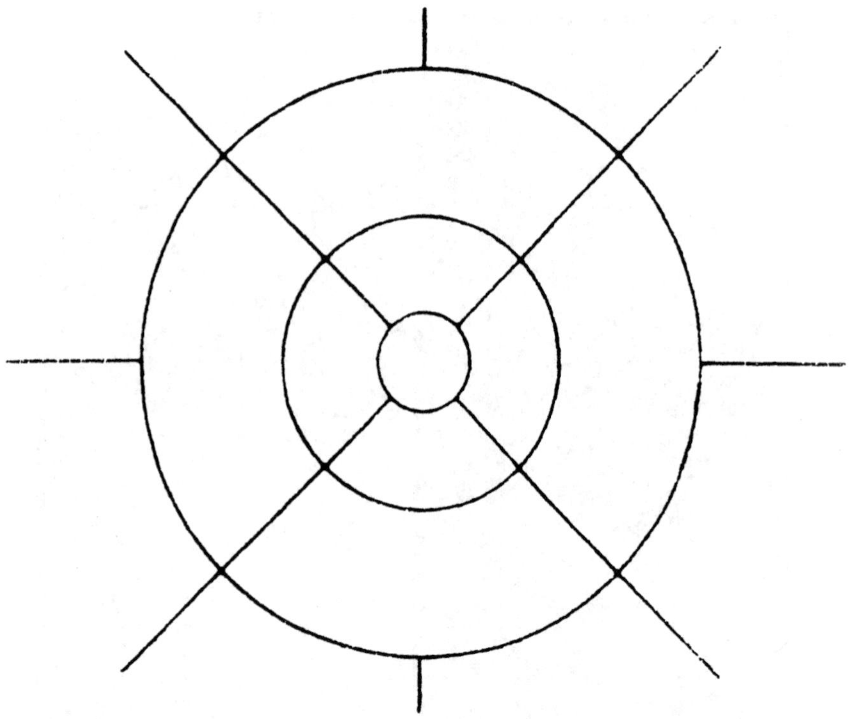

Fig. 2. Standard grid for ARM classification for a 30° fundus camera. The diameter of the central, middle and outer circle is, respectively, 1000, 3000 and 6000 μm. These circles represent, respectively, the central, middle and outer subfield. The midperipheral subfield is outside the outer circle within field 2. The spokes may be of help in centering the grid on the macula and in estimating the length of a lesion. (Reprinted courtesy of Ophthalmology from Klein R. et al. The Wisconsin age-related maculopathy grading system. *Opthhalmology* 98: 1128-1134, 1991.)

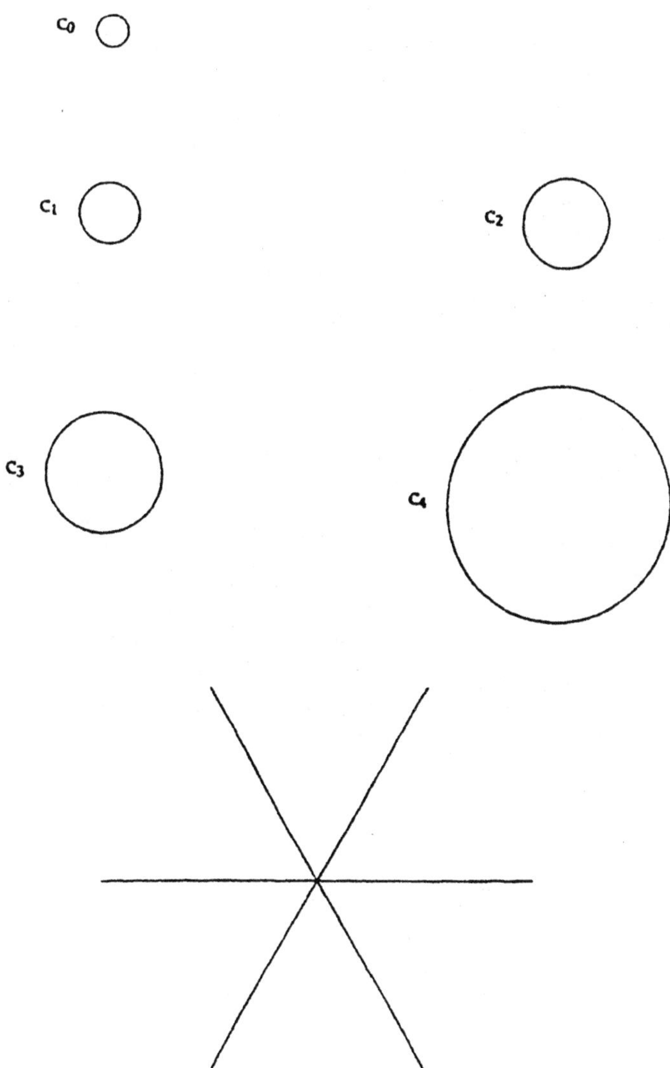

Fig. 3. Standard circles for grading of ARM-related fundus changes. The circles C_0, C_1, C_3 and C_4 are used for subfields. The circles should be reduced on a transparent sheet, according to the fundus camera used, so that they are 1/24, 1/12, 1/8.6, 1/6 and 1/3 disk diameter resulting in approximate diameters in the average fundus of 63 µm, 125 µm, 175 µm, 250 µm, and 500 µm. Note that the diameter of circle C4 is half the diameter of the inner circle on Figure 2. All circles may be used for estimation of drusen size. Circle C_0 differentiates small from large drusen. Circles C_1 and C_2 may be used for grading area involved by increased pigmentation or RPE depigmentation; C_2 for minimum area of geographic atrophy; and Circles C_2 and C_4 for area of geographic atrophy or neovascular AMD. (Reprinted courtesy of *Ophthalmology* from Klein R. et al. The Wisconsin Age-Related Maculopathy Grading System. *Ophthalmol*ogy 98: 1128-1134, 1991.)

2. Drusen Type

Grade 0=hard indistinct, 1=hard distinct drusen, 2=soft indistinct, 3=soft indistinct, 4=reticular, 5=faded, 7=cannot grade due to obscuring lesion, 8=cannot grade due to photographic quality. The type of drusen is classified mostly by the drusen size. Drusen which are less than 63 μm in diameter are classified as hard. Drusen which are 63 μm-124 μm or greater are classified as soft. There is no size requirement for faded or reticular drusen. Drusen are separated into hard-distinct and hard-indistinct. Standard photographs are used for comparison of questionable the drusen into the appropriate type. Faded drusen are classified as areas from which all the drusen material disappeared; they are distinguished from RPE degeneration by the spacing and the round or oval shape. However, if patches of confluent drusen fade, they leave larger areas called RPE degeneration.

3. Drusen Area

The drusen area is estimated in the Wisconsin system. Soft drusen is a confluent condition of the pigment epithelium-choriocapillaries complex. Therefore, the area occupied by drusen is the most important parameter to measure. Area estimation is done by percentage of the subfield 1.5 as follows: less than 10%; less than 25%; less than 50% and over 50% of the area which is occupied by drusen (Table 1). Other parameters to be graded in a qualitative way are the absence/presence and location of the hyperpigmentation or hypopigmentation (Table 2). Geographic atrophy is graded for its presence, location and the area covered by it (Table 3). Neovascular macular degeneration is graded by its presence, typical features, location and the area involved (Table 4).

Table 1
Grading of Drusen

1.1 *Drusen morphology grade highest no. present within outer circle*
- 0) absent
- 1) questionable
- 2) hard drusen (<C_1, 125 μm)
- 3) intermediate, soft drusen (>$C_0 \leq C_1$; >63 μm ≤ 125 μm)
- 4) large, soft distinct drusen (>C_0, 125μm)
- 5) large, soft indistinct drusen (>C_1, 125μm)
  - 5a) cystalline/calcified/glistening
  - 5b) semisolid
  - 5c) serogranular
- 7) cannot grade due to obscuring lesions
- 8) cannot grade due to poor photo quality

1.2 *Predominant drusen type within outer circle*
- 0) absent
- 1) questionable
- 2) hard drusen (<C_1, 125 μm)
- 3) intermediate, soft drusen (>$C_0 \leq C_1$; >63 μm ≤ 125 μm)
- 4) large, soft distinct drusen (>C_1, 125 μm)
- 5) large, soft indistinct drusen (>C_1, 125 μm)
  - 5a) crystalline/calcified/glistening
  - 5b) semisolid
  - 5c) serogranular
- 7) cannot grade due to obscuring lesions
- 8) cannot grade due to poor photo quality

1.3 *Number of drusen*
- 0) absent
- 1) questionable
- 2) 1-9
- 3) 10-19
- 4) ≥ 20
- 7) cannot grade due to obscuring lesions
- 8) cannot grade due to poor photo quality

1.4 *Drusen size*
- 1) <C_0 (<63μm)
- 2) ≥C_0 < C_1 (≥63 μm, <125 μm)
- 3) ≥ C_1 < C_2 (≥125 μm, <175 μm)
- 4) ≥ C_2 < C_3 (≥175 μm, < 250 um)
- 5) ≥ C_3 (≥250μm)
- 7) cannot grade due to obscuring lesions
- 8) cannot grade due to poor photo quality

Table 1 (continued)

1.5 *Main location of drusen.* Drusen may not be central to indicated subfield, but may be more to periphery.

- 1) outside outer circle (mid-peripheral subfield)
- 2) in outer subfield
- 3) in middle subfield
- 4) in central subfield
  - 4a) outside fovea (center point)
  - 4b) in fovea
- 7) cannot grade due to obscuring lesions
- 8) cannot grade due to poor photo quality

1.6 *Area covered by drusen in subfield 1.5*

- 1) <10%
- 2) <25%
- 3) <50%
- 4) ≥50%
- 7) cannot grade due to obscuring lesions
- 8) cannot grade due to poor photo quality

Tables 1-4 were reproduced courtesy of *Survey Ophthalmology* from An International Classification and Grading System for Age- Related Maculopathy and Age-Related Macular Degeneration. *Survey Ophthalmol.* 39, 367-374, 1995.

Table 2
Hyperpigmentation and Hypopigmentation of the Retina

Hyperpigmentation

0) absent
1) questionable
2) present < C_0 (< 63 µm)
3) present ≥ C_0 (≥63 µm)
7) cannot grade due to obscuring lesions
8) cannot grade due to poor photo quality

Hypopigmentation

0) absent
1) questionable
2) present < C_0 (<63µm)
3) present ≥ C_0 (≥ 63µm)
7) cannot grade due to obscuring lesions
8) cannot grade due to poor photo quality

Main location hyper/hypopigmentation. This may not be central to indicated subfield, but may be more to periphery. Choose most central location

1) outside outer circle (mid-peripheral subfield)
2) in outer subfield
3) in middle subfield
4) in central subfield
    4a) outside fovea (center point)
    4b) in fovea
7) cannot grade due to obscuring lesions
8) cannot grade due to poor photo quality

Table 3
Geographic Atrophy

Presence
- 0) absent
- 1) questionable
- 2) present $\geq C_2$
- 7) cannot grade due to obscuring lesions
- 8) cannot grade due to poor photo quality

Location. Choose most central location
- 1) outside outer circle (mid-peripheral subfield)
- 2) in outer subfield
- 3) in middle subfield
- 4) in central subfield
    - 4a) not in fovea (center point)
    - 4b) in fovea
- 7) cannot grade due to obscuring lesions
- 8) cannot grade due to poor photo quality

Area covered
- 1) $\geq C_2 < C_3$ ($\geq$175 μm<250 μm)
- 2) $\geq C_3 < C_4$ ($\geq$250 μm<500 μm)
- 3) $\geq C_4$ and <1000 μm and <3000 μm (~central circle of grid)
- 4) $\geq$1000 μm and <3000 μm (~middle circle)
- 5) $\geq$3000 μm and <6000 μm (~outer circle)
- 6) >6000 μm
- 7) cannot grade due to obscuring lesions
- 8) cannot grade due to poor photo quality

Table 4
Neovascular AMD

Presence
- 0) absent
- 1) questionable
- 2) present
- 7) cannot grade due to obscuring lesions
- 8) cannot grade due to poor photo quality

Typifying features
- 1) hard exudates
- 2) serous neuroretinal detachment
- 3) serous RPE detachment
- 4) hemorrhagic RPE detachment
- 5) retinal hemorrhage
  - 5a) subretinal
  - 5b) in plane of retina
  - 5c) subhyaloid
  - 5d) intravitreal
- 6) scar/glial/fibrous tissue
  - 6a) subretinal
  - 6b) preretinal
- 7) cannot grade due to obscuring lesions
- 8) cannot grade due to poor photo quality

Location. Choose most central location
- 1) outside outer circle (mid-peripheral subfield)
- 2) in outer subfield
- 3) in middle subfield
- 4) in central subfield
  - 4a) not underlying (in) fovea (center point)
  - 4b) underlying (in) fovea
- 7) cannot grade due to obscuring lesions
- 8) cannot grade due to poor photo quality

Area covered
- 1) $\geq C_2 < C_3$ (≥ 175 μm <250 μm)
- 2) $\geq C_3 < C_4$ (≥ 250 μm <500 μm)
- 3) $\geq C_4$ and <1000 μm (~central circle of grid)
- 4) ≥ 1000 μm and <3000 μm (~middle circle)
- 5) ≥ 3000 μm and <6000 μm (~outer circle)
- 6) >6000 μm
- 7) cannot grade due to obscuring lesions
- 8) cannot grade due to poor photo quality

IV. SUMMARY

The Wisconsin classification is the most comprehensive and reproducible system currently available. However, it is still semi-quantitative, thus leaving gaps for estimation and inter-observer variability. This complicated grading should be done by experienced graders in one center where the margin of disagreement is rather low. In the age of digital imaging and computing, it seems useful to identify some of those parameters which are considered pathognomonic for age-related maculopathy and try to use digital techniques to achieve a more quantitative method. The system should be constructed based on known clinical histopathological correlations so as to approximate the real nature of the pathological process rather than its most obvious manifestations such as the drusen which actually represents a widespread pathological process of the sub-retinal region. It is possible that, with more advanced visualization techniques such as Indocyanin Green Angiography, Optical Coherent Tomography or Confocal Microscopy, the underlying process can be visualized better than with conventional fundus photographs. Those techniques provide digital output that could be analyzed directly. Information which is associated with AMD will be visualized and analyzed by different diagnostic modalities, and the sum of the information will have to be integrated in a universal computerized system that will advance our knowledge of the pathogenesis, natural history and effect of treatments on the disease process.

V. REFERENCES

1. **Evans K, Gregory CY, Wijesariya SD, Kermani S, Jay ME, Plant C, Bird AC,** Assessment of the Penotypic ranges seen in Doyne Honeycomb Retina Dystrophy, *Arch. Ophthalmol.*, 115, 904-910, 1997.
2. **Heon E, Piguet B, Munier F, Need SR, Morgan CM, Forni S, Pescia G, Schorderet D, Taylor CM, Streb LM, Wiles CB, Nishimura DY, Sheffield VC, Stone EM,** Linkage of autosomal dominant radial drusen (Malattia Leventinese) to chromosome 2p 16-21, *Arch. Ophthalmol.,* 114, 193-198, 1996.
3. **Allikmets R, Schroyer NF, Singh N, Seddon JM, Lewis RA, Bernstein PS, Peiffer A, Zabriskie NA, Li Y, Hutchinson A, Dean M, Lupski JR, Leppert M,** Mutation of the Stargardts disease gene (ABCR) in age-related macular degeneration, *Science,* 277, 1805-1807, 1997.
4. **Gass DM,** Drusen and disciform macular detachment and degeneration, *Arch. Ophthalmol.*, 90, 206-217, 1973.
5. **Melrose MA, Magragal LE, Lucier AC,** Identical twins with subretinal neovascularization complicating senile macular degeneration, *Ophthalmic Surg.*, 16, 648-651, 1985.
6. **Meyers SM, Zachary AA,** Monozygotic twins with age-related macular degeneration, *Arch. Ophthalmol.*, 106, 651-653, 1988.

7. **Klein ML, Maudlin WM, Stoumbos VD,** Heredity and age-related macular degeneration: Observation in monozygotic twins, *Arch. Ophthalmol.*, 112, 932-937, 1994.
8. **Meyers SM, Green T, Gutman, FA,** A twin study of age-related macular degeneration, *Am. J. Ophthalmol.,* 120, 757-766, 1995.
9. **Heiba IM, Elston RC, Klein BEK, Klein R,** Sibling correlations and segregation analysis of age-related maculopathy. The Beaver Dam Eye Study, *Genet. Epidemiol.*, 11, 51-17, 1994.
10. **DeLa Paz MD, Fericak-Vance MA, Hains JL, Seddon JM,** Phenotypic heterogeneity in families with age-related macular degeneration, *Am. J. Ophthalmol.,*124, 331-343, 1997.
11. **Seddon JM, Ajani VA, Mitchell BD,** Familial aggregation of age-related maculopathy, *Am. J. Ophthalmol.*, 124, 199-206, 1997.
12. **Sarks SH,** Council Lecture: Drusen and their relationship to senile macular degeneration, *Aust. NZ J. Ophthalmol.*, 8, 117-130, 1980.
13. **Green WR, Enger C,** Age-related macular degeneration histopathologic studies, *Zimmerman Lecture, Ophthalmology*, 100, 1519-1535, 1993.
14. **Smiddy WE, Fine SL,** Prognosis of patients with bilateral macular drusen, *Ophthalmology*, 91, 271-277, 1984.
15. **Peli E, Lahav M,** Drusen measurement from fundus photographs using computer image analysis, *Ophthalmology*, 93, 1575-1580, 1986.
16. **Sebag M, Peli E, Lahav M,** Image analysis of changes in drusen area, *Acta Ophthalmol.*, 69, 603-610, 1991.
17. **Bressler NM, Bressler SB, West SK, Fine SL, Taylor HR,** The grading and prevalence of macular degeneration in Chesapeake Bay Watermen, *Arch. Ophthalmol.*, 107, 847-856, 1989.
18. **Mares-Perlman SA, Brady WE, Klein R, Klein BEK, Bolvea P, Stacewicz-Sapuntzakis M, Palta N,** Serum antioxidants and age-related macular degeneration in a population-based case-control study, *Arch. Ophthalmol.*, 113, 1518-1523, 1995.
19. **Klein R, Davis, MD, Maglis ML, Segal P, Klein BEK, Hubbard L,** The Wisconsin age-related maculopathy grading system, *Ophthalmology*, 98, 1128-1134, 1991.
20. **The International ARM Epidemiological Study Group,** An international classification and grading system for age-related maculopathy and age-related macular degeneration, *Survey Ophthalmol.*, 39, 367-374, 1995.

Chapter 11

DIET AND AGE-RELATED MACULAR DEGENERATION

Julie A. Mares-Perlman and Ronald Klein

I. INTRODUCTION

Age-related macular degeneration (ARMD) is a degenerative condition of the outer layers of the region of the retina that is responsible for central vision (the macula). The later stages of the condition are associated with atrophy and death of photoreceptors and sometimes the formation and leakage of new blood vessels. The late stages of this condition have been estimated to affect 640,000 Americans over 75 years of age.[1] At present, medical interventions are of limited value to persons with late stage ARMD and cannot prevent the eventual loss of vision or provide a cure. The burden of ARMD to individuals and society is expected to rise as more people survive into their seventh, eighth and ninth decades of life.[2]

Modification of diet is one of several possible lifestyle changes with the potential to delay the onset and progression of this condition. There is increasing evidence for genetic predisposition in ARMD,[3-5] which appears to be higher in prevalence in white, compared with some other non-white, populations.[6,7] However, the possibly increasing prevalence of ARMD in Japan[8] may indicate a role for dietary or environmental factors as well. This chapter will review the proposed roles for dietary factors in the pathogenesis of ARMD and discuss evidence from animal, clinical and epidemiologic research to support these roles. In order to consider roles of nutrients in the pathophysiology of ARMD, the structure of the macula and current thoughts regarding pathophysiologic changes that accompany ARMD are discussed first.

A. STRUCTURE OF THE MACULA

Lesions of ARMD occur between the layer of the retina that contains the rod and cone cells and the vascular layer in the choroid (Figure 1). The rods and cones have stacks of lipid-rich disks or outer segments that extend back into the microvillous processes of a single layer of cells that compose the retinal pigment epithelium (RPE). The photoreceptors regularly shed the disk materials, which are engulfed and digested by the RPE. The rate of digestion of these materials is high. It has been estimated that the RPE phagocytizes more than 2000 photoreceptor disk membranes daily.[9]

0-8493-8565-2/99/$0.00+$.50

Nutrients and waste products are exchanged between the RPE and its blood supply at the choriocapillaris through Bruch's membrane. Bruch's membrane, together with the RPE, serves as the blood-retinal barrier. Thus, the RPE and Bruch's membrane are important in maintaining retinal integrity.

B. CLINICAL FEATURES OF AGE-RELATED MACULAR DEGENERATION

At this time, the pathogenesis of ARMD is unknown. Theories of the pathogenesis have largely evolved from clinical and histological studies in which the pathologic features of the lesions that accompany ARMD at various stages in its natural history are described. Observations from epidemiological studies of the correlates of the incidence and progression of these lesions, and manipulations which produce similar lesions in experimental animals, have also provided further understanding of the pathogenesis of this disease.

Many of the histopathologic lesions which frequently accompany ARMD[10-15] are illustrated in Figure 2. They include (1) thickening and degenerative changes in Bruch's membrane, including the accumulation of basal laminar deposits and drusen, (2) pigmentary disturbances of the RPE, (3) atrophy of the RPE and overlying photoreceptors, and (4) neovascularization. Basal laminar deposits, which are frequently seen in the histopathological study of the eyes of patients with ARMD,[13,14] may increase with age rather than be specific to ARMD.[16] These deposits reside between the RPE and its basal lamina and are composed of amorphous and filamentous material of unknown composition.

Drusen are extracellular masses that clinically vary in size, shape, and composition. They are round, yellow to whitish-yellow deposits that are located between the basal lamina of the RPE and the inner collagenous membrane of Bruch's membrane. It is theorized that drusen result from the incomplete transport of metabolic end products from the RPE to the choriocapillaris due to one or more pathogenic mechanisms that are discussed in the following sections. While small, hard drusen are a common feature of aging and appear to be benign, large, soft, and confluent drusen are both more common with increasing age[1] and more frequently observed in patients with ARMD.[11,12,14] The presence of large, soft, and confluent drusen was observed to increase the risk for developing more severe ARMD in patients[17] and in the general population.[18] However, only some people who have large, soft drusen will ultimately develop ARMD. Drusen may also disappear.[18,19] It is not known whether this is the result of a repair process or an indicator of more severe disease.

Pigmentary disturbances that are observed in patients with ARMD include depigmentation of the RPE and hyperpigmentation, often around the periphery of depigmented zones. The presence of pigmentary change is associated with increased risk for late macular degeneration.[18,19]

Atrophy of the RPE and the overlying photoreceptors is a late stage of ARMD that is referred to as "dry" ARMD or geographic atrophy. These lesions are sometimes accompanied by the development of new blood vessels in the choroid that penetrate Bruch's membrane. Leakage from these vessels may result in the choroid that penetrate Bruch's membrane. Leakage from these vessels may result

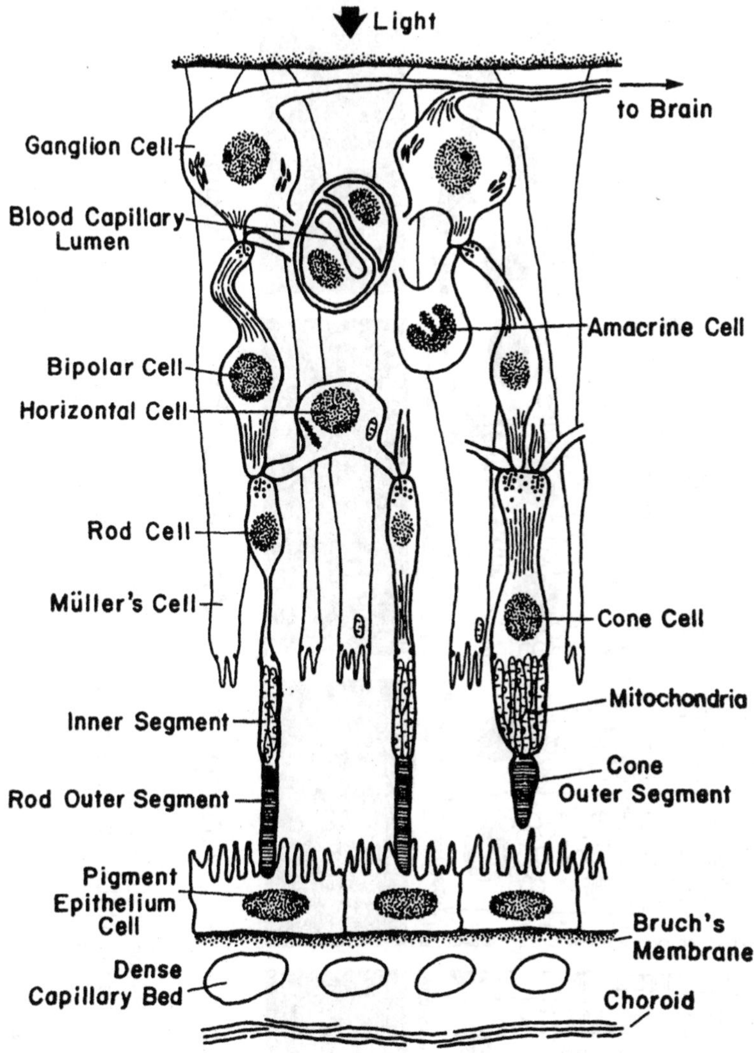

Figure 1. Simplified diagram of the cellular structures of the retina. Lesions of ARMD involve the photoreceptor layer (which includes rod and cone cells), the retinal pigment epithelium cells (RPE), Bruch's membrane and the choroidal capillaries. (From Handelman, G. J., and Dratz, E. A., The Role of Antioxidants in the Retina and Retinal Pigment Epithelium and the Nature of Prooxidant-Induced Damage in *Advances in Free Radical Biology & Medicine*, Vol. 2, Pergamon Press Ltd., Elmsford, NY, 1986.)

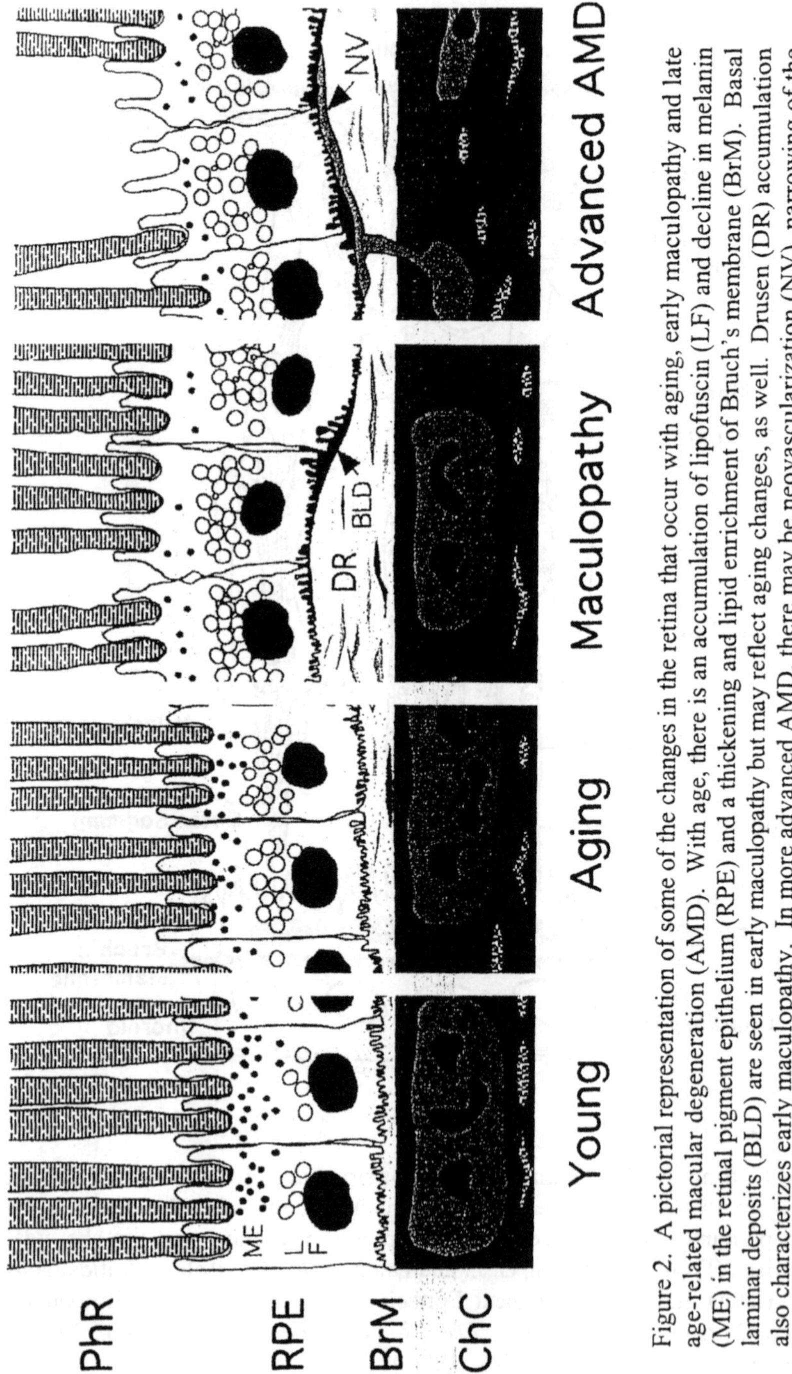

Figure 2. A pictorial representation of some of the changes in the retina that occur with aging, early maculopathy and late age-related macular degeneration (AMD). With age, there is an accumulation of lipofuscin (LF) and decline in melanin (ME) in the retinal pigment epithelium (RPE) and a thickening and lipid enrichment of Bruch's membrane (BrM). Basal laminar deposits (BLD) are seen in early maculopathy but may reflect aging changes, as well. Drusen (DR) accumulation also characterizes early maculopathy. In more advanced AMD, there may be neovascularization (NV), narrowing of the choriocapillaris (ChC), and photoreceptor (PhR) atrophy. (Reprinted with permission from Delori, F.C., Dorey, C.K., Scheppens Eye Institute, Boston, MA.)

in the detachment of the sensory retina, hemorrhage, and, ultimately, scar tissue development.

Thus, there are a variety of different lesions that are associated with age-related maculopathy. Nutrition may influence one or several of the processes that lead to the development of these lesions. Theories which link the development of these lesions into proposed sequences and indicate specific roles of nutrients in the pathogenesis of ARMD are described next.

C. THE NATURAL HISTORY AND ETIOLOGY OF AGE-RELATED MACULAR DEGENERATION

The natural history of ARMD is still under study. Most observations have been made in specialty clinics, where late stages of the disease predominate so that little is known about the progression of earlier lesions. Clinically, soft drusen, which are thought to originate from the RPE, and pigmentary abnormalities of the RPE are often observed prior to the development of atrophy of the RPE and neovascular macular degeneration.[10,17] The causes of these early lesions are likely to provide keys to the pathogenesis of ARMD. Currently, there are three main theories regarding the primary causes of the extracellular accumulation of large, soft drusen and pigmentary changes in the RPE: (1) the oxidative stress theory, (2) the impairment in choroidal circulation theory, and (3) the degradation of Bruch's membrane theory. The basis for these theories and the implications for roles of nutrients in the pathogenesis of ARMD are discussed in the following sections.

1. Oxidative Stress Theory

It has been suggested that the primary defect of ARMD is associated with an age-related disorder of the RPE. Age-related changes observed in the RPE support this hypothesis. Some changes in the RPE with age include alterations in the microvilli and basal enfoldings of the RPE cells and a thickening of their basal lamina.[20] Another age-related change is the accumulation of lipofuscin in the RPE.[20,21] Lipofuscin is thought to be composed of indigestible residues that result from the large volume of lipid-rich photoreceptor outer segments and other cellular materials that are phagocytized in the RPE. The extracellular deposits characteristic of ARMD (drusen) are thought to contain these and other RPE-derived residues. One piece of evidence in support of their RPE origin is the observation of lysosomal enzymes (of the RPE) in Bruch's membrane in eyes from persons over 80 years of age.[22] Second, the lipid content of Bruch's membrane from older adults more closely parallels that in the RPE than in the blood.[23] The accumulation of the lipid-rich residues in Bruch's membrane is hypothesized to interfere with the ability of the RPE to exchange nutrients with the choroidal capillaries, resulting in the eventual death of the RPE cells and the photoreceptors they support.

Oxidative stress is one mechanism that can lead to the accumulation and shedding of indigestible lipid-rich residues by the RPE. Oxidative stress can be induced by several factors that produce free radicals, including light exposure and oxidative metabolism. These reactive molecules, such as singlet oxygen and superoxide radicals, have an unpaired electron and need to remove an electron from other cell molecules in order to achieve a more stable state (see Chapter 2 by Varma). Protein and lipid molecules that are damaged as a result of attack by free radicals are theorized to impair the ability of RPE cells to phagocytize photoreceptor membranes and other cell substances. Mitochondrial DNA deletions due to free radical damage may also contribute to RPE malfunction.[24]

The theory that oxidative stress contributes to ARMD is based on several lines of evidence from animal and human studies. Oxidative stress is likely to occur in the macula, a structure that is particularly vulnerable to this type of damage because of its high exposure to light and the high rate of oxidative metabolism.[25] There is a high concentration of polyunsaturated fatty acids [26] which, because of the presence of double bonds, are particularly likely to participate in free radical reactions.

Evidence of retinal damage caused by light exposure is also consistent with the notion that oxidative stress contributes to ARMD. Noell[27] proposed a role for lipid oxidation in light-induced damage to the retina after observing that rat retinas can be damaged with moderate-intensity light exposure. Light exposure produces free radicals from oxygen species and other molecules.[28] Also, end products of lipid peroxidation have been observed in animal retinas exposed to intense light.[29] Chronic or intense light exposure in monkeys produces RPE and photoreceptor atrophy [30,31] and, in some cases,[30] subretinal neovascularization, which are lesions similar to those observed with ARMD. However, it is also possible that light can damage the retina via mechanisms that are independent of oxidative stress such as by thermal stress.

Several factors that are thought to increase oxidative stress have been associated with increased risk for ARMD in some epidemiologic studies. These include light exposure,[32,33] lack of pigmentation (which may protect against oxidative stress),[34-36] and smoking [35,37-42] (see Chapter 8 by H. Taylor and Chapter 9 by S. West). However, these findings, with the exception of cigarette smoking, have been inconsistent.

The theory that oxidative stress contributes to the development of ARMD is also supported by observations in animals who are deficient in nutrients with known ability to protect against oxidative stress. Deficiency of vitamin E has been shown to increase retinal damage due to light exposure,[43,44] while supplementation with or injections of vitamin C[45-47] or synthetic antioxidants[48,49] have been shown to reduce retinal damage.Lower levels of antioxidant enzymes havebeen observed in the red blood cells (superoxide dismutase and glutathione peroxidase)[50] or RPE cells (catalase)[51] of people with ARMD compared to similarly aged people without ARMD. Calorie restriction, which is theorized to reduce oxidative stress by lowering the rate of oxidative metabolism, also results in a decline in lipofuscin accumulation in the rat retina.[52]

Thus, several factors which are associated with increased oxidative stress are also associated with increased short-term light damage to the retina in experimental animals and/or risk for ARMD in humans. Consequently, nutrients with roles in protection against oxidative stress are hypothesized to protect against ARMD. However, to date, there are no direct measures of oxidative stress and its relationship to the onset of ARMD. At this time, the relationship between oxidative stress and ARMD remains unproven.

2. Impairment in Choroidal Circulation Theory

As early as 1937, Verhoeff and Grossman[53] proposed that sclerotic disturbance of the choriocapillaris in the macular region contributed to ARMD. Friedman[64] suggests that age-related arteriosclerotic processes lead to hemodynamic changes in the choroidal circulation that may initiate RPE degeneration by reducing the ability to dispose of metabolic waste. Thus, nutrients which protect against arteriosclerotic or capillary degeneration might also protect against ARMD. Changes in the choriocapillaris have been observed in patients with ARMD and include a thickening of the intercapillary septa and a narrowing of the lumen of capillaries.[55] Duke-Elder [55] theorized that narrowing of the choriocapillaris, due to arteriosclerotic changes similar to those that occur with cardiovascular disease, limited the exchange of nutrients between the RPE and its blood supply. This theory is supported by evidence of delayed choroidal perfusion in some patients with ARMD[57] and the recent observation of almost 5 times higher risk for ARMD in persons with atherosclerotic plaques on the bifurcation of the carotid artery.[58] It is also supported by observations of higher rates of ARMD among people with a history of stroke in some studies[35,59] and among people with risk factors for cardiovascular disease such as smoking,[35,37-41] high blood cholesterol,[60] and low estrogen exposure. [60] However, data from epidemiologic studies are not consistent in this regard.[61-64]

The possibility that changes in the choriocapillaris are initiating events in ARMD has also been called into question. Garner[65] suggests that degradation of the choriocapillaris occurs secondarily to RPE degeneration rather than as a primary initiating event in ARMD. Glaser[66] observed that a growth factor produced by the RPE modulates the structure and function of the choriocapillaris. Deposits and thickening of Bruch's membrane could limit the diffusion of this growth factor to the choroid, leading to sclerosis of the choriocapillaris. Regardless of whether blood vessel degeneration is a primary initiating event or a contributing event, nutrients which influence integrity of the choroidal vasculature may influence the development of ARMD by influences on vascular pathology.

3. Degradation of Bruch's Membrane Theory

A third theory for the pathogenesis of ARMD is that degradative changes in Bruch's membrane compromise retinal integrity and initiate or contribute to ARMD. With age, Bruch's membrane thickens, especially on the choroidal side. Abnormal collagen formations, calcification, and hyalinization of Bruch's membrane are observed.[67,68] There is an increase in the quantity of lipids in Bruch's membrane with age[23,69] and a higher concentration in the macular area[23] where photoreceptors are concentrated compared with more peripheral areas of the retina.

These changes are hypothesized to contribute to the decrease in the hydraulic permeability of Bruch's membrane with age and may compromise the exchange of nutrients, fluids, and metabolic end-products between the RPE and choroid.[70] These age-related changes may play a role in the pathogenesis of ARMD.

The appearance of leukocytes, macrophages or multi-nucleated giant cells in relation to Bruch's membrane in patients with ARMD[71-74] has led to the theory that cells of the immune system contribute to the degradation of Bruch's membrane and also to subretinal neovascularization. It has been proposed that macrophages which are attracted to debris may accumulate as a reaction to the accumulation of lipids and metabolic end-products from the RPE.[74] The secretion of collagenase and elastase by macrophages[75] may contribute to the erosion of this membrane that is rich in collagen and elastin. The eroded membrane may permit the entry of larger destructive molecules, interfere with nutrient and oxygen exchange and/or establish a break for subretinal neovascularization. These changes in Bruch's membrane have been suggested[71] to alter the balance of angiogenic promoting and inhibiting factors, possibly leading to neovascularization, which is characteristic of later stages of some types of ARMD. Evidence for the involvement of the immune system in neovascularization also includes the recent observation of an increase in major histocompatibility complex class II immunoreactivity on retinal vascular elements in aged eye donors, particularly in those with ARMD, compared with younger donors.[76]

It has been suggested that ARMD etiology is multifactorial.[30] Several factors, including oxidative stress to the RPE, damage to choroidal circulation and age-related degradation of Bruch's membrane, are likely to contribute to the pathogenesis of ARMD through damage to both the RPE and choriocapillaris. The heterogeneity of the histopathologic features of ARMD[12] is consistent with a multifactorial condition. Observations that nutrients and other diet components may influence a variety of these processes that could increase risk for ARMD provide evidence of biologic plausibility for a role of nutrients in the prevention of several lesions associated with this condition. The following section describes evidence for specific nutrients.

II. EVIDENCE FOR ROLE OF DIETARY FACTORS IN THE PATHOGENESIS OF AGE-RELATED MACULAR DEGENERATION

A. SCIENTIFIC APPROACHES TO UNDERSTANDING ROLES OF NUTRITIONAL FACTORS IN AGE-RELATED MACULAR DEGENERATION

The evidence to support possible roles of nutritional factors comes primarily from two types of scientific inquiry: experimental studies in animals and epidemiologic studies in people. Experiments on the effects of changing nutrient availability on short-term retinal change in animals or cultured retinal cells provide proof of biologic mechanisms by which nutrients may exert protective effects.

The following discussion will describe animal studies that have demonstrated that changes in nutrient availability can alter short-term light damage or biochemical mechanisms integral to the proper function of the RPE and Bruch's membrane. However, the potential impact of these nutrients on the long-term development of ARMD in people is difficult to evaluate for several reasons. Adaptive mechanisms may result in physiologic differences between short-term effects observed in experimental animals and long-term effects which result in the development of ARMD over several decades. Evidence of such adaptive mechanisms has been demonstrated in rats raised under bright light. In this condition, levels of the fatty acid most vulnerable to oxidative stress are decreased in photoreceptor outer segments and levels of antioxidants and antioxidant enzymes are increased.[77]

An additional aspect of animal experiments that limits the ability to generalize to the human condition is the use of extremely high or low levels of antioxidants administered in the diet or intraperitoneally. The effects of extreme variations in antioxidant availability may not parallel the effects of more moderate variations in antioxidant variability that are likely through dietary variations in the human population. A final consideration is that there is no direct evidence that the physiologic changes and anatomic lesions that are studied in animals are similar to those that lead to late ARMD in humans. While there is a population of free-ranging rhesus monkeys with age-related drusen in whom one case of late-stage ARMD was recently reported,[78] models of late-stage ARMD are not generally available.

For these reasons, epidemiologic studies are a critical complementary approach to understanding the relationship of nutrition to ARMD in people. The characteristics of the larger observational studies which evaluate nutritional factors and the occurrence of ARMD[59,79-85] are indicated in Table 1. Due to the greater possibility for false-positive and false-negative results in smaller studies, studies with fewer than 100 people were not included.

It is important to evaluate epidemiologic evidence across several studies rather than from single studies alone. Relationships of specific nutrient factors to ARMD that are consistent across studies that utilize different populations and study different ARMD lesions are less likely to be the result of chance or bias. This is because the types of bias that could influence results of single studies are often not similar across different studies. In case-control studies, selection bias can result if controls have diets that differ from the general population. Recall bias can also result in cohort studies of prevalent or existing ARMD if patients with this condition remember their long-term diets differently than those without this condition. Results of cohort studies, in which diet is assessed before newly developing ARMD, are prone to the fewest of these types of biases but can be biased if people who drop out over time had different diets and rates of ARMD than those who remain. To date, there are only data from one such prospective study (Beaver Dam)[85] where the relationship of diet to the development of early ARMD, over five years, was assessed. The ability to generalize the results of this study is limited by its short-term nature and the insufficient number of people who develop late-stage ARMD, limiting the evaluation of the long-term consequences of diet factors that were related to earlier stages of ARMD. Thus, it is important to evaluate a body of evidence from multiple studies to gain reliable insights about roles of diet in ARMD.

The body of epidemiologic evidence that has accumulated to date is not yet large. Therefore, the overall evidence should be considered to be preliminary. Nevertheless, observational studies conducted to date have provided some interesting insights about the potential relationships of diet to ARMD, particularly when integrated with biologic mechanisms for nutrient action suggested by animal experiments. Data from both types of scientific inquiries will be discussed in the following paragraphs.

B. DIETARY COMPONENTS WITH ROLES IN OXIDATIVE STRESS

There are three groups of diet components that may affect oxidative stress in the retina. One group is composed of nutrients and non-nutritive food components that can scavenge reactive oxygen molecules and other free radicals and convert them to nonreactive compounds. These are referred to as antioxidants. A second class of diet components includes certain carotenoid plant pigments that comprise macular pigment that may reduce oxidative stress by absorbing blue light and reducing the number of reactive oxygen species formed. A third group includes dietary fatty acids that could influence susceptibility to oxidative stress. Long-chain polyunsaturated fatty acids that are present in photoreceptor outer segments and other membranes are susceptible to attack by free radicals and further the generation of reactive species because of the presence of double bonds. Evidence to support a relationship of these groups of food components to ARMD is discussed next.

Table 1. Epidemiologic Studies of Associations Between Nutrition and Age-Related Macular Degeneration (ARMD).

Design	Study	Sample	Age Range at Baseline	ARMD Endpoints	Nutrition Data
Case-Control	Eye Disease Case-Control Study (EDCCS)[59,79]	421 recruited cases, 615 controls, matched on age, sex, clinic	55-80	Newly diagnosed neovascular/exudative macular degeneration assessed in fundus photographs	Serum carotenoids, vitamins C, E and Zinc
Case-Control	Eye Disease Case-Control Study (EDCCS)[80]	356 cases and 520 age, sex, and clinic matched controls who completed diet questionnaires	55-80	Neovascular/exudative macular degeneration assessed from fundus photographs	Diet assessed from a 66-item food frequency questionnaire
Case-Control	United Kingdom (UK)[81]	65 randomly selected cases, 65 age and sex matched controls	66-87	Any ARMD (mostly early) assessed in fundus exams	Serum carotenoids and α-tocopherol
Cohort Study of Existing ARMD	First National Health & Nutrition Examination Survey (NHANES I)[58]	3,082 persons from a national probability sample who underwent ocular examinations	45-74	Any ARMD assessed in ocular exams	Diet vitamin A and C assessed with food frequency questions and 24-hour recall
Cohort Study of Existing ARMD	Baltimore Longitudinal Study of Aging (BLSA)[82]	827 volunteers	40 +	Any ARMD and late ARMD assessed in fundus exams	Plasma β-carotene, vitamin E, vitamin C (collected 2 or more years before eye exams)
Cohort Study of Existing ARMD	Beaver Dam Nutritional Factor in Eye Disease Study (BDES)[83,143]	1,968 randomly selected participants from the Beaver Dam Eye Study population-based cohort	45-86	Any early ARMD, soft, indistinct drusen, pigmentary abnormalities, and any late ARMD assessed from fundus photographs	Diet in distant past assessed retrospectively with a 100-item food frequency questionnaire
Nested Case-Control Study of Existing ARMD	Beaver DamNutritional Factor in Eye Disease Study (BDES)[84]	167 randomly relected cases with pigment abnormalities and soft drusen or worse ARMD, and controls matched on age, sex, and current smoking status	43-86	Any ARMD (mostly early) assessed from fundus photographs	Nonfasting blood level of individual carotenoids, γ-tocopherol and α-tocopherol
Prospective Cohort	Beaver Dam Nutritional Factor in Eye Disease Study (BDES)[85]	1,586 persons in baseline diet study who participated in 5-year follow-up eye examinations	43-86	Incident early ARMD, large drusen, and pigmentary abnormalities assessed from fundus photographs	Dietary intake at baseline and distant past assessed from a 100-item food frequency questionnaire

1. Antioxidants

Some nutrients can directly quench free radicals (vitamins C and E and carotenoids). While many non-nutritive plant constituents can also be antioxidants,[86] there are no data regarding the existence of non-nutritive food chemicals in the retina. Antioxidant nutrients that predominate in lipid-rich segments of the cell include vitamin E[87-89] and carotenoids.[90-91] Vitamin C is abundant in the retina, although more so in the inner neural retina than in RPE cells.[92] The consequences of manipulating the availability of these compounds on retinal lesions in animals are described below.

a. *Vitamin E*

The concentration of vitamin E in the retina is high,[87] particularly in the rod outer segments[88,89] and RPE.[89] Furthermore, vitamin E intake in the rat results in increased vitamin E concentration in retinal photoreceptors.[89] The degree to which the availability of vitamin E influences light-induced or long-term retinal damage in experimental animals is inconsistent. Rats deficient in vitamin E show evidence of more retinal damage than those supplied with vitamin E in some,[43] but not all, studies.[93,94] Dogs [95] and monkeys [44] fed vitamin E deficient diets for several years accumulate lipofuscin in the RPE and show photoreceptor loss. These are lesions that are also associated with ARMD in humans, although it is not clear that the pathologic conditions in these animals are identical to those observed in humans with ARMD. While retinal damage is often observed with vitamin E deficiency, vitamin E supplementation did not protect against light damage in one study in rats.[93]

An increase in vitamin E levels in the retina or rod outer segments[96] has been observed in response to a period of constant light exposure. This suggests that the retina may have the ability to modulate the concentration of vitamin E to protect against light damage. This may explain some inconsistency in relationships between vitamin E status and light damage in experimental animal studies.

Vitamin E may influence longer-term degenerative changes in humans by influencing other processes that lead to degradation of Bruch's membrane or the retinal vasculature. For example, the adhesion of monocytes to vascular endothelium in people treated with alpha-tocopherol is less than the adhesion of monocytes in untreated subjects.[97] Thus, one could speculate that vitamin E may influence the adhesion of immunologic cells which can degrade Bruch's membrane or vascular endothelium.

A link between retinal degeneration and vitamin E availability, suggested by studies of people with an inherited defect in the synthesis of beta-lipoproteins (abetalipoproteinemia), has been previously discussed by Handelman and Dratz.[98] In this condition, fat-soluble vitamins are not transferred efficiently into the intestinal lymph for absorption. This disease, if untreated, results in changes in the retina in which lipofuscin deposits have been observed in the macula.[99] Supplements containing vitamin E [100,101] prevented chronic retinal degeneration in patients with this condition. However, supplements containing other fat-soluble vitamins without vitamin E did not prevent retinal degeneration.[100] This suggests a role for vitamin E in preventing one type of non-age-related retinal degeneration in humans.

The majority of epidemiologic studies of relationships between vitamin E and ARMD[79-85] have observed a lower risk for ARMD associated with higher levels of this vitamin in the diet or serum,[79,82-85] although these relationships were often not statistically significant (Figure 3). There has been only one study in which higher levels of vitamin E was significantly related to lower risk for ARMD.[82]

Although significant inverse relationships with dietary vitamin E have not been reported in epidemiologic studies to date, several features of dietary vitamin E and its measurement could have contributed to a difficulty in detecting potentially important relationships. For example, the long-term intake of oils, in which the vitamin E content varies considerably, is difficult to determine with diet questionnaires. Change in cooking oils used is common and people are often unaware of changes in oils in processed foods made by the food industry. Also, bioavailability of vitamin E in supplements, which contributes to the total vitamin E intake, varies considerably.[102] Both of these factors could contribute to misclassification of vitamin E intake which may attenuate risk estimates. Larger studies (which lessen the impact of measurement error) and attempts to minimize misclassification are needed to better evaluate relationships of vitamin E status to the development of ARMD.

In future studies, an ability to detect potentially important relationships of vitamin E intake to ARMD may be increased by the use of strategies to take into account exposure to different types of vitamin E compounds. Vitamin E in foods is largely in the form of gamma-tocopherol, whereas that in supplements is usually alpha-tocopherol. Simply totaling the alpha-tocopherol equivalents of vitamin E from two sources may contribute to inaccuracies in assessing the relationship between vitamin E and ARMD. Recent evidence suggests that gamma-tocopherol may have greater activity in some physiologic functions than alpha-tocopherol[103] and that high intake of alpha-tocopherol (such as in a supplement) could reduce the concentration of gamma tocopherol in plasma and tissues.[104] Therefore, dietary estimates which simply sum dietary alpha-tocopherol equivalents (from both alpha- and gamma-tocopherols) and supplemental sources of alpha-tocopherol may not accurately reflect exposure to all protective vitamin E compounds. Consistent with this, VandenLangenberg et al.[85] observed that after excluding people who do not use supplements (which minimizes potential misclassification of vitamin E exposure in supplement users), past dietary vitamin E was related to lower incidence of large drusen, one early macular lesion that increases risk for developing late-stage ARMD (odds ratio [OR]: 0.4; 95% confidence interval [CI] = 0.2-0.9; p-trend = 0.04) for highest versus lowest quintile. A weaker and non-significant association was observed if people who took vitamin E in supplements were included and intake of vitamin E from both sources was summed (OR: 0.6; CI = 0.3-1.2; p-trend = 0.16). This difference may reflect inaccuracies resulting from simple summation of the alpha-tocopherol equivalents of different vitamin E compounds in food and supplements. Because of the different biologic activities of different tocopherol compounds, the measurement of exposure to different dietary tocopherols may be enhanced by considering intakes of different tocopherol sources separately, when possible.

An adjustment for overall intake of polyunsaturated fats may also be important to accurately assess vitamin E exposure. This is because the need for vitamin E depends, in part, on the amount of polyunsaturated fatty acids in the diet.[105] The association between the intake of dietary vitamin E and the incidence of large drusen was strengthened, in the Beaver Dam Eye Study,[85] by adjusting for the intake of linoleic acid, a major source of polyunsaturated fat in the diet (OR for high versus low quintiles: 0.4; CI = 0.2-0.9 compared with 0.2; CI = 0.1-0.6 after the adjustment for linoleic acid, a major source of polyunsaturated fat).

Thus, in summary, the overall support for a relationship between vitamin E intake and ARMD in epidemiologic studies is, to date, somewhat consistent (in direction) but weak. However, this may be due, in part, to the difficulty in assessing exposure to vitamin E compounds using traditional approaches. Future epidemiologic studies may increase the opportunity to assess the potentially important relationships of vitamin E intake to ARMD by separately considering the exposure to different types of vitamin E compounds and by adjusting for the overall intake of polyunsaturated fat.

b. *Vitamin C*

Evidence that vitamin C may protect against light damage has been provided in studies of animals that were supplemented with vitamin C. Several studies have shown that supplementing rats with vitamin C both increases the retinal level of vitamin C and decreases the amount of light-induced retinal damage relative to unsupplemented rats.[45-47] There is very little evidence of the specific mechanisms by which vitamin C may prevent oxidant damage in the retina. Vitamin C may participate with other antioxidants such as vitamin E[106] or melanin[107] in electron transfer reactions that reduce oxidative stress.

Significant associations between vitamin C in the diet or serum and ARMD have not been observed in epidemiologic studies[59,79,80,82,83,85] to date. The observation of consistent inverse, but non-significant associations (Figure 4), suggests the possibility that associations with vitamin C, if they exist, may be too weak to detect with the current smaller sizes of populations studied. Larger studies need to be conducted before an inverse relationship with vitamin C can be dismissed.

c. *Carotenoids*

Two of the six carotenoids that are abundant in human plasma are concentrated in the retina. The carotenoid lutein is spread diffusely throughout the macula, whereas its stereoisomer, zeaxanthin, is concentrated in the fovea center.[90] Carotenoids, besides those comprising macular pigments, are not normally detectable in the retina.[91]

Nevertheless, high-dose oral supplements of beta-carotene have been observed to increase retinal levels in one study.[108] In this study, beta-carotene supplements did not reduce photoreceptor loss in light exposed rats but appeared to reduce RPE destruction.

The xanthophyll carotenoids (lutein and its stereoisomer zeaxanthin) comprise macular pigment,[109] the yellow spot located at the macula. They are two of several pigments in the retina that can absorb blue light.[110] They also quench reactive oxygen species after light exposure.[111] It is currently hypothesized that the concen-

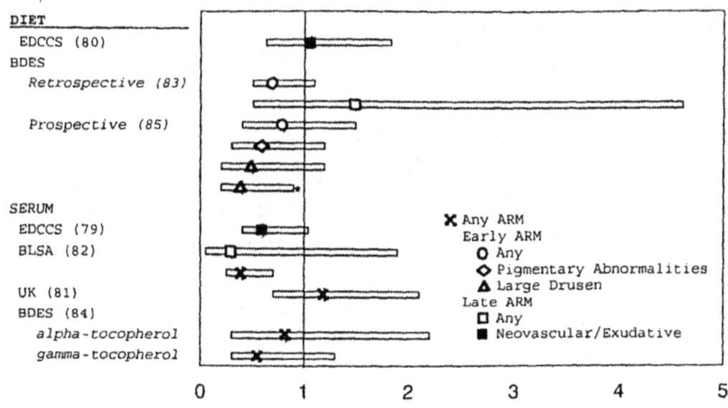

Figure 3. Summary of adjusted odds ratios and 95% confidence intervals for age-related macular degeneration among persons with high versus low vitamin E in diet or serum in epidemiologic studies (listed in Table 1). Vitamin E levels in the diet reflect α-tocopherol equivalents of all dietary and supplemental tocopherols. Vitamin E levels in the serum reflect α-tocopherol only unless otherwise specified.

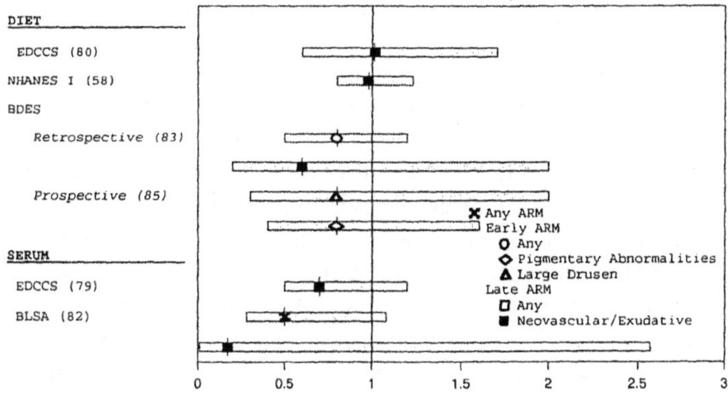

Figure 4. Summary of adjusted odds ratios and 95% confidence intervals for age-related macular degeneration among persons with high versus low vitamin C in diet or serum in epidemiologic studies (listed in Table 1).

trations of these pigments in the retina can influence risk for ARMD. (See Chapter 12 for a more detailed discussion of carotenoids in the retina and Chapter 13 for a discussion of methods to quantify these constituents).

The first research that suggested that carotenoid pigment could influence retinal damage that is characteristic of ARMD was conducted in macaque monkeys fed diets devoid of plant pigments.[112] Feeding these diets for almost six years resulted in diminished macular pigment and the accumulation of drusen. The degree to which these diet changes promote ARMD characterized by progressive photoreceptor loss and neovascularization cannot be determined in experimental animals because this late-stage condition is, to date, unique to humans. Furthermore, because the carotenoid-free diets fed were also high in vegetable fat, it is not possible to distinguish between the effects of these two dietary changes in this experiment.

A protective role of the macular pigment is suggested by maculopathies in humans such as bull's eye maculopathy, caused by intake of the drug chloroquinine, which acts as a photosensitizer. In this condition[113] and in light-exposed monkeys,[31] the fovea which contains macular pigment is spared the degenerative changes that are noted in more peripheral areas of the retina.

Evidence that genetic or environmental factors may influence macular pigment density is provided by observations that the level of lutein and zeaxanthin in human autopsy specimens[90] and monkeys[114] varies considerably among individuals, although it is fairly constant between fellow eyes. Hammond et al. observed that macular pigment density varied among monozygotic twins,[115] suggesting that environmental or dietary factors may influence macular pigment density.

Several recent studies suggest that diet can alter macular pigment density in people. Landrum and Bone demonstrated increases in macular pigment density with high-dose lutein supplements for 140 days.[116] The intake of foods that are high in lutein can also increase macular pigment levels.[117] However, variability among individuals in the enhancement of macular pigment with diet intake in this study suggests that other factors may determine the ability to concentrate these carotenoids in the macula.

Relationships between ARMD and one or more carotenoids in the diet or blood have been investigated in five different epidemiology study samples[59,79-85] (Figure 5, Figure 6, and Figure 7). The pro-vitamin A carotenoids, alpha- and beta-carotene and cryptoxanthin, are hydrocarbon carotenoids that can be converted in the body to vitamin A. One or more of these carotenoids have been related to ARMD in each of the three populations[59,80,83,85] in which relationships of these components in diets to ARMD were investigated. This is despite the fact that these carotenoids cannot be found in the macula.[91] Therefore, any protective effects, if present, would most likely be exerted by their influence on systemic factors, such as on oxidant stress in the blood. Goldberg et al.[58] first identified a 40% lower estimated risk of ARMD among persons in the NHANES I cohort eating more than seven fruits and vegetables rich in vitamin A per week, compared with those eating these foods less than once per week. Pro-vitamin A carotenoids were related to the five-year incidence of specific macular lesions in the Beaver Dam Eye Study.[85] High intake of these carotenoids was related to a two-fold lower incidence of large drusen over

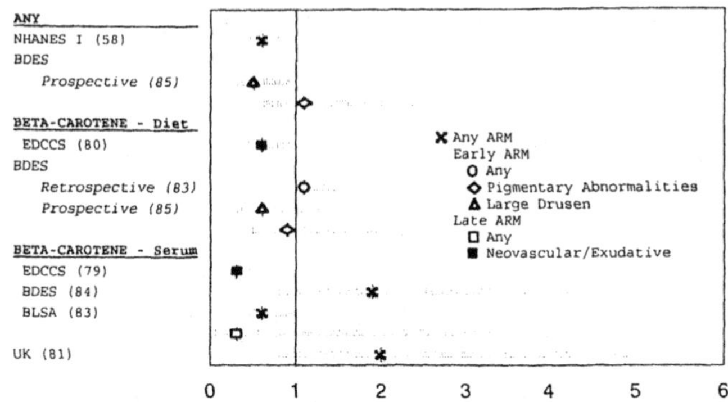

Figure 5. Summary of adjusted odds ratios and 95% confidence intervals for age-related macular degeneration among persons with high versus low levels of pro-vitamin A carotenoids in diet or serum in epidemiologic studies (listed in Table 1).

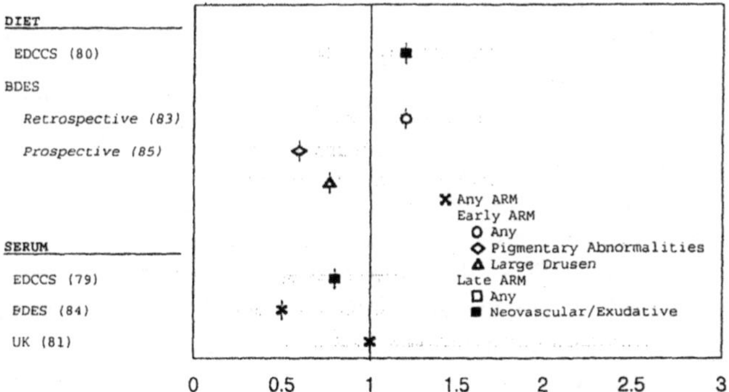

Figure 6. Summary of adjusted odds ratios and 95% confidence intervals for age-related macular degeneration amonpersons with high versus low levels of lycopene in diet or serum in epidemiologic studies (listed in Table 1).

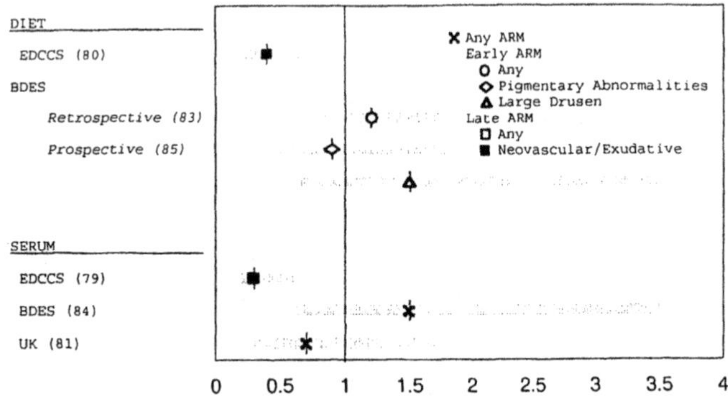

Figure 7. Summary of adjusted odds ratios and 95% confidence intervals for age-related macular degeneration among persons with high versus low levels of lutein/zeaxanthin in diet or serum in epidemiologic studies (listed in Table 1).

five years. Because retinol (pre-formed vitamin A) was not related to this (or to any form of ARMD), this relationship with pro-vitamin A carotenoids probably does not reflect a protective association with vitamin A, per se, but with these individual carotenoids or other diet or non-dietary factors related to their intake. The association between incident large drusen and pro-vitamin A carotenoids was weakened after adjusting for the frequency of fruits and vegetables consumed. Similarly, relationships with single pro-vitamin A carotenoids and ARMD that were observed in the EDCCS[80] did not persist after adjustment for dietary levels of macular carotenoids, lutein, and zeaxanthin. This indicates that associations with pro-vitamin A carotenoids in some studies may reflect protective influences of other diet constituents.

The measurement of serum levels of carotenoids has some advantages in epidemiologic studies because it bypasses the need to estimate the carotenoid composition of foods using incomplete databases[118] and accounts for the large variability in the degree to which dietary carotenoids are absorbed among people.[119] However, associations between pro-vitamin A carotenoids in the serum and ARMD are even less consistent than associations with diet (Figure 5). Levels of beta-carotene in the serum have been related to both higher[81,84] and lower[79,82] rates of ARMD in epidemiologic studies. These results were not statistically significant except in one case-control study.[79] The instability of these relationships might be explained by the study design. Higher (non-significant) blood levels of carotenoids were associated with higher risk for ARMD only in those studies in which levels

ARMD in epidemiologic studies. These results were not statistically significant except in one case-control study.[79] The instability of these relationships might be explained by the study design. Higher (non-significant) blood levels of carotenoids were associated with higher risk for ARMD only in those studies in which levels in serum were assessed at the same time as ARMD was assessed.[81,84] Because levels of carotenoids in blood reflect recent, rather than long-term intake, the direct associations could reflect a greater likelihood of people with ARMD to have recently increased their intake of fruits and vegetables.

In future studies, it may be possible to evaluate whether carotenoids protect against only certain stages or types of ARMD. In the Beaver Dam population, the intake of pro-vitamin A carotenoids was related to the incidence of large drusen but not to the incidence of pigmentary abnormalities[85] or to overall prevalent early or late ARMD[83] (Figure 5). Few other published papers report associations of diet with specific lesions of ARMD. Thus, little is known about the relationships of diet to specific types or stages of ARMD.

Because lycopene is better able than other carotenoids to quench singlet oxygen (a reactive-oxygen species prevalent in light-exposed tissues like the retina),[120] a protective relationship between lycopene intake and ARMD could be hypothesized. However, lycopene has not been detected in the human retina.[91] A higher risk for ARMD was observed among a sample of Beaver Dam Eye Study participants below the 20th percentile for serum lycopene compared with those above that level.[84] However, a statistically significant association with lycopene was not observed when comparing those in the highest versus lowest quintile and was not observed in other studies[79-81,83-85] (Figure 6).

Relationships between the intake of carotenoids that compose macular pigment and ARMD have been inconsistent in epidemiologic studies[79-81,83-85] (Figure 7). An association between the dietary intake [80] and serum levels[79] of lutein and ARMD was first observed in a large case-control study of newly diagnosed neovascular ARMD. This association has not been observed in the Beaver Dam Eye Study[83-85] or in the small case-control eye study in the United Kingdom.[81] The inconsistency among studies may be due to different ranges in carotenoid intakes between samples. The intakes or serum levels of controls in the EDCCS were higher than in the Beaver Dam or United Kingdom populations. The inconsistency among studies may also be due to the stage of ARMD studied. Late neovascular, exudative macular degeneration was studied in the EDCCS, and earlier stages of ARMD predominated in the Beaver Dam and United Kingdom samples.

d. *Nutrient Cofactors of Antioxidant Enzymes*

In addition to the role of nutrients as direct antioxidants, other nutrients including essential minerals (i.e., zinc, copper, selenium, iron, and riboflavin) may influence oxidative stress indirectly by their involvement in oxidant defense enzyme systems. A simplified diagram of these interrelated enzyme systems is given in Figure 8. These enzyme systems work in concert to quench free radicals and other reactive oxygen species such as superoxide anion free radical ($O_2^{\bullet -}$) and hydrogen peroxide (H_2O_2) that are produced as a result of energy metabolism and light exposure.

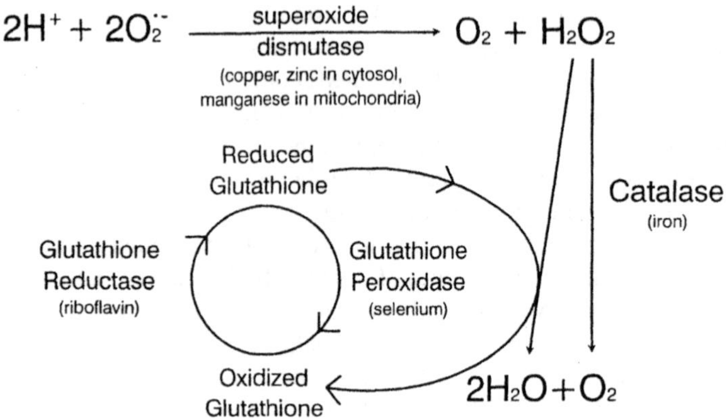

Figure 8. A simplified description of the roles of key enzymes of oxidant defense and nutrients which influence their activity. Superoxide radical ($O_2^{\cdot -}$) and hydrogen peroxide (H_2O_2) are some of the reactive oxygen molecules that are formed from light exposure and oxidative metabolism that are quenched by an interrelated series of antioxidant enzymes (superoxide dismutase, catalase, glutathione peroxidase and glutathione reductase) shown in this diagram. Activity of these enzymes require adequate levels of the indicated nutrient cofactors indicated in parentheses.

Superoxide dismutase catalyzes the quenching of superoxide anion free radicals. Two forms of superoxide dismutase are found in human RPE, including the cytosolic form that requires zinc and copper as cofactors, and the mitochondrial form that requires manganese.[121] The quenching of superoxide anions in these reactions forms H_2O_2 as a product.

Two enzymes convert H_2O_2 to nontoxic products. These include catalase and glutathione peroxidase. Catalase activity is high in the RPE and declines with age.[51] Catalase requires iron as a cofactor. Furthermore, adequate diet levels of zinc and copper are required for proper functioning of this enzyme.[122] Glutathione peroxidases in the retina can also convert hydrogen peroxide to nontoxic products. All of the glutathione peroxidase activity of the human retina is dependent on selenium.[123] The hydrogen for this reaction is donated by glutathione, a molecule made from amino acids. Regeneration of reduced glutathione requires another enzyme, glutathione reductase, which requires riboflavin as a cofactor.

Deficiency of these nutrient cofactors of antioxidant enzymes may result in a lower ability to quench free radicals by these systems. While nutrients cofactors or components of antioxidant enzymes need to be present at certain baseline levels to permit enzyme activity, higher levels of nutrient cofactors do not influence enzyme activity. Therefore, if adequate levels of these nutrients are available in the diet, additional levels (such as by supplementation) will not confer additional protection through this mechanism.

To date, studies of the retinal content of nutrient cofactors of enzymes and the consequences of low intake have mainly focused on zinc. Zinc, which is a cofactor for cytosolic superoxide dismutase and is required for optimal catalase activity,[124] has a concentration in the retina and choroid that exceeds those elsewhere in the body.[125] However, this mineral has numerous biochemical roles besides those in oxidant defense. For example, zinc is involved in the activity of alpha-mannosidase, a lysosomal enzyme of the retinal pigment epithelium,[124] and retinal dehydrogenase,[126] which catalyzes the interconversion of retinal and retinaldehyde in visual pigment recycling associated with dark vision.

The retina appears to be sensitive to changes in zinc availability. The zinc content of melanosomes of the retinal pigment epithelium can be altered in pigs by feeding low zinc diets.[127] Humans fed parenterally with solutions devoid of zinc develop abnormal electroretinographic patterns that are reversed when zinc is added to the solution.[128] Short-term zinc depletion in cultured retinal pigment epithelium cells results in decreased activities of catalase and alpha-mannosidase.[124] Extreme deficiencies of zinc in rats result in marked ultrastructural alterations in the retinal pigment epithelium and degeneration of photoreceptor outer segments and lipid inclusion bodies in the retinal pigment epithelium.[129]

Epidemiologic investigations of the intake or blood levels of mineral cofactors for antioxidant enzymes have been primarily focused on zinc. One randomized clinical trial raised interest in the potential role of zinc supplementation when results demonstrated that large quantities of supplement-al zinc sulphate, taken over two years, modestly reduced the decrease in visual acuity in patients with macular degeneration.[130] However, a subsequent trial using a similar dose and duration failed to replicate this finding.[131] In the EDCCS, levels of zinc in the serum were not related to incident neovascular or exudative macular degeneration.[60] However, levels of zinc in the diet were related to both prevalent[83] and newly developed[85] macular pigmentary abnor-malities in the Beaver Dam population. Intakes of zinc (from diet and supplements) in the highest versus lowest quintiles of intake ten years before baseline studies were related to a 40% lower odds for existing pigment abnormalities at baseline and 60% lower odds for newly developed pigment abnormalities after five years of follow-up. Because associations with diet zinc have only been evaluated in a limited number of studies, the possible associations between zinc and ARMD require further evaluation.

Copper, which is a cofactor for the cytosolic form of the oxidant defense enzyme superoxide dismutase, is also concentrated in the retina and choroid, as well as in other ocular structures.[132] In addition to its role as a component in this enzyme of oxidative defense, copper is a component of a metalloenzyme which functions in melanin formation and in the cross-linking of collagen and elastin.[133] As a component of cytochrome oxidase,[134] copper could also conceivably play a role in the waste disposal system of the retinal pigment epithelium.[132] Rosenthal and Eckhert[132] suggest that copper may be involved in the pathogenesis of ARMD because of copper's involvement in the metabolism of the RPE and structural proteins in Bruch's membrane. However, there have been no studies in humans or animals which investigate a role of copper in this condition with one exception. Newsome et al.[135] noted levels of the main copper-carrying protein in plasma, ceruloplasmin, in patients with ARMD that were higher than controls. The elevation in the blood may signal abnormalities in copper metabolism that could be associated with lower levels in certain tissues like the retina or any other number of acute and chronic conditions that elevate ceruloplasmin, such as infection.

e. *Summary*

Thus, sufficient availability of several nutrients, which either directly quench free radicals or are components of enzyme systems which quench free radicals, may prevent oxidative stress to the RPE and associated retinal structures which support the health of photoreceptors. Evidence was given that several nutrients with roles in defense against oxidative stress protect against retinal pathology that may contribute to ARMD. Some nutrients, such as zinc and copper that are concentrated in the retina, may also have roles in protecting against retinal degeneration by mechanisms that do not involve oxidative stress.

While animal studies suggest that deficiency or supplementation with antioxidant nutrients can alter short-term retinal damage, epidemiologic studies have not yet provided conclusive support for a protective role of any single antioxidant nutrient. The inconsistent results of epidemiologic studies to date may reflect differences in the susceptibility of the populations studied (due to genetic predisposition or environmental exposures), differences in the effect of nutrients at different stages in the pathogenesis of ARMD or variations in the accuracy of measurements of exposure to specific nutrients in different studies. Larger samples and long-term follow-up will be useful in further evaluating relationships with specific maculopathy lesions in future studies.

2. Fatty Acids

The retina contains high levels of long-chain polyunsaturated fatty acids.[26] The polyunsaturated fatty acid content of the retina has been thought to be relatively resistant to dietary alterations in fat.[136] However, there is recent evidence that diet alterations can influence retinal lipids. Compromised retinal accumulation of polyunsaturated n-3 fatty acids over 20 carbons in length was observed in piglets fed diets devoid of these long-chain polyunsaturated fatty acids despite adequate levels of shorter-chain (18 carbon) precursors.[137] Feeding fish oils in rats can also alter the level of some long-chain fatty acids.[138] The fatty acid content of the rod outer segments can also be affected by nondietary factors, such as the exposure to bright light.[139]

Because of the large number of double bonds, which are targets for the attack by reactive oxygen species, polyunsaturated fatty acids could increase susceptibility to light damage. Consistent with this, retinal light damage in rats has been observed to be higher in rats fed one type of polyunsaturated fat (linseed oil)[141] and lower in rats fed diets deficient in long-chain fatty acids.[140] However, feeding fish oils, which are longer in length and contain more double bonds than other polyunsaturated fats, was found to protect against light-induced damage despite evidence for higher susceptibility to lipid peroxidation.[138] The authors suggest that a mechanism for the protective effect of fish oils could involve their ability to influence the types of eicosanoids synthesized and the resultant anti-inflammatory effect.

There are few epidemiologic studies of relationships between dietary fatty acids and ARMD. Consistent with studies in animals, diets high in polyunsaturated fatty acids are sometimes related to higher rates of ARMD. In the EDCCS, preliminary data indicated that a higher intake of vegetable fat (which in the U.S. is high in linoleic acid) was related to a higher risk for neovascular or exudative macular degeneration.[142] A similar but nonsignificant relationship of linoleic acid to early ARMD was observed among women (OR: 1.4; CI = 0.8-2.4) but not among men (OR: 0.7; CI = 0.4-1.2) in retrospective dietary studies in the Beaver Dam population.[143] The intake of fish or fish oils was non-significantly related to lower rates of ARMD in both the EDCCS[142] and Beaver Dam studies. (However, the low fish consumption in the Beaver Dam population[143] may limit the ability to detect statistically significant associations.) Fatty acids in serum were not related to early ARMD in the UK case-control study.[81] Thus, while results of some epidemiologic studies are consistent with results of animal studies, which indicate adverse influences of diets high in polyunsaturated fats less than 20 carbons in length and protective influences of longer chain fish oils, results are still inconsistent in the few studies that have evaluated these associations.

Saturated fat intake may influence risk for ARMD, as well. Intakes of saturated fats were related to an 80 percent higher risk for early ARMD in the Beaver Dam population[143] (OR: 1.8; CI = 1.2-2.7). This association may reflect the influence on cardiovascular risk (see next section) rather than susceptibility to oxidative stress. The continued study of relationships between the intakes of specific types of fat and ARMD in populations with widely varying intakes will facilitate the further evaluation of these relationships in human populations.

C. DIETARY COMPONENTS WITH ROLES IN CARDIOVASCULAR DISEASE

Speculation from early clinical reports about vascular changes in ARMD[53,55] and the observation of relationships between cardiovascular disease or its risk factors and ARMD[35,37-39,58,59] have led to the hypotheses that dietary factors may influence ARMD either by indirectly influencing atherosclerosis, which may in turn influence choroidal circulation, or by directly influencing retinal circulation or metabolism in a fashion parallel to that observed in the process of developing atherosclerosis. One of several ways that antioxidants have been hypothesized to influence the process of atherosclerosis is by reducing the oxidation of low-density lipoproteins (LDL), which are thought to be more atherogenic than non-oxidized low-density lipoproteins (reviewed in Diaz et al.[144]). Oxidized lipoproteins might also affect the retina. Receptors to take up damaged lipoproteins (scavenger receptors) have been observed in RPE cells.[145] However, a role in RPE cells for oxidized lipoproteins has not been determined. Antioxidants may also inhibit atherosclerosis by several mechanisms independent of LDL oxidation.[144]

As summarized above, higher intakes of vitamin E have been related to lower rates of ARMD in some, but not all, previous epidemiologic studies. It is possible that these associations reflect systemic factors, such as atherosclerotic or arteriosclerotic change, rather than direct retinal effects.

The intake of saturated fats is known to promote the process of atherosclerosis. The presumed mechanism is by increasing the concentration of low-density lipoproteins in the blood, which in turn increases the propensity for atherosclerotic lesions to develop. There have been no animal studies that link the intake of saturated fat to the development of lesions that predispose to ARMD. As previously discussed, a high past intake of saturated fat in the Beaver Dam population was related to an 80 percent higher risk for prevalent early ARMD.[143] A higher intake of total fat was related to incident neovascular or exudative macular degeneration in the EDCCS.[142] Polyunsaturated fats which are generally thought to lower risk for high blood cholesterol were related to higher, rather than lower, risk for ARMD in the EDCCS and in women in the Beaver Dam Eye Study (although the relationship was not statistically significant in the latter study). The relationship between fat intake and ARMD may be complex.

While it remains feasible that diet may affect the development of ARMD indirectly through an influence on cardiovascular disease and its risk factors, this possibility remains speculative until a direct link between cardiovascular disease processes and ARMD can be demonstrated. Both animal and human studies of retinal changes associated with atherosclerosis are needed to establish this link.

As discussed earlier in the chapter, there is increasing evidence for a role in immunologic events in the development of ARMD. Nutritional factors such as zinc (reviewed by Keen and Gershwin[147]) and vitamin E [97,148,149] play a role in various immunologic processes that could conceivably influence ARMD. However, specific roles for these nutrients in immunologic events that lead to macular degeneration have not been explored.

III. SUMMARY AND FUTURE DIRECTIONS

Data regarding the role of nutritional factors in the development of ARMD are accumulating. Significant questions remain regarding mechanisms by which specific nutrients play a role and the overall importance of nutritional factors in influencing the development of ARMD. Current theories of the pathogenesis of ARMD suggest possible roles for nutrients that function in a variety of systems that may influence ARMD. These include systems that protect against oxidative stress, atherosclerosis, or other types of vascular damage. Recent evidence that cells of the immune system may be involved in the pathogeneses of ARMD permits further speculation of roles for nutrients in the modulation of the impact of immunologic events, as well.

Animal and clinical studies of nutrient deficiencies or supplementation suggest that nutrient availability can influence retinal pathology that may be involved in ARMD. Epidemiologic evidence is inconsistent regarding these potential relationships but this inconsistency may reflect limitations associated with the study design or the measurement and/or classification of macular lesions or nutrient status. The inconsistency in epidemiologic studies, to date, may also reflect the complexity of relations of diet to ARMD. These relationships may be influenced by the stage of ARMD, by a genetic predisposition to ARMD, or by the presence of other risk factors (such as smoking). New data from ongoing prospective cohort studies and clinical trials should provide greater insights regarding the possible impact of dietary factors in preventing or slowing the development of ARMD.

IV. REFERENCES

1. **Klein, B. E. K., Klein, R., Linton, K. L. P.,** Prevalence of age-related lens opacities in a population. The Beaver Dam Eye Study, *Ophthalmology*, 99, 546, 1992.
2. **Treas, J.,** Older Americans in the 1990s and Beyond. *Population Bulletin*, Population Reference Bureau, Inc. Washington, D.C., vol 50, no. 2, May 1995.
3. **Heiba, I. M., Elston, R. C., Klein, B. E. K., Klein, R.,** Sibling correlations and segregation analysis of age-related maculopathy: the Beaver Dam Eye Study, *Genet Epidemiol*, 11, 51, 1994.
4. **Allikmets, R., Shroyer, N. F., Singh, N., Seddon, J. M., Lewis, R. A., Bernstein, P. S., Peiffer, A., Zabriskie, N. A., Li, Y., Hutchinson, A., Dean, M., Lupski, J. R., Leppert, M.,** Mutation of the Stargardt disease gene (ABCR) in age-related macular degeneration, *Science*, 277, 1805, 1997.
5. **Klein, M. L., Mauldin, W. M., Stoumbos, V. D.,** Heredity and age-related degeneration observations in monozygotic twins, *Arch Ophthalmol*, 112, 932, 1994.
6. **Cruickshanks, K. J., Hamman, R. F., Klein, R., Nondahl, D.M., Shetterly, S. M.,** The prevalence of age-related maculopathy by geographic region and ethnicity. The Colorado-Wisconsin study of age-related maculopathy, *Arch Ophthalmol*, 115, 242, 1997.
7. **Schachat, A. P., Hyman, L., Leske, M. C., Connell, A. M., Wu, S. Y.,** Features of age-related macular degeneration in a black population, *Arch Ophthalmol*, 113, 728, 1995.
8. **Maruo, T., Ikebukuro, N., Kawanabe, K., Kubota, N.,** Changes in causes of visual handicaps in Tokyo, *Jpn J Ophthalmol*, 35, 268, 1991.
9. **Young, R. W.,** The renewal of rod and cone outer segments in the rhesus monkey, *J Cell Biol*, 49, 303, 1971.
10. **Sarks, J. P., Sarks, S. H., Killingsworth, M. C.,** Evolution of geographic atrophy of the retinal pigment epithelium, *Eye*, 2, 552, 1988.
11. **Burns, R. P., Feeney-Burns, L.,** Clinico-morphologic correlations of drusen of Bruch's membrane, *Trans Am Ophthalmol Soc*, 78, 206, 1980.
12. **Green, W. R., Enger, C.,** Age-related macular degeneration histopathologic studies. The 1992 Lorenz E. Zimmerman Lecture, *Ophthalmology*, 100, 1519, 1993.
13. **Sarks, S. H.,** Ageing and degeneration in the macular region: a clinico-pathological study, *Br J Ophthalmol*, 60, 324, 1976.

14. **Sarks, S. H.,** Drusen patterns predisposing to geographic atrophy of the retinal pigment epithelium, *Aust J Ophthalmol*, 10, 91, 1982.
15. **Bressler, N. M., Silva, J. C., Bressler, S. B., Fine, S. L., Green, W. R.,** Clinicopathologic correlation of drusen and retinal pigment epithelial abnormalities in age-related macular degeneration, *Retina*, 14, 130, 1994.
16. **van der Schaft, T. L., de Bruijn, W. C., Mooy, C. M., Ketelaars, D. A., de Jong, P. T.,** Is basal laminar deposit unique for age-related macular degeneration?, *Arch Ophthalmol*, 109, 420, 1991.
17. **Bressler, S. B., Maguire, M. G., Bressler, N. M., Fine, S. L.,** Relationship of drusen and abnormalities of the retinal pigment epithelium to the prognosis of neovascular macular degeneration, *Arch Ophthalmol*, 108, 1442, 1990.
18. **Klein, R., Klein, B. E. K., Jensen, S. C., Meuer, S. M.,** The five-year incidence and progression of age-related maculopathy: The Beaver Dam Eye Study, *Ophthalmology,* 104, 7, 1997.
19. **Bressler, N. M., Muñoz, B., Maguire, M. G., Vitale, S. E., Schein, O. D., Taylor, H. R., West, S. K.,** Five-year incidence and disappearance of drusen and retinal pigment epithelial abnormalities. Waterman Study, *Arch Ophthalmol*, 113, 301, 1995.
20. **Katz, M. L., Robison, Jr., W. G.,** Age-related changes in the retinal pigment epithelium of pigmented rats, *Exp Eye Res*, 38, 137, 1984.
21. **Delori, F. C., Dorey, C. K., Staurenghi, G., Arend, O., Goger, D. G., Weiter, J. J.,** In-vivo fluorescence of the ocular fundus exhibits RPE lipofuscin characteristics, *Invest Ophthalmol Vis Sci*, 36, 719, 1995.
22. **Feeney-Burns, L., Gao, C-L., Tidwell, M.,** Lysosomal enzyme cytochemistry of human RPE, Bruch's membrane and drusen, *Invest Ophthalmol Vis Sci*, 28, 1138, 1987.
23. **Holz, F. G., Sheraidah, G., Pauleikhoff, D., Bird, A. C.,** Analysis of lipid deposits extracted from human macular and peripheral Bruch's membrane, *Arch Ophthalmol*, 112, 402, 1994.
24. **Barreau, E., Brossas, J-Y, Courtois, Y., Tréton, J. A.,** Accumulation of mitochondrial DNA deletions in human retina during aging, *Invest Ophthalmol Vis Sci*, 37, 384, 1996.
25. **Sickel, W.,** Retinal metabolism in dark and light, in *Handbook of Sensory Physiology*, Vol. 7, Fuortes, M. G. F., Ed., Berlin; NewYork:Springer-Verlag, 1972, part 2, p 667.
26. **Fliesler, S. J., Anderson, R. E.,** Chemistry and metabolism of lipids in the vertebrate retina, *Progr Lipid Res*, 22, 79, 1983.
27. **Noell, W. K., Walker, V. S., Kang, B. S., Berman, S.,** Retinal damage by light in rats, *Invest Ophthalmol*, 5, 450, 1966.
28. **Dayhaw-Barker, P.,** Ocular photosensitation, *Photochem Photobiol*, 46, 1051, 1986.
29. **Wiegand, R. D., Giusto, N. M., Rapp L. M., Anderson, R. E.,** Evidence for rod outer segment lipid peroxidation following constant illumination of the rat retina, *Invest Ophthal Vis Sci*, 24, 1433, 1983.
30. **Tso, M. O. M.,** Pathogenetic factors of aging macular degeneration,

Ophthalmology, 92, 628, 1985.

31. **Borges, J., Li, Z-Y., Tso, M. O. M.,** Effects of repeated photic exposures on the monkey macula, *Arch Ophthalmol,* 108, 727, 1990.
32. **Taylor, H. R., West, S., Muñoz, B., Rosenthal, F. S., Bressler, S. B., Bressler, N. M.,** The long-term effects of visible light on the eye, *Arch Ophthalmol*, 110, 99, 1992.
33. **Cruickshanks, K. J., Klein, R., Klein, B. E. K.,** Sunlight and age-related macular degeneration: The Beaver Dam Eye Study, *Arch Ophthalmol*, 111, 514, 1993.
34. **Gregor, Z., Joffe, L.,** Senile macular changes in the black African, *Br J Ophthalmol*, 62, 547, 1978.
35. **Hyman, L., Lilienfeld, A., Ferris III., F. L., Fine, S.,** Senile macular degeneration: A case-control study, *Am J Epidemiol,* 118, 213, 1983.
36. **Weiter, J. J. C., Wing, G. L., Fitch, K. A.,** Relationship of senile macular degeneration to ocular pigmentation, *Am J Ophthalmol*, 99, 185, 1985.
37. **Paetkau, M., Boyd, T., Grace, M., Bach-Mills, J., Winshop, B.,** Senile disciform macular degeneration and smoking, *Can J Ophthalmol*, 13, 67, 1978.
38. **Seddon, J. M., Willett, W. C., Speizer, F. E., Hankinson, S.E.,** A prospective study of smoking and age-related macular degeneration, *JAMA*, 276, 1141, 1996.
39. **Christen, W. G., Glynn, R. J., Manson, J. E., Ajani, U. A., Buring, J. E.,** A prospective study of cigarette smoking and risk of age-related macular degeneration in men, *JAMA*, 276, 1147, 1996.
40. **Vingerling, J. R., Hofman, A., Grobbee, D. E., de Jong, P. T. V. M.,** Age-related macular degeneration and smoking. The Rotterdam Study, *Arch Ophthalmol*, 114, 1193, 1996.
41. **Klein, R., Klein, B. E. K., Moss, S. E.,** The relation of smoking to the incidence of age-related maculopathy. The Beaver Dam Eye Study, *Am J Epidemiol,*147, 103, 1998.
42. **Klein, R., Klein, B. E. K.,** Smoke gets in your eyes too, *JAMA*, 276[Editorial], 1178, 1996.
43. **Katz, M. L., Parker, K. R., Handelman, G. J., Bramel, T. L., Dratz, E. A.,** Effects of antioxidant nutrient deficiency on the retina and retinal pigment epithelium of albino rats: a light and electron microscopic study, *Exp Eye Res*, 34, 339, 1982.
44. **Hayes, K. C.,** Retinal degeneration in monkeys induced by deficiency of vitamin E or A, *Invest Ophthalmol Vis Sci*, 13, 499, 1974.
45. **Organisciak, D. T., Want, H. M., Li, Z., Tso, M. O. M.,** The protective effect of ascorbate in retinal light damage of rats, *Invest Ophthalmol Vis Sci*, 26, 1580, 1985.
46. **Organisciak, D. T., Jiang, Y. L., Wang, H. M., Bicknell, I.,** The protective effect of ascorbic acid in retinal light damage of rats exposed to intermittent light, *Invest Ophthalmol Vis Sci*, 31, 1195, 1990.
47. **Li, Z. Y., Tso, M. O. M., Wang, H. M., Organisciak, D. T.,** Ameliora-

tion of photic injury in rat retina by ascorbic acid: a histopathologic study, *Invest Ophthalmol Vis Sci*, 26, 1589, 1985.

48. **Lam, S., Tso, M. O. M., Gurne, D., H.,** Amelioration of retinal photic injury in albino rats by dimethylthiourea, *Arch Ophthalmol*, 108, 1751, 1990.
49. **Organisciak, D. T., Darrow, R. M., Jiang, Y. L., Marak, G. E., Blanks, J. C.,** Protection by dimethylthiourea against retinal light damage in rats, *Invest Ophthalmol Vis Sci*, 33, 1599, 1992.
50. **Prashar, S., Pandav, S. S., Gupta, A., Nath, R.,** Antioxidant enzymes in RBCs as a biological index of age related macular degeneration, *Acta Ophthalmologica*, 71, 214, 1993.
51. **Liles, M. R., Newsome, D. A., Oliver, P. D.,** Antioxidant enzymes in the aging human retinal pigment epithelium, *Arch Ophthalmol*, 109, 1285, 1991.
52. **Katz, M. L., White, H. A., Gao, C-L., Roth, G. S., Knapka, J. J., Ingram, D. K.,** Dietary restriction slows age pigment accumulation in the retinal pigment epithelium, *Invest Ophthalmol Vis Sci*, 34, 3297, 1993.
53. **Verhoeff, F. H., Grossman, H. P.,** Pathogenesis of disciform degeneration of the macula, *Arch Ophthalmol*, 18, 561, 1937.
54. **Kornzweig, A. L.,** Changes in choriocapillaris associated with senile macular degeneration, *Ann Ophthalmol*, 9, 753, 1977.
55. **Duke-Elder, S., Perkins, S. S.,** System of ophthalmology, in *Diseases of the Uveal Tract*, Vol. IX, Kimpton, H., Ed., C. V. Mosby, St. Louis, 1966, p 610.
56. **Pauleikhoff, D., Chen, J. C., Chisholm, I. H., Bird, A. C.,** Choroidal perfusion abnormality with age-related Bruch's membrane change, *Am J Ophthalmol*, 109, 211, 1990.
57. **Vingerling, J. R., Dielemans, I., Bots, M. L., Hofman, A., Grobbee, D. E., de Jong, P. T. V. M.,** Age-related macular degeneration is associated with atherosclerosis. The Rotterdam Study, *Am J Epidemiol*, 142, 404, 1995.
58. **Goldberg, J., Flowerdew, J., Smith, E., Brody, J. A., Tso, M. O. M.,** Factors associated with age-related macular degeneration: an analysis of data from the First National Health and Nutrition Examination survey, *Am J Epidemiol*, 128, 700, 1988.
59. **Eye Disease Case-Control Study Group,** Risk factors for neovascular age-related macular degeneration, *Arch Ophthalmol*, 110, 1701, 1992.
60. **Klein, R., Klein, B. E. K., Franke, T.,** The relationship of cardiovascular disease and its risk factors to age-related maculopathy. The Beaver Dam Eye Study, *Ophthalmology*, 100, 406, 1993.
61. **Klein, B. E. K., Klein, R., Jensen, S.C., Ritter, L. L.,** Are sex hormones associated with age-related maculopathy in women? The Beaver Dam Eye Study, *Trans Am Ophthalmol Soc*, 92, 289, 1994.
62. **Kahn, H. A., Liebowitz, H. M., Ganley, J. P., Kini, M. M., Colton, T., Nickerson, R. S., Dawber, T. R.,** The Framingham Eye Study. II. Association of ophthalmic pathology with single variables previously

measured in the Framingham Heart Study, *Am J Epidemiol*, 106, 33, 1977.

63. **Maltzman, B. A., Mulvihill, M. N., Greenbaum, A.**, Senile macular degeneration and risk factors: a case-control study, *Ann Ophthalmol*, 11, 1197, 1979.

64. **Friedman, E.**, A hemodynamic model of the pathogenesis of age-related macular degeneration, *Am J Ophthalmol*, 124, 677, 1997.

65. **Garner, A., Sarks, S., Sarks, J. P.**, in *Pathobiology of Ocular Disease. A Dynamic Approach*, 2nd Edition, Marcel Dekker, Inc., New York, 1994, Chap. 20.

66. **Glaser, B. M.**, Extracellular modulating factors and the control of intraocular neovascularization, *Arch Ophthalmol*, 106, 603, 1988.

67. **Hogan, M. J., Alvarado, J.**, Studies on the human macula. IV. Aging changes in Bruch's membrane, *Arch Ophthalmol*, 77, 410, 1967.

68. **Feeney-Burns, L., Ellersieck, M.R.**, Age-related changes in the ultrastructure of Bruch's membrane, *Am J Ophthalmol*, 100, 686, 1985.

69. **Sheraidah, G., Steinmetz, R., Maguire, J., Pauleikhoff, D., Marshall, J., Bird, A. C.**, Correlation between lipids extracted from Bruch's membrane and age, *Ophthalmology*, 100, 47, 1993.

70. **Moore, D. J., Hussain, A. A., Marshall, J.**, Age-related variation in the hydraulic conductivity of Bruch's membrane, *Invest Ophthalmol Vis Sci*, 36, 1290, 1995.

71. **Dastgheib, K., Green, R.**, Granulomatous reaction to Bruch's membrane in age-related macular degeneration, *Arch Ophthalmol*, 112, 813, 1994.

72. **Penfold, P. L., Provis, J. M., Billson, F. A.**, Age-related macular degeneration: ultrastructural studies of the relationship of leucocytes to angiogenesis, *Graefe's Arch Ophthalmol*, 225, 70, 1987.

73. **Gehrs, K. M., Heriot, W. J., De Juan Jr., E.**, Transmission electron microscopic study of a subretinal choroidal neovascular membrane due to age-related macular degeneration, *Arch Ophthalmol*, 110, 833, 1992.

74. **Killingsworth, M. C., Sarks, J. P., Sarks, S. H.**, Macrophages related to Bruch's membrane in age-related macular degeneration, *Eye*, 4, 613, 1990.

75. **Jones, P. A., Werb, Z.**, Degradation of connective tissue matrices by macrophages. II. Influence of matrix composition on proteolysis of glycoproteins, elastin, and collagen by macrophages in culture, *J Exp Med*, 152, 1527, 1980.

76. **Penfold, P. L., Liew, S. C. K., Madigan, M. C., Provis, J. M.**, Modulation of major histocompatibility complex class II expression in retinas with age-related macular degeneration, *Invest Ophthalmol Vis Sci*, 38, 2125, 1997.

77. **Penn, J. S., Anderson, R. E.**, Effects of light history on the rat retina, in *Progress Retinal Research*, Osborne, N., Chader, G., Eds., Pergamon Press, New York, vol 11, 1992, p 75.

78. **Hope, G. M., Dawson, W. W., Engel, H. M., Ulshafer, R. J., Kessler, M. J., Sherwood, M. B.**, A primate model for age-related macular drusen,

Br J Ophthalmol, 76, 11, 1992.

79. **Eye Disease Case-Control Study Group**. Antioxidant status and neovascular age-related macular degeneration, *Arch Ophthalmol*, 111, 104, 1993.

80. **Seddon, J. M., Ajani, U. A., Sperduto, R. D., Hiller, R., Blair, N., Burton, T. C., Farber, M. D., Gragoudas, E. S., Haller, J., Miller, D. T., Yannuzzi, L. A., Willett, W., for the Eye Disease Case-Control Study Group**, Dietary carotenoids, vitamins A, C, and E, and advanced age-related macular degeneration. Eye Disease Case-Control Study Group, *JAMA*, 272, 1413, 1994.

81. **Sanders, T. A. B., Haines, A. P., Wormald, R., Wright, L. A., Obeid, O.,** Essential fatty acids, plasma cholesterol, and fat-soluble vitamins in subjects with age-related maculopathy and matched control subjects, *Am J Clin Nutr*, 57, 428, 1993.

82. **West, S., Vitale, S., Hallfrisch, J., Muñoz, B., Muller, D., Bressler, S., Bressler, N. M.,** Are antioxidants or supplements protective for age-related macular degeneration?, *Arch Ophthalmol*, 112, 222, 1994.

83. **Mares-Perlman, J. A., Klein, R., Klein, B. E. K., Greger, J. L., Brady, W. E., Palta, M., Ritter, L.,** Association of zinc and antioxidant nutrients with age-related maculopathy, *Arch Ophthalmol*, 114, 991, 1996.

84. **Mares-Perlman, J. A., Brady, W. E., Klein, R., Klein, B. E. K., Bowen, P., Stacewicz-Sapuntzakis, M., Palta, M.,** Serum antioxidants and age-related macular degeneration in a population-based case-control study, *Arch Ophthalmol*, 113, 1518, 1995.

85. **VandenLangenberg, G. M., Mares-Perlman, J. A., Klein, R., Klein, B. E. K., Brady, W. E., Palta, M.,** Associations between antioxidant and zinc intake and the 5-year incidence of early age-related maculopathy in the Beaver Dam Eye Study, *Am J Epidemiol*, 148, 204, 1998.

86. **Steinmetz, K. A., Potter, J. D.,** Vegetables, fruit, and cancer. II. Mechanisms, *Cancer Cause Control*, 2, 427, 1991.

87. **Friedrichson, T., Kalbach, H. L., Buck, R., van Kuijk, F. J. G. M.,** Vitamin E in macular and peripheral tissues of the human eye, *Curr Eye Res*, 14, 693, 1995.

88. **Hunt, D. F., Organisciak, D. T., Wang, H. M., Wu, R. L. C.,** α-Tocopherol in the developing rat retina: a high pressure liquid chromatographic analysis, *Curr Eye Res*, 3, 1281, 1984.

89. **Stephens, R. J., Negi, D. S., Short, S. M., van Kuijk, F. J., Dratz, E. A., Thomas, D. W.,** Vitamin E distribution in ocular tissues following long-term dietary depletion and supplementation as determined by microdissection and gas chromatography-mass spectrometry, *Exp Eye Res*, 47(2), 237, 1988.

90. **Bone, R. A., Landrum, J. T., Fernandez, L., Tarsis, S. L.,** Analysis of the macular pigment by HPLC: retinal distribution and age study, *Invest Ophthalmol Vis Sci,* 29, 843, 1988.

91. **Handelman, G. J., Dratz, E. A., Reay, C. C., van Kuijk, F. J. G. M.,** Carotenoids in the human macular and whole retina, *Invest Ophthalmol*

Vis Sci, 29, 850, 1988.

92. **Tso, M. O. M., Woodford, B. J., Lam, K. W.,** Distribution of ascorbate in normal primate retina and after photic injury: a biochemical, morphological correlated study, *Curr Eye Res*, 3, 181, 1983.

93. **Katz, M. L., Eldred, G. E.,** Failure of vitamin E to protect the retina against damage resulting from bright cyclic light exposure, *Invest Ophthalmol Vis Sci*, 30, 29, 1989.

94. **Stone, W. L., Katz, M. L., Lurie, M., Marmor, M. F., Dratz, E. A.,** Effects of vitamin E and selenium deficiency on light damage to the rat retina, *Photochem Photobiol*, 29, 725, 1979.

95. **Hayes, K. C., Rousseau, J. E., Hegsted, D. M.,** Plasma tocopherol concentrations and vitamin E deficiency in dogs, *J Am Vet Med Assoc*, 157, 640, 1970.

96. **Wiegand, R. D., Joel, C. D., Rapp, L. M., Nielsen, J. C., Maude, M. B., Anderson, R. E.,** Polyunsaturated fatty acids and vitamin E in rat rod outer segments during light damage, *Invest Ophthalmol Vis Sci*, 27, 727, 1986.

97. **Devaraj, S., Li, D., Jialal, I.,** The effects of alpha tocopherol supplementation on monocyte function. Decreased lipid oxidation, interleukin 1 beta secretion, and monocyte adhesion to endothelium, *J Clin Invest*, 98, 756, 1996.

98. **Handelman, G. J., Dratz, E. A.,** The role of antioxidants in the retina and retinal pigment epithelium and the nature of prooxidant-induced damage, *Adv Free Rad Biol Med*, 2, 1, 1986.

99. **Sobrevilla, L. A., Goodman, M. L., Kane, C. A.,** Demyelinating central nervous system disease, macular atrophy and acanthocytosis (Bassen-Kornzweig Syndrome), *Am J Med*, 37, 821, 1964.

100. **Muller, D. P. R., Lloyd, J. K., Wolff, O. H.,** Vitamin E and Neurological Function; Abetaliproteinemia and Other Disorders of Fat Absorption, in *Biology of Vitamin E*, Porter, R., Whelan, J., Eds., Pitman, London, 1983.

101. **Bishara, S., Merin, S., Cooper, M., Azizi, E., Delpre, G., Deckelbaum, R. J.,** Combined vitamin A and E therapy prevents retinal electrophysiological deterioration in abetalipoproteinemia, *Br J Ophthalmol*, 66, 767, 1982.

102. **Acuff, R. V., Thedford, S. S., Hidiroglou, N. N., Papas, A. M., Odom Jr., T. A.,** Relative bioavailability of RRR-and all-rac-α-tocopheryl acetate in humans: studies using deuterated compounds, *Am J Clin Nutr*, 60, 397, 1994.

103. **Christen, S., Woodall, A. A., Shigenaga, M. K., Southwell-Keely, P. T., Duncan, M. W., Ames, B. N.,** γ-Tocopherol traps mutagenic electrophiles such as NO_x and complements α-tocopherol: Physiological implications, *Proc Natl Acad Sci*, 94, 3217, 1997.

104. **Handelman, G. J., Machlin, L. J., Fitch, K., Weiter, J. J., Dratz, E. A.,** Oral α-tocopherol supplements decrease plasma γ-tocopherol levels in humans, *J Nutr*, 115, 807, 1985.

105. **Dam, H.,** Interrelations between vitamin E and polyunsaturated fatty acids in animals, *Vit Horm*, 20, 527, 1962.

106. **Niki, E., Saito, T., Kawakami, A., Kamiya, Y.,** Inhibition of oxidation of methyl linoleate in solution by vitamin E and vitamin C, *J Biol Chem*, 259,4177, 1984.

107. **Rozanowska, M., Bober, A., Burke, J. M., Sarna, T.,** The role of retinal pigment epithelium melanin in photoinduced oxidation of ascorbate, *J Photochem Photobiol*, 65, 472, 1997.

108. **Rapp, L. M., Fisher, P. L., Suh, D. W.,** Evaluation of retinal susceptibility to light damage in pigmented rats supplemented with beta-carotene, *Curr Eye Res*, 15(2), 219, 1996.

109. **Bone, R. A., Landrum, J. T., Tarsis, S. L.,** Preliminary identification of the human macular pigment, *Vision Res*, 25, 1531, 1985.

110. **Kirschfeld, K.,** Carotenoid pigments: their possible role in protecting against photooxidation in eyes and photoreceptor cells, *Proc R Soc Lond [Biol]*, 216, 71, 1982.

111. **Mathews-Roth, M. M., Wilson, T., Fujimori, E., Krinsky, N. I.,** Carotenoid chromophobe length and protection against photosensitization, *Photochem Photobiol*, 19, 217, 1974.

112. **Malinow, M. R., Feeney-Burns, L., Peterson, L. H., Klein, M. L., Neuringer, M.,** Diet-related macular anomalies in monkeys, *Invest Ophthalmol Vis Sci*, 19, 857, 1980.

113. **Bernstein, H. N., Ginsberg, G.,** The pathology of chloroquine retinopathy, *Arch Ophthalmol*, 71, 238, 1964.

114. **Handelman, G. J., Snodderly, D. M., Krinsky, N. I., Russett, M. D., Adler, A. J.,** Biological control of primate macular pigment, *Invest Ophthalmol Vis Sci*, 32, 257, 1991.

115. **Hammond Jr., B. R., Fuld, K., Curran-Celentano, J.,** Macular pigment density in monozygotic twins, *Invest Ophthalmol Vis Sci*, 36, 2531, 1995.

116. **Landrum, J. T., Bone, R. A., Joa, H., Kilburn, M. D., Moore, L. L., Sprague, K. E.,** A one year study of macular pigment modification: the effect of 140 days of lutein supplement, *Exp Eye Res*, 65, 57, 1997.

117. **Hammond, Jr., B. R., Johnson, E. J., Russell, R. M., Krinsky, N. I., Yeum, K. J., Edwards, R. B., Snodderly, D. M.,** Dietary modification of human macular pigment density, *Invest Ophthalmol Vis Sci*, 38, 1795, 1997.

118. **Mangels, A. R., Holden, J. M., Beecher, G. R., Forman, M. R., Lanza, E.,** Carotenoid content of fruits and vegetables: an evaluation of analytic data, *J Am Diet Assoc*, 93, 284, 1993.

119. **Carughi, A., Hooper, F. G.,** Plasma carotenoid concentrations before and after supplementation with a carotenoid mixture, *Am J Clin Nutr*, 59, 896, 1994.

120. **Dimascio, K. S., Sies, H.,** Lycopene as the most efficient biologic carotenoid singlet oxygen quencher, *Arch Biochem Biophys*, 274, 1, 1989.

121. **Oliver, P. D., Newsome, D. A.,** Mitochondrial superoxide dismutase in mature and developing human retinal pigment epithelium, *Invest Ophthalmol Vis Sci*, 33, 1909, 1992.

122. **Taylor, C. G., Bettger, W. J., Bray, T., M.,** Effect of dietary zinc or

copper deficiency on the primary free radical defense system in rats, *J Nutr*, 118, 613, 1988.

123. **Singh, S. V., Dao, D. D., Srivastava, S. K., Awasthi, Y. C.,** Purification and characterization of glutathione S-transferase in human retina, *Curr Eye Res*, 3, 1273, 1984.

124. **Tate, D.J., Miceli, M.V., Newsome, D.A., Alcock, N.W., Oliver, P.D.,** Influence of zinc on selected cellular functions of cultured human retinal pigment epithelium, *Curr Eye Res,* 14, 897, 1995.

125. **Karcioglu, Z. A.,** Zinc in the eye, *Surv Ophthalmol*, 27, 114, 1982.

126. **Lion, F., Rotmans, J. P., Daemen, F. J., Bonting, S. L.,** Biochemical aspects of the visual process. XXVII. Stereospecificy of ocular retinal dehydrogenases and the visual cycle, *Biochem Biophys Acta*, 384, 283, 1975.

127. **Samuelson, D. A., Smith, P., Ulshafer, R. J., Hendricks, D. G., Whitley, R. D., Hendricks, H., Leone, N. C.,** X-ray microanalysis of ocular melanin in pigs maintained on normal and low zinc diets, *Exp Eye Res*, 56, 63, 1993.

128. **Vinton, N. E., Heckenlively, J. R., Laidlaw, S. A., Martin, D. A., Foxman, S. R., Ament, M. E., Kopple, M. E.,** Visual function in patients undergoing long-term total parenteral nutrition, *Am J Clin Nutr*, 52, 895, 1990.

129. **Leure-duPree, A.E., McClain, C.J.,** The effect of severe zinc deficiency on the morphology of the rat retinal pigment epithelium, *Invest Ophthalmol Vis Sci*, 23, 425, 1982.

130. **Newsome, D. A., Swartz, M., Leone, N. C., Elston, R. C., Miller, E.,** Oral zinc in macular degeneration, *Arch Ophthalmol*, 106, 192, 1988.

131. **Stur, M., Tittl, M., Reitner, A., Meisinger, V.,** Oral zinc and the second eye in age-related macular degeneration, *Invest Ophthalmol Vis Sci*, 37(7), 1225, 1996.

132. **Rosenthal, A. R., Eckhert, C.,** Copper and zinc in ophthalmology, *Zinc and Copper in Medicine*, Karcioglu, Z. A., Sarper, R. M., Eds., Springfield, IL, Charles C. Thomas, 1980.

133. **Dowdy, R. P.,** Copper metabolism, *Am J Clin Nutr*, 22, 887, 1969.

134. **Griffiths, D. E., Wharton, D. C.,** Purification and properties of cytochrome oxidase, *Biochem Biophys Res Commun*, 4, 151, 1961.

135. **Newsome, D. A., Swartz, M., Leone, N. C., Hewitt, A. T., Wolford, F., Miller, E. D.,** Macular degeneration and elevated serum ceruloplasmin, *Invest Ophthalmol Vis Sci*, 27(12), 1675, 1986.

136. **Futterman, S., Downer, J. L., Hendrickson, A.,** Effect of essential fatty acid deficiency on the fatty acid composition, morphology and electroretinographic response of the retina, *Invest Ophthalmol,* 10, 151, 1971.

137. **Hrboticky, N., MacKinnon, M. J., Innis, S. M.,** Retina fatty acid composition of piglets fed from birth with a linoleic acid-rich vegetable-oil formula for infants, *Am J Clin Nutr*, 53, 483, 1991.

138. **Remé, C. E., Malnoë, A., Jung, H. H., Wei, Q., Munz, K.,** Effect of

dietary fish oil on acute light-induced photoreceptor damage in the rat retina, *Invest Ophthalmol Vis Sci*, 35, 78, 1994.

139. **Penn, J. S., Anderson, R. E.,** Effect of light history on rod outer-segment membrane composition in the rat, *Exp Eye Res*, 44, 767, 1987.

140. **Bush, R. A., Reme, C. E., Malnoe, A.,** Light damage in the rat retina; the effect of dietary deprivation of n-3 fatty acids on acute structural alterations, *Exp Eye Res*, 53, 741, 1991.

141. **Koutz, C. A., Wiegand, R. D., Rapp, L. M., Anderson, R. E.,** Effect of dietary fat on the response of rat retina to chronic and acute light stress, *Ex Eye Res*, 60, 307, 1995.

142. **Seddon, J., Ajani, U., Sperduto, R., Yannuzzi, L., Burton, T., Haller, J., Blair, N., Farber, M., Miller, D., Gragoudas, E., Willett, W., and the EDCCS Group,** Dietary fat intake and age-related macular degeneration, *Invest Ophthalmol Vis Sci*, 35(Abs), 2003, 1994.

143. **Mares-Perlman, J. A., Brady, W. E., Klein, R., Vanden-Langenberg, G. M., Klein, B. E. K., Palta, M.,** Dietary fat and age-related maculopathy, *Arch Ophthalmol*, 113, 743, 1995.

144. **Diaz, M. N., Frei, B., Vita, J. A., Keaney, J. F.,** Antioxidants and atherosclerotic heart disease, *N Eng J Med*, 337, 408, 1997.

145. **Hayes, K. C., Lindsey, S., Stephan, Z. F., Brecker, D.,** Retinal pigment epithelium possesses both LDL and scavenger receptor activity, *Invest Ophthalmol Vis Sci*, 30, 225, 1989.

146. **Reaven, P. D., Khouw, A., Beltz, W. F., Parthasarathy, S., Witztum, J. L.,** Effect of dietary antioxidant combinations in humans: protection of LDL by vitamin E but not beta-carotene, *Arterioscler Thromb*, 13, 590, 1993.

147. **Keen, C. L., Gershwin, M. E.,** Zinc deficiency and immune function, *Ann Rev Nutr*, 10, 415, 1990.

148. **Gogu, S. R., Blumberg, J. B.,** Vitamin E enhances murine natural killer cell cytotoxicity against YAC-1 tumor cells, *J Nutr Immunol*, 1, 31, 1992.

149. **Meydani, S. N., Barklund, M. P., Liu, S., Meydani, M., Miller, R. A., Cannon, J. G., Morrow, F. D., Rocklin, R., Blumberg, J. B.,** Vitamin E supplementation enhances cell-mediated immunity in healthy elderly subjects, *Am J Clin Nutr*, 52, 557, 1990.

Chapter 12

THE CAROTENOIDS OF THE HUMAN RETINA

Wolfgang Schalch, Pierrette Dayhaw-Barker, and Felix M. Barker, II

I. INTRODUCTION

A. MACULA LUTEA

In the late 18th century, the presence of a "yellow spot" within the area centralis of the human retina (Figure 1) was described in post-mortem eyes and was subsequently termed the "macula lutea" [1]. It was much later, in 1945, that its chemical composition was identified as a "leaf xanthophyll" carotenoid [2]. Research has since concentrated on the chemistry, anatomy and physiology of the macula lutea carotenoids, particularly with respect to their uptake, metabolism and physiological role in retinal tissue.

The retina has a central area of maximal visual acuity, called the macula, which is dedicated to high resolution tasks and detailed color discrimination. The structure of the macula (Figure 1 [3]) is very specifically adapted to its visual function. Located within the greater area centralis of the retina, the macula is subdivided into a central foveola surrounded by the foveal and parafoveal areas. The macula has the highest density of cone photoreceptors: unlike the more peripherally-located rod photoreceptors, cones have the overlying neurons pushed aside at their central, most dense concentration, the fovea. Therefore, in comparison to other retinal areas, fewer cell layers lie between the incoming light and the photoreceptors, one of the reasons which makes the macula photoreceptors more vulnerable. On the other hand, the greater resolving ability of the macula is at least partly attributable to this anatomical alteration, since the lack of the inner neural layers minimizes distortion of the incident optical image focused upon the macular cone photoreceptors. Furthermore, the high cone density in the macula is amplified by projection to a disproportionately large area of the visual cortex. Thus diseases of the macula such as age-related macular degeneration (AMD) usually produce devastating visual loss: AMD is estimated to affect almost 30 % of those over 75 years of age as estimated in a compilation of 9 AMD prevalence/incidence studies carried out in the U.S., New Zealand, the U.K., Iceland, Denmark and The Netherlands, which have investigated a total of slightly more than 20,000 subjects [4].

0-8493-8565-2/99/$0.00+$.50

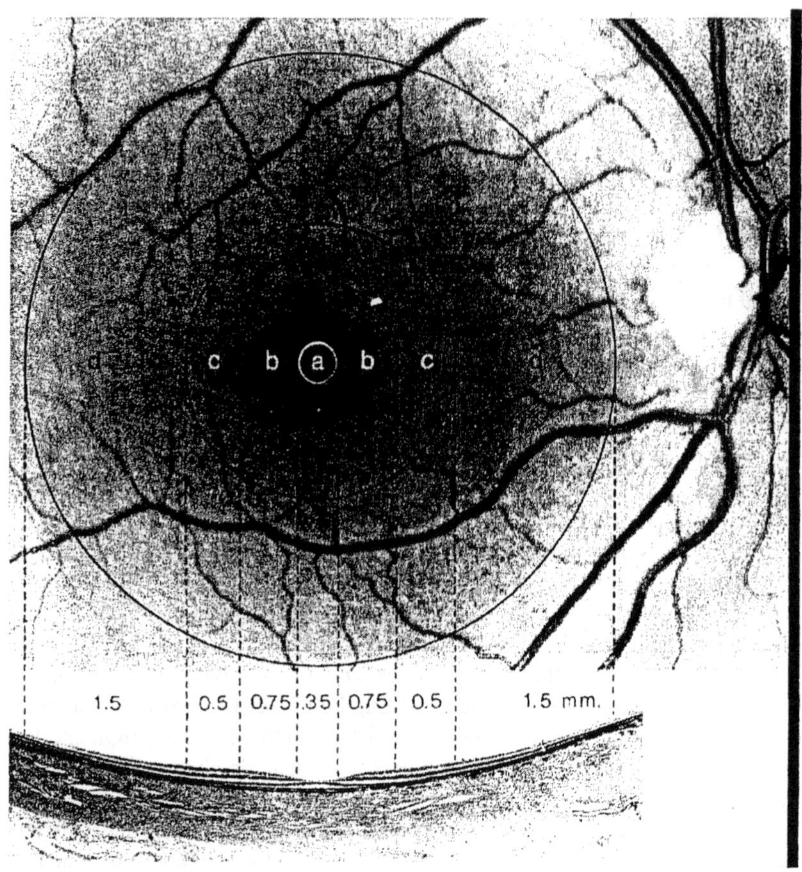

Figure 1. The human macula. Photograph of the fundus (top) matched with a meridional light micrograph of the macular region (bottom). The macula lutea ("yellow spot") is located in the center of the area centralis (largest circle comprising the foveola a, ≅ 1.2°, fovea b, ≅ 6°, parafoveal area c, ≅ 9.3°, and peri-foveal region d, ≅ 18°), and varies in size but normally covers at least the fovea. Reproduced with permission from Hogan et al., 1971 [3].

B. MACULAR YELLOW PIGMENT

Snodderly et al. [5,6,7] located the macular yellow pigment within Henle's fiber layer (Figure 2). The chemical components of the macular pigment were identified as the carotenoids lutein and zeaxanthin by Bone et al. [8] and Handelman et al. [9]. Later, the macular zeaxanthin was itself shown to comprise two stereoisomers: 3R,3′R-zeaxanthin and 3R,3′S-(=*meso*)-zeaxanthin [10]. Figure 3 shows the structural formulas of the three most important macular carotenoids in comparison to other carotenoids.

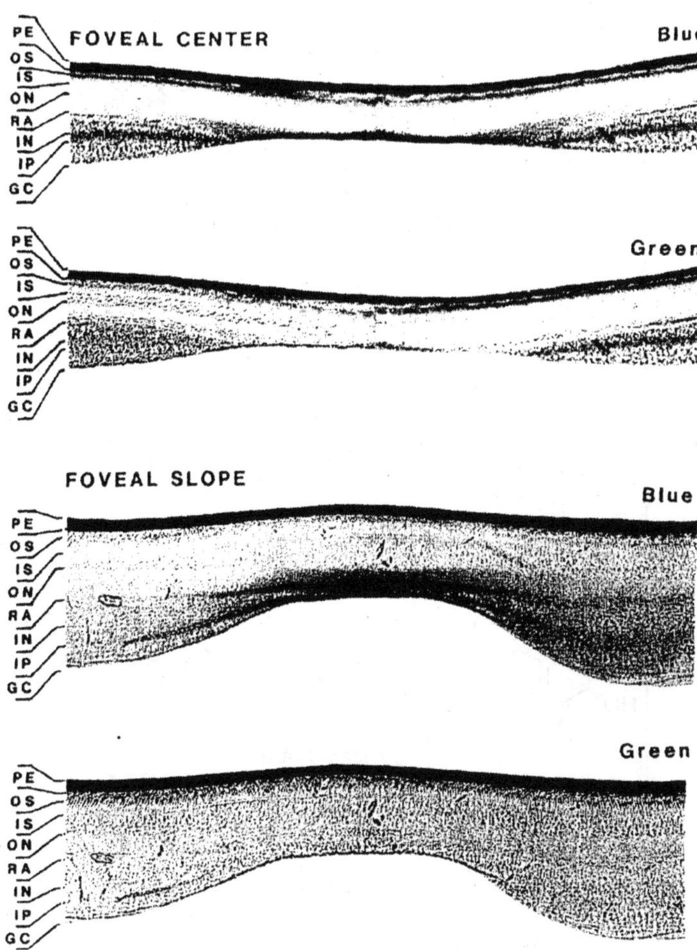

Figure 2. The vertical distribution of carotenoids within the fovea. Microphotographs taken in monochromatic blue or green light of unstained frozen sections through the fovea of *M. fascicularis* monkeys. The macular yellow pigment appears dark in blue light due to the absorbance of blue light by the yellow carotenoids, while in green light no absorbance is seen. Retinal layers are: retinal pigment epithelium (PE), photoreceptor outer segments (OS), photoreceptor inner segments (IS), outer nuclear layer (ON), receptor axons (RA, or Henle's fiber layer), inner nuclear layer (IN), inner plexiform layer (IP) and ganglion cell layer (GC). Reproduced with permission from Snodderly et al., 1984 [5].

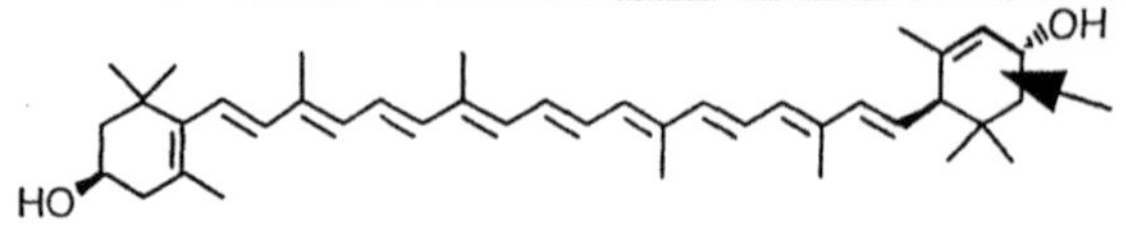

3,R,3′R,6′R-lutein

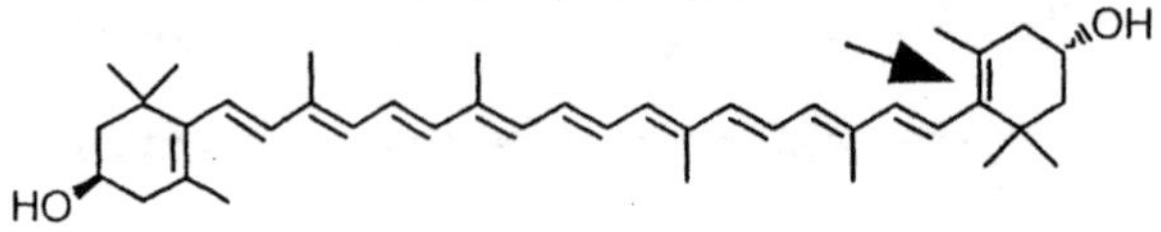

3R,3′S-(*meso*)-zeaxanthin

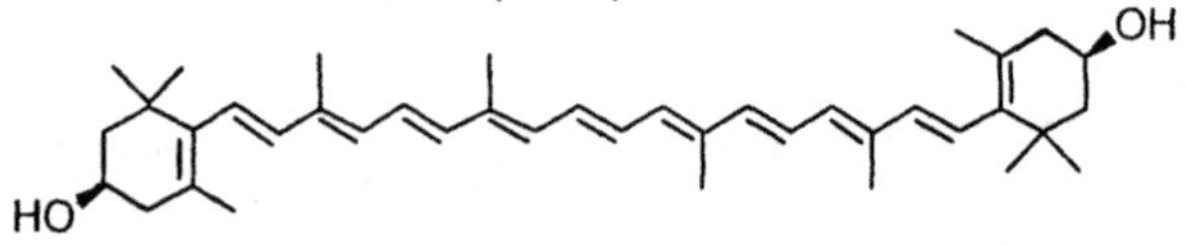

3R,3′R-zeaxanthin

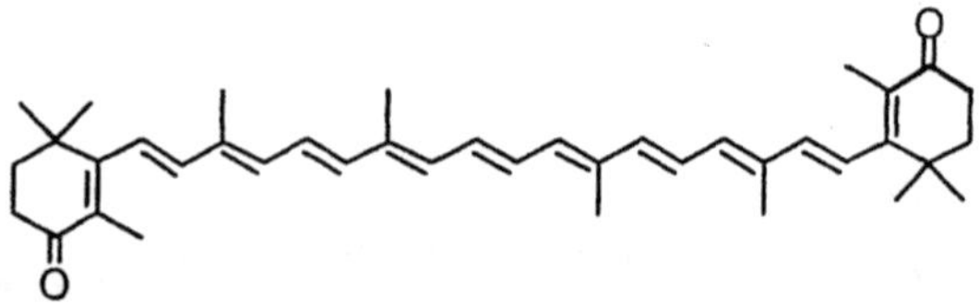

Canthaxanthin

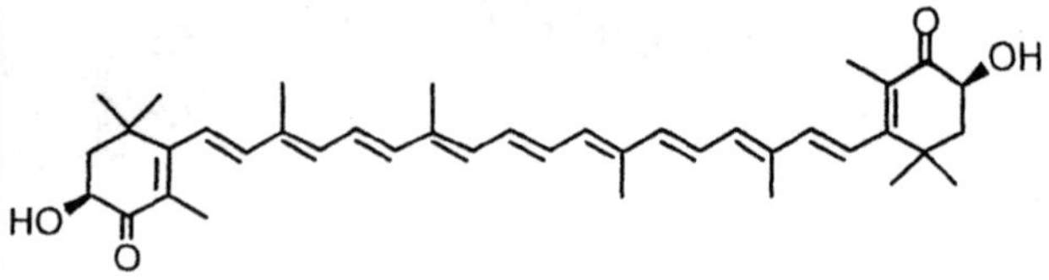

Astaxanthin

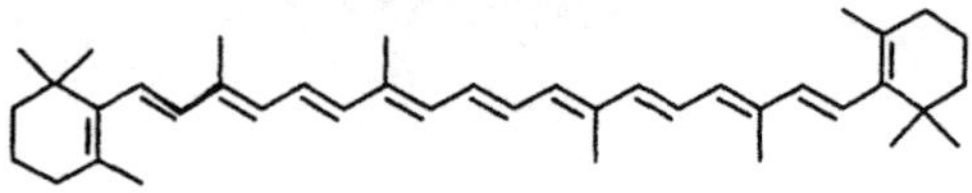

β-carotene

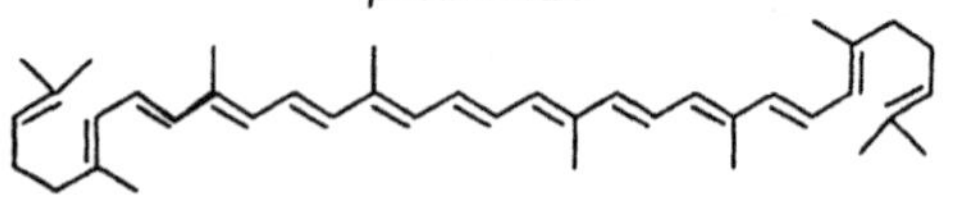

Lycopene

Figure 3. Structural formulas of the retinal xanthophylls: lutein, *meso*-zeaxanthin, and 3R,3′R-zeaxanthin, and of the naturally occurring xanthophylls canthaxanthin and astaxanthin, in comparison with β-carotene and lycopene. Note the shift of the double bond (arrowed) in lutein and *meso*-zeaxanthin. 3R,3′R-zeaxanthin and *meso*-zeaxanthin differ only in the stereochemistry of the hydroxyl group at the 3′-position.

C. MACULAR YELLOW PIGMENT FUNCTION

The macular yellow spot was traditionally believed to aid visual resolution in the macula by filtering out the shorter wavelength blue light that is more easily scattered and which is normally focused slightly on the myopic side of the retinal surface due to chromatic aberration [11]. More recently, this filtration effect has been considered as directly protective against blue light retinal damage [12,13] or as indirectly protective given that these carotenoids are able to quench singlet oxygen and scavenge various excited-state species [14,15]. The retinal carotenoids may also enhance cellular gap junction communication [16], though whether this is relevant to their role in the retina remains to be demonstrated. Their other putative function, given that many carotenoids are metabolized to vitamin A, would be to store vitamin A within the macula. However, provitamin A activity of carotenoids was investigated [17,18] using a rat model of epithelial protection [19]. Lutein and zeaxanthin were found to have only a fraction of the vitamin A activity of β-carotene (Table 1). They therefore cannot be viewed as contributing significantly to the retinol requirements of the retina.

Table 1[a]
Relative Provitamin A Activity of Selected Carotenoids Measured Using the Epithelial Protection Test in Rats [19]

Carotenoid	Relative vitamin A activity (%)
β-carotene	100
Canthaxanthin	5.2
Zeaxanthin	4.2
Lycopene	3.1
Lutein	2.6

[a]: adapted from Weiser et al., 1993 [17,18].

II. NUTRITIONAL SUPPLY, TRANSPORT, AND METABOLISM

It has been known for some time that pro-vitamin A carotenoids are an essential dietary constituent, but this was recognized largely due to the serious repercussions of vitamin A deficiency. Many studies from 1930 to 1980 were designed to establish recommended daily allowances for vitamin A. These vary between countries (reviews in [20,21]). The U.S. recommends 1000 μg retinol equivalents for men and 800 μg for pregnant and non-pregnant women. However, there are no recommended daily allowances for lutein and zeaxanthin and other non-pro-vitamin A carotenoids.

A. NUTRITIONAL ASPECTS

The best dietary sources for carotenoids in general are dark-green leafy vegetables and yellow/red fruits; carrots are the best source of β-carotene and tomatoes of lycopene (review in [22]). Specific information on the lutein and zeaxanthin contents of foodstuffs was hard to find as the two compounds were usually totaled, until separate values were recently reported for a reasonably large number of vegetables and fruits [23] (Table 2). Zeaxanthin is the dominant carotenoid in only a few vegetables such as orange pepper and sweet corn, while most other vegetables such as cabbage, spinach, and watercress are rich in lutein and/or β-carotene.

Table 2[a]
Vegetables and Fruits High in Carotenoids (μg/100 g)

	Z	L	β-C	α-C	Lyc
Vegetables (raw)					
Orange pepper	1608	503	219	167	n.d.
Sweet corn, frozen	522	437	45	60	n.d.
Cabbage	n.d.	14457	10020	n.d.	n.d.
Spinach	n.d.[b]	5869	3397	n.d.	n.d.
Watercress	n.d.	10713	4777	n.d.	n.d.
Carrots	n.d.	283	10800	3610	n.d.
Tomatoes	n.d.	78	415	n.d.	2937
Fruits					
Mandarins	142	50	274	12	n.d.
Apple peel	16	434	190	n.d.	n.d.
Apricots, fresh	31	101	1458	37	n.d.
Satsumas	41	44	23	n.d.	n.d.

[a]: adapted from [23];
[b]: other source reports Z content [51];
Z = zeaxanthin, L = lutein, β-C = β-carotene, α-C = α-carotene,
Lyc = lycopene; n.d. = not detectable;
shaded: carotenoid with highest values in respective vegetable/fruit category.

Thus it is not surprising that the average dietary intake (mg/day) of zeaxanthin is much lower than that of lutein: 0.14 (range: 0.02-0.69) and 0.97 (range: 0.19-2.9), respectively [24], i.e., approximately 7-fold less. This is consistent with earlier figures of 0.3 and 2.3 mg/day, respectively, which assumed a high fruit and vegetable diet [25]. Total daily carotenoid intake averages 6 mg in U.S. men [26]. An important point is that the stereochemistry of retinal zeaxanthin and lutein is 3R,3′R and 3R,3′R,6′R, respectively; this is highly indicative of a dietary origin because the same configuration is found in the naturally occurring lutein [27] and zeaxanthin [28] in food of plant origin. The situation is different with *meso*-zeaxanthin which has the 3R,3′S conformation. This stereoisomer does not occur in plant food [28] and is probably formed in the retina by an as yet unidentified metabolic process (see below).

B. CIRCULATING CAROTENOIDS

The intake of zeaxanthin-rich fruits and/or vegetables is lower than that of the more abundant lutein-rich sources, resulting in serum levels of zeaxanthin which are up to 7 times lower than those of lutein (Tables 3a and 3b).

Table 3a[a]
Serum Carotenoid Values

Carotenoid	Typical serum values μmol/L
Lutein (L)	0.19 [37]
	0.28 [26]
	0.29 [38]
	0.48[44]
Zeaxanthin (Z)	0.04 [38]
	0.06 [37]
	0.07 [26]
β-carotene	0.22 [37]
	0.46 [26]
Lycopene	0.35 [37]
	0.82 [26]

Table 3b[a]
Lutein (L) / total Zeaxanthin (Z_T) Ratios in Serum and Retina[b] Sections

Serum	Retina Sections [39]
3.2 [37]	inner: 0.7 [c]
4.0 [26]	medial: 1.3 [c]
7.3 [38]	outer: 1.9 [c]

[a]: adapted from various sources as indicated.
[b]: pooled samples.
[c]: inner, medial, and outer retina sections: refer to Figures 4a and 4b.

However, the retina seems to concentrate zeaxanthin in the center of the macula where the ratio of lutein to total zeaxanthin becomes 0.7 (Table 3b). Therefore, the key questions are how are the macular carotenoids selected from the approximately 50 different carotenoids found in foodstuffs and the approximately 20 carotenoids in the blood and how are they transported into and metabolized in the retina?

The gastrointestinal absorption of carotenoids has several specific characteristics [29]: (1) absorption decreases with increases in available carotenoid concentration; (2) there is some evidence that various carotenoids may inhibit the absorption of other carotenoids [30], although this is disputed; and (3) the diet must contain a minimum of fat to permit micelle formation given that mucosal cells absorb β-carotene from lipid micelles [31].

Of primary interest are the concentrations of lutein and zeaxanthin relative to other carotenoids and the effects that one carotenoid may have on another. Gärtner et al.. [32] analyzed a natural carotenoid mixture derived from algae containing 0.5% lutein, 0.8% zeaxanthin, 3.6% α-carotene, 70.3% all-trans β-carotene, 22.7% cis isomers of β-carotene, 2.1% unidentified carotenoids, and no lycopene. Uptake into chylomicrons was 14-fold and 4-fold greater with lutein and zeaxanthin, respectively, than their relative contents in the mixture. The serum levels of α-carotene were proportional to the source content while those of all-trans β-carotene were lower. Gärtner et al. concluded that lutein and zeaxanthin are preferentially absorbed into chylomicrons even in the presence of high amounts of β-carotene. This contrasts with an earlier report of impaired lutein absorption in the presence of high intake levels of β-carotene [33].

This issue was recently addressed in a study of carotenoid serum values in a group of 237 subjects who had ingested 20 mg per day of β-carotene for an average of almost 7 years. Of all carotenoids studied, only the serum levels of lutein were reduced, by 11% [34]. Another smaller study also indicated a reduction of lutein serum values. In this study, 90 subjects receiving β-carotene 18 mg, vitamin E 600 mg, and vitamin C 750 mg daily [35] for 3 years showed a statistically significant reduction of lutein serum values after 2 and 3 years [36] with average serum β-carotene levels of 4.9 μmol/L.

C. BINDING PROTEINS AND METABOLISM

While a number of studies have quantified plasma carotenoid concentrations in relation to their absorption from the gastrointestinal tract, the exact mechanisms of uptake into the retina have remained elusive. Two groups recently reported carotenoid binding proteins in the retina [40,41]. The first group isolated a protein with a molecular weight of approximately 40 kD, while the second group described two proteins, 28 kD and 38 kD, respectively. It has also been suggested that intracellular carotenoid binding is mediated by retinal tubulin located in the receptor axon layer of the fovea (i.e., in Henle's fiber layer) [42]. The authors postulate that tubulin may "stabilize" the zeaxanthin and lutein in the fovea just as actin stabilizes astaxanthin in salmon muscle fibers.

Though in the serum the lutein/zeaxanthin (L/Z) ratio varies widely, it does not seem to fall below 2-3, i.e., serum contains at least 2-3 times more lutein than zeaxanthin (Tables 3a and 3b). This is consistent with the greater abundance of dietary lutein. However, in the central retina, the L/Z ratio changes to 0.7, with zeaxanthin becoming the dominant carotenoid (Table 3b). Only in the peripheral retina does lutein remain dominant, with a L/Z ratio of 1.9, approximating the minimum ratio in serum [39]. The retinal distribution of zeaxanthin thus seems to parallel that of the cone photoreceptors, the density of which is high in the central macula but rapidly decreases with higher eccentricities. Bone et al. [39,43] have therefore hypothesized that both lutein and zeaxanthin are taken up by the retina in proportion to their blood concentrations and that a cone-specific enzyme catalyses migration of the double bond to convert lutein to *meso*-zeaxanthin, thus accounting for the higher relative concentration of zeaxanthin and its stereoisomers in the macula. The purported enzyme is thought to mature during development [39], explaining why the infantile retina contains more lutein and less zeaxanthin than in adults. However, there are numerous other factors that can influence the availability and accumulation of zeaxanthin and lutein in the retina. The wide variability in the amount of macular pigment present in different individuals is therefore not surprising (see below).

III. QUANTITATION AND TOPOGRAPHICAL DISTRIBUTION OF RETINAL LUTEIN AND ZEAXANTHIN

Carotenoids may be crucial to macula health and hence vision. For this reason many methods have been developed to determine their concentration, chemical composition and distribution in the retina, both *in vivo* and *postmortem*. Some of these techniques and their results are described below.

A. SPECTROPHOTOMETRY

The earliest attempt to map the yellow macular pigment within the retina was by Snodderly et al. who analyzed dissected unfixed monkey retinae by microspectrography and microdensitometry [5-7]. They determined the absorption maximum of macular pigment at 460 nm, with an interindividual optical density range of 0.6-1.2; two other pigments were observed absorbing at 410 and 435 nm. The macular pigment was identified within Henle's fiber layer of the macula photoreceptor axons (Figure 2), decreasing markedly with increasing retinal eccentricity out to approximately 4°. Its distribution displayed a trimodal distribution profile in some of the monkeys [6].

B. HPLC

Bone et al. [8] and Handelmann et al. [9] used HPLC and showed that the two carotenoids extracted from excised human maculae were lutein and zeaxanthin. Using a micro-trephine technique, it was suggested that within the central 2.3 mm of the macula, zeaxanthin was more concentrated than lutein [43]. Bone et al. [10] also identified a third major macular carotenoid as a stereoisomer of zeaxanthin namely, 3R,3′S-(*meso*)-zeaxanthin (Figure 3). They subsequently described the retinal distribution of the two zeaxanthin stereoisomers and of lutein [39] by dissecting human retinae obtained through eye banks (Figure 4a, legend). The sections prepared were extracted and analyzed using reversed-phase HPLC. Zeaxanthin predominates centrally, while lutein is more abundant in the outer annulus (Figure 4a). Using a chiral column and chemical derivatization they were also able to resolve the total zeaxanthin peak (Z_T): in the central disk, total zeaxanthin (the sum of all its stereoisomers) is represented by roughly equal amounts of 3R,3′R-zeaxanthin and 3R,3′S-(=meso)-zeaxanthin, and very minor amounts of the tentative 3S,3′S-zeaxanthin (Figure 4b), while peripherally, the amount of *meso*-zeaxanthin relative to 3R,3′R-zeaxanthin gradually decreases. *Meso*-zeaxanthin is thus specifically concentrated in the center of the macula, while lutein is relatively more abundant in the periphery.

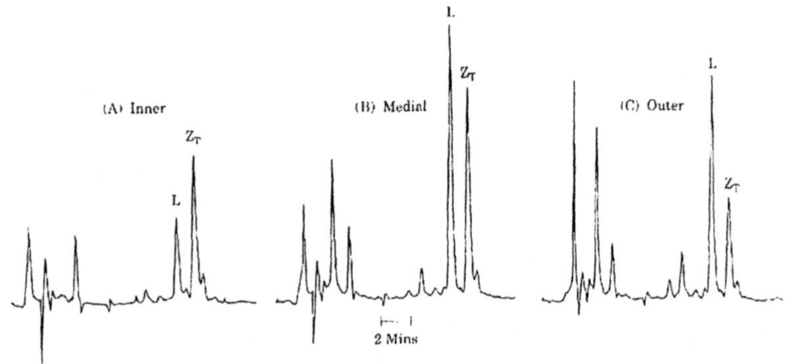

Figure 4a. HPLC chromatograms (reversed phase) from three different regions of a single human retina. (A) Inner - 7.1 mm^2 disk centered on the fovea obtained with 3 mm trephine. (B) Medial - 93 mm^2 annulus obtained with 3 and 11 mm trephines. (C) Outer - 343 mm^2 annulus obtained with 11 and 21 mm trephines. L = lutein, Z_T = total zeaxanthin stereoisomers. Reproduced with permission from Bone et al., 1997 [39].

Further evidence that lutein predominates peripherally was suggested by the finding that subretinal fluid extracts from patients with rhegmatogenous retinal detachment, a disease which primarily involves the peripheral retina, shows only retinol and lutein on HPLC analysis [45]. In a study of macular carotenoid pigment distribution in postmortem human eyes, van Kuijk et al. [46] found lutein to be the predominant carotenoid associated with the rod photoreceptors, residing primarily in the retinal periphery and accounting for 30-40% of the total carotenoid content of the retina, while only 10% was accounted for by the choroid. However, as the cone photoreceptors were destroyed in the rod isolation process, they could not determine cone carotenoid content.

As the above analytical methods require the retina to be excised, they are only applicable postmortem. However, given the possible role of carotenoids for the health of the retina and the potential for augmenting retinal carotenoid levels by diet or supplementation (see below), especially in individuals at increased risk for macular disease, methods have also been developed for the noninvasive *in vivo* measurement of intramacular carotenoid levels. These have been used in various studies, and the results correlated with a number of other ocular and physical parameters (see below).

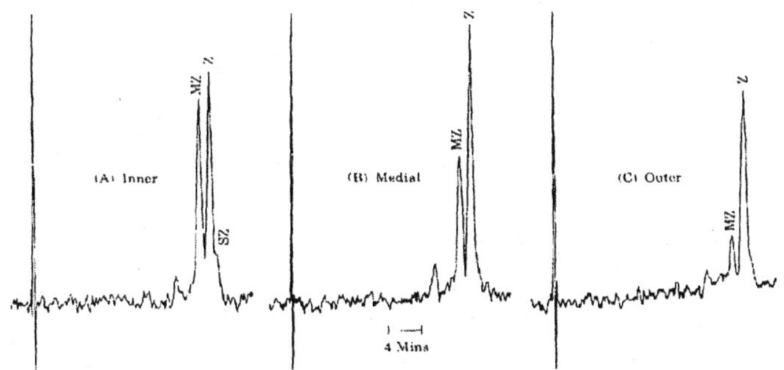

Figure 4b. HPLC chromatograms (chiral column) of pooled extracts from 10 retinas resolving the total zeaxanthin (Z_T) peak. In order of elution, the stereoisomers are *meso*-zeaxanthin (MZ), zeaxanthin (Z), and (3S,3′S)-zeaxanthin (SZ). (A), (B), and C) are the three regions defined in Figure 4a. Reproduced with permission from Bone et al., 1997 [39].

C. HETEROCHROMATIC FLICKER PHOTOMETRY

A standard technique of measuring and quantifying macular pigment in human subjects is heterochromatic flicker photometry. This psychophysical method is described in chapter 13 in more detail. In brief, subjects view a narrow spot of light whose color alternates between blue and green (460 nm and 550 nm, respectively, the maximum and minimum absorbances of the macular yellow pigment). When the spot of light falls within the area of the macula lutea, the blue light is absorbed by the yellow macular pigment and therefore attenuated, while the green light is not. This results in a difference in luminance which in turn causes the light impression to flicker. The flicker can be eliminated by manually increasing the luminance of the attenuated blue light until it matches the luminance of the non-attenuated green light. When corrected by the luminance at a parafoveal location (usually at around 5.5°), where it is assumed that no macular pigment is present, the increment in luminance is a measure of the relative optical density of the macular yellow pigment at the location targeted by the light spot.

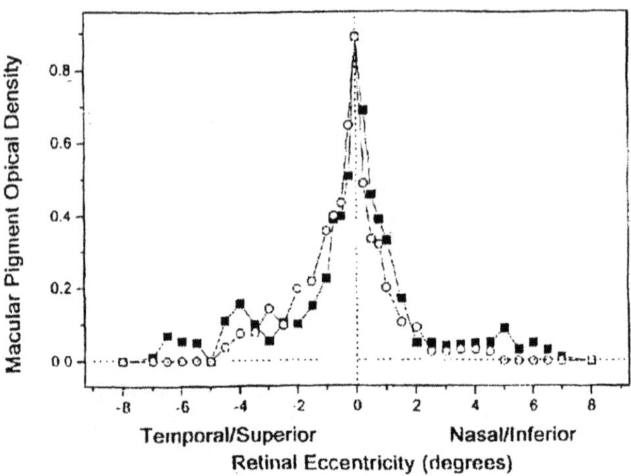

Figure 5. Macular pigment distribution in a single subject measured along the horizontal (filled squares) and vertical (open circles) meridians of the retina. The close correspondence between the two curves suggests a symmetric distribution. Reproduced with permission from Hammond et al., 1997 [52].

Using this technique, Bone and Sparrock [47] reconstructed a detailed absorbance spectrum of yellow macular pigment showing a maximum at 460 nm with an optical density range of 0.3 to 0.7. Werner et al. [11] used a flickering 1° spot at 460 nm comparing the fovea with a 5° parafoveal position in 50 subjects (age range 10-90 years). The mean optical density was 0.39 but there were substantial individual differences from 0.10-0.80 that were not systematically related to age.

In their studies of the effects of gender [48], smoking [49], iris color [50] and diet [51], Hammond et al. also used a flicker technique to measure macular pigment optical density. The test stimulus was a 1° spot presented near the center of a 10° background comparison field. Measurements were made at the center of the fovea and at a 6° paracentral location. Most recently, in a population of 32 subjects, they used smaller stimuli (12' and 20' instead of 1°) to enhance resolution in mapping the distribution of macular carotenoid pigment [52]. The 12' stimulus detected mean peak macular pigment densities (optical density range: 0.18 to 1.35) within the foveola 40% higher than those detected using the 20' stimulus. Results from a typical subject nicely illustrate the symmetrical distribution of macular yellow pigment (Figure 5). In the same work, Hammond *et al.* also found that an exponential decay function with eccentricity modeled the yellow pigment decline toward the periphery better than a Gaussian curve and they gave a formula to estimate macular pigment density across the retina from data at only one point. At higher macular pigment peak densities, the distribution of carotenoids is wider, resulting in higher carotenoid concentrations in the more peripheral retina. This in turn can lead to an underestimation of the peak density, because the assumption of no macular pigment at the reference point for the flicker measurements is no longer valid in such cases.

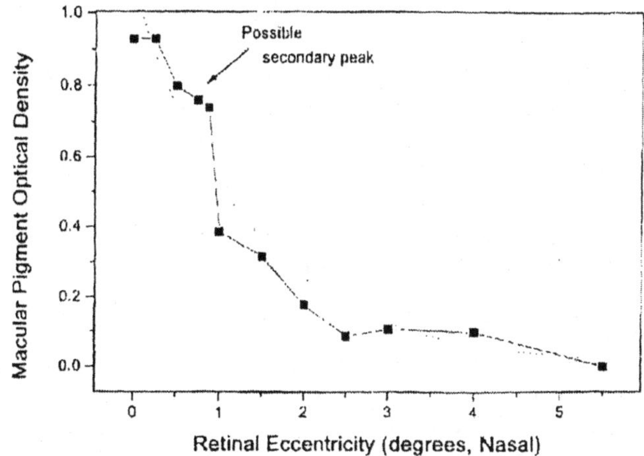

Figure 6. Macular pigment distribution measured in a different subject than in Figure 5. The use of 8' stimuli gave exceptionally high resolution distribution maps suggesting a secondary peak between 0.5 and 1°. The dotted curve shows the best-fitting exponential. Reproduced with permission from Hammond *et al.*, 1997 [52].

In 40% of their subjects, Hammond et al. [52] suggested the existence of secondary "flanking peaks" in the decline of macular yellow pigment density (Figure 6), indicating that macular pigment in humans may also have a trimodal distribution, as described by Snodderly et al. in monkeys [6]. The apparent parafoveal variability in macular pigment density may also be significant in macular degenerative disease as it is the 2-4° region of eccentricity from the fovea which is thought to be most vulnerable in the onset of AMD [15,53].

D. MACULAR PIGMENT POLARIZATION

Based on the polarization properties of the macular yellow pigment, Bone described a "dichroic ratio" measured by the orthogonal comparison of polarized light extinction [54]. This ratio correlates positively with other measures of macular pigment density including the flicker technique.

E. LIPOFUSCIN FLUORESCENCE

A different new method of measuring macular pigment density using lipofuscin fluorescence has been described by Delori *et al.* [55]. Upon excitation with wavelengths of 470, 510 or 550 nm the lipofuscin in the RPE fluoresces as orange and red light [56], and this fluorescence is not absorbed by the macular pigment. Thus only the excitation is affected by macular pigment absorption. A comparison of the fluorescence excited at 470 and 550 nm in the fovea and at a location where no macular pigment is present provides a single pass measure of the density of the macular pigment. Their results using this method showed good correlation with psychophysical methods and confirmed that macular pigment density was lower in smokers ($p = 0.008$) and higher in subjects with dark irises ($p = 0.02$). They also were able to reproduce the finding that females tended to have lower macular pigment densities. This fluorescence technique appears to offer the future possibility of a rapid and reliable objective assessment technique, therefore making it also attractive for the clinical determination of macular pigment density. Furthermore, the method is applicable to autofluorescence imaging techniques allowing the derivation of detailed distribution maps of the macular pigment.

F. RAMAN SPECTROSCOPY

Bernstein et al. used resonance Raman spectroscopy for the noninvasive measurement of carotenoid distribution, physical state and concentration in whole mounted human retinae [57]. The technique utilizes the fact that zeaxanthin and lutein exhibit strong resonance-enhanced Raman spectra when excited by visible light. The excitatory light is generated by an argon ion laser and the scattered light analyzed by a Raman spectrometer. In their prototype system, Bernstein et al. demonstrated an extraordinarily high correlation in macular carotenoid values between HPLC and Raman spectroscopy, making the technique a viable candidate for complementing other *in vivo* noninvasive assessment methods for macular pigment.

IV. MACULAR PIGMENT OPTICAL DENSITY: INTERINDIVIDUAL DIFFERENCES AND EFFECTS OF GENDER, SMOKING, AND OTHER FACTORS

Regardless of the measurement method utilized, interindividual macular pigment density values reported in the literature vary 4- to 10-fold. In monkeys, Snodderly et al. found that histological microdensity maps varied substantially and were specific to each individual [5,6]. In humans, even homozygous twins demonstrate noticeable differences in macular pigment density [58]. That these interindividual differences are genuine is suggested by the matching bilateral results for eyes from the same individual [59,60]. But the issue remains unresolved as exemplified by Hammond and Fuld who found substantial intraindividual variation on retesting subjects in a psychophysical study [60].

Like Werner et al. [11], Bone et al. [43] looked at age as a determinant of interindividual differences in macular carotenoid content. HPLC analysis of 87 trephined donor specimens, however, demonstrated no age-related difference in macular lutein or zeaxanthin density in the range 3-95 years; however, below 2 years of age lutein was the predominant central macular carotenoid, being replaced by zeaxanthin only in specimens of older donors.

Macular yellow pigment density is also influenced by a number of other factors including sex [48], smoking history [49], iris color [50] and diet [51]. Hammond et al. found 38% higher values in males *vs* females ($p<0.001$) despite similar plasma carotenoid concentrations and dietary intake (except for fats) [48]. Pigment density is also significantly lower in blue/gray *vs* brown/black eyes ($p<0.01$); there are no significant differences with green/hazel eyes or any other iris color [50]. The differences do not correlate with plasma concentrations or with the dietary intake of carotenoids or fat. As a result, the authors suggest that macular pigment density may be linked to the inheritance of other traits but it is also possible that with blue irises transmitting increased levels of light, the "photo-oxidant load" might decrease the macular pigment density in these individuals. Thus these data expand on the body of evidence that there are individual variations a) in peak macular pigment density and b) across the spatial distribution of the macular pigment.

A prospective study of macular degeneration in twins should help to resolve this question of interindividual differences and genetic factors. Seddon et al. [61] will be studying several etiological factors including serum lutein and zeaxanthin levels in subjects recruited from a pool of 14,000 twins.

V. PRINCIPLES UNDERLYING THE PHYSIOLOGICAL SIGNIFICANCE OF THE MACULAR CAROTENOIDS

The roles played by the macular carotenoids have not been fully characterized nor conclusively verified experimentally. Nonetheless we can theorize about their putative functions by extrapolating from their known photochemical and biological properties. These functions center on the yellow color of the pigment which confers the ability to absorb high-energy blue light and on the general quenching capability which the macular carotenoids share with most other carotenoids. Both properties may be important in reducing the risk of AMD.

A. BLUE LIGHT FILTRATION

The radiation incident upon the human eye is filtered by the various ocular tissues anterior to the retina. Thus the cornea absorbs UV-B and the lens absorbs UV-A while transmitting blue light. This blue light has the potential to damage the retina as has been detailed by a number of findings. Ham and Mueller [12] introduced the blue light hazard function to characterize the potential for damage semiquantitatively. It describes the extent of macular damage as dependent on wavelength and peaks at around 430 nm, thereby overlapping significantly with the absorbance spectrum of the macular yellow pigment [13]. Experiments with rabbit retinas have shown that exposure to blue light (400-520 nm) induces dysfunction of the blood-retinal barrier at the retinal pigment epithelium 30 times more effectively than the longer wavelength fraction of white light [56]. Also lipofuscin, which accumulates during aging in the retinal pigment epithelium, can increase the susceptibility to blue light [63]. By virtue of their yellow color the macular carotenoids have the capability to absorb blue light [13] and could thus reduce the potential hazard caused by blue light.

It has been known for some time that the human lens changes in transmittance, absorbing more shorter wavelength visible light as it ages [64]. In the most detailed study to date, total transmittance of postmortem human lenses was measured over the age range between birth and 90 years [65]. At birth the lens is already pale yellow in color. Its filtering capability, however, is smaller than in later years. Thus in childhood and adolescence (< 20 years), much more blue range energy reaches the retina than in later life, when lenticular short wavelength absorbance increases with the yellowing of the lens. In fact, around 60 years of age, the lens affords nearly as much blue light protection as does the macular pigment [13]. This means that the young are at higher risk of macular exposure to blue light. This may be a significant risk factor for later retinal disease in genetically predisposed individuals or in conditions where dietary or other factors decrease carotenoid levels in the macular pigment. Lutein and zeaxanthin were recently reported to be the most abundant carotenoids in breast milk [38]. This may be relevant in terms of retinal protection from blue light by ensuring the provision of yellow macular carotenoids to the newborn and infant during a period when the lens is virtually transparent to blue light.

In investigating the correlation between lenticular optical density and macula carotenoid levels, an inverse relationship between macular pigment density and lens opacity was recently found in older but not younger subjects, meaning that older people with a high amount of macular pigment appear to have less lens opacities [66]. The investigators suggested that macular lutein and zeaxanthin could serve as markers for lenticular carotenoid levels, which cannot be satisfactorily measured *in vivo*. In fact, they proposed macular lutein and zeaxanthin levels as a general biomarker of ocular health, lens included. This idea is partly supported by findings of three independent research groups, which have identified lutein and zeaxanthin as occurring in the human lens to the exclusion of other carotenoids [67-69].

B. ANTIOXIDANT ACTION

Through thermal effects and photooxidation, radiation can produce both acute and chronic retinal lesions [70]. Absorption of short wavelengths in the ultraviolet and blue range especially by endogenous and exogenous photosensitizers results in the immediate formation of excited species termed singlet state molecules. These short-lived molecules form photoproducts, fluoresce or give rise to the generation of triplet state molecules by intersystem crossing. Excited triplet state molecules are longer-lived than singlet state molecules, and react with neighboring molecules, especially oxygen, to produce free radicals such as the oxygen free radicals superoxide and the hydroxyl radical, or give rise to potentially destructive singlet oxygen via type II reactions. The excited oxygen moieties thus produced can, in turn, oxidize many cellular targets. They may interact with polyunsaturated fatty acids in a chain-like series of reactions collectively referred to as lipid peroxidation. Cellular structures containing large amounts of polyunsaturated fatty acids, such as the retinal photoreceptor outer segments [71], are especially vulnerable to these excited molecules [72,73].

The carotenoids have two important and well-documented properties: their singlet oxygen quenching capability [71,75,76] and their ability to scavenge other reactive oxygen species [77-79]. Quenching potentials differ between carotenoids: the *in vitro* quenching rate constant increases with the number of conjugated double bonds present in the molecule [80,81]. It has long been known that lycopene (Figure 3) is the most effective singlet oxygen quencher among the carotenoids [74,78]. It is followed by β-carotene, canthaxanthin, and the zeaxanthin stereoisomers which are virtually identical in their *in vitro* singlet oxygen quenching capability as shown by recent data for *meso*-zeaxanthin (Table 4 [82]).

Table 4 [a]
Repair of the α-Tocopheryl Radical Cation and Quenching of Singlet Oxygen by Different Carotenoids

Carotenoid	Tocopheryl radical cation[b]	Singlet oxygen[c]
Zeaxanthin	26.4	12.6
Meso-zeaxanthin	23.3	12.2
Lycopene	13.5	16.8
ß-carotene	10.2	13.5
Canthaxanthin	8.8	13.2
Lutein	5.3	6.6
Astaxanthin	not measured	11.3

[a]: adapted from personal communication, Truscott, 1997 [82].
[b]: generated by pulse radiolysis [83], 2nd order rate constant, $M^{-1}s^{-1}$, in hexane.
[c]: generated by laser photoexcitation [78], 2nd order rate constant, $M^{-1}s^{-1}$, in benzene.

The situation is different regarding the quenching of the α-tocopheryl radical cation (Table 4). In this system, zeaxanthin and *meso*-zeaxanthin are the best *in vitro* quenchers among the carotenoids. Though these are *in vitro* experiments which cannot readily be extrapolated to *in vivo* situations, α-tocopherol has for some time been known to occur in the retina [84]. It is thus theoretically possible that the α-tocopheryl radical cation is generated somewhere deep within the cell membranes of the retina and then quenched by the xanthophylls, which are thought to span the membrane. The resulting xanthophyll radical cations could in turn be repaired by ascorbic acid, also known to exist in the retina [85], and this reaction would then regenerate the parent xanthophylls [86].

Whatever the physiological validity of such speculation, the quenching data unanimously support the theory that the carotenoids are present in the retina at least in part because of their antioxidative functions. If singlet oxygen and radical quenching is important in the retina, the incorporation of the more efficient molecule(s) appears logical. Crabtree and Adler [87] recently hypothesized that lycopene, the most effective quencher [74], would have been the better choice in the retina. Yet this non-polar carotenoid has not been identified in a human retina [9]. The polarity of the carotenoids may therefore be crucial for transport into the retina. Thus β-carotene, another non-polar carotenoid, was not even detected in a postmortem retina from a subject who had been taking very high doses of a combination of β-carotene and canthaxanthin [88]; the highly polar canthaxanthin, on the other hand, was present in substantial amounts.

Quenching capability is measured *in vitro* using organic solvents and some caution is needed in extrapolating to *in vivo* systems. Nonetheless, the singlet oxygen quenching and radical scavenging capabilities of the carotenoids were the major reason why β-carotene, for example, was suggested for the treatment of erythropoietic protoporphyria [89], a genetically determined disease with abnormal high sensitivity to light.

The antioxidant activities of the carotenoids may also be regulated by their cellular distribution. As recently demonstrated [79] in an *in vitro* system, β-carotene is effective in inhibiting lipid peroxidation of liposomes, but only when it has been previously incorporated into the liposomal bilayer membranes; it has little antioxidant effect when added to preformed liposomes in solution. Other carotenoids are also capable of inhibiting membrane peroxidation [90]. This function is extremely attractive in trying to explain the role of the retinal carotenoids because the concentration of polyunsaturated fatty acids and the incident visible light has been repeatedly reported to induce lipid peroxidation [91].

While blue light filtration may be of particular importance in youth, the antioxidant properties of lutein and zeaxanthin may become more important in later life due to age-related deterioration in the antioxidant enzymatic system, at least in the rat [92]. A study in patients aged 7-85 years concluded that, except for superoxide dismutase which declined in the peripheral retina but not in the macular region, age did not appear to affect antioxidant enzyme activity [93]; however, there was considerable interindividual variability. This study made some important observations: 1) the activity of retinal antioxidant enzymes, i.e., superoxide dismutase, catalase, glutathione peroxidase and glutathione reductase, was verified and quantitated over a large part of the human life span; 2) the usual complement of antioxidant enzymes is present and the enzymes are active within the macula and retinal tissues; 3) there appears to be no "preferential" distribution of these enzymes or at least none was reported; 4) age does not affect macular activity, suggesting a sustained need for protection; and 5) the large interindividual variability is common to both carotenoids and these antioxidant enzymes. Perhaps they should be grouped together to ascertain whether decreases in concentration and/or activity correlate with an increased risk of AMD.

Khachik *et al.* recently described the existence of putative oxidation products of both zeaxanthin and lutein in 58 pairs of postmortem human retinae and one pair of monkey retinae, namely 3R,6′R-hydroxy-β,ϵ-carotene-3′-one (A) and 3R,3′S,6′R-(=3′-epi-)lutein (B), respectively [94]. They suggest that (A) could have been formed directly from lutein, while (B) could have been generated through a cascade of oxidation/reduction sequences coupled with double bond isomerisations either from lutein or from zeaxanthin.

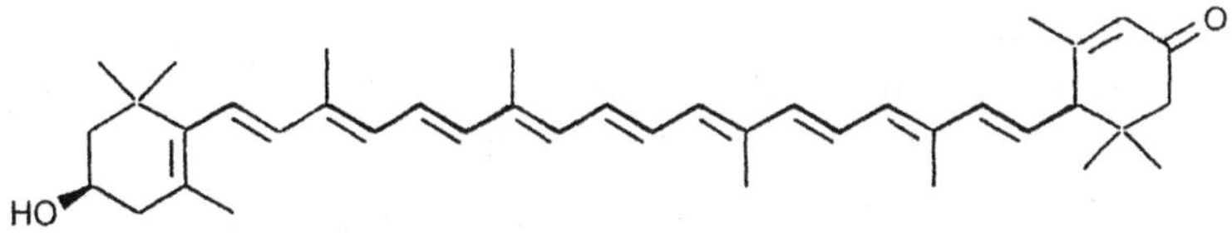

HO O

(3R,6'R)-3-hydroxy-β,ε-carotene-3'-one (A)

HO OH

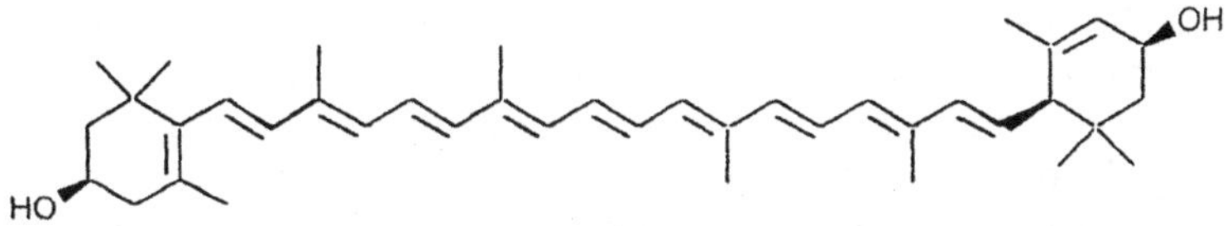

(3R,3'S,6'R)-lutein (= 3'-epi-lutein) (B)

The amount of (A) – up to 24% of total retinal lutein – suggests that it could be a major oxidative metabolite of lutein, while only minor amounts of (B) were identified. However, as Khachik et al. point out, the possibility cannot be excluded that these metabolites were formed in serum, where they have already been identified [94], and that they were only subsequently transported passively into the retina. Should the production of the carotenoid oxidation products, however, be verified as occurring in the retina, then it would be the first direct demonstration of those substances in the retina, which would lend considerable additional support to their antioxidant action *in vivo*.

VI. RISK REDUCTION IN AGE-RELATED MACULAR DEGENERATION (also see Chapter 11)

A. GENERAL

AMD is a devastating degenerative condition of the macula and in the western world it is the main cause of irreversible blindness among the elderly [4]. It occurs in two forms: a "dry" atrophic form, and a "wet" form characterized by the presence of neovascularization causing fluid accumulation and eventually loss of sight due to hemorrhagic maculopathy. AMD is significantly associated with increasing age. In the Blue Mountain Eye Study, it was present in 1.9% of the overall population; it was absent below 55 years of age, but present in 18.5% of those aged ≥ 85 years [95]. Distributions were similar in the Framingham Eye Study [96], Beaver Dam Study [97], and in the Finnish Oulu county study [98].

While Caucasians have long been known to be at greater risk, a recent study found wet AMD to be rare in Hispanic vs non-Hispanic whites, probably due to an important genetic determinant [99]. Other studies [100-102] have reported a family history of the condition as a risk factor.

Other AMD susceptibility variables reviewed in [15] include gender: women are at greater risk than men. This may in part be related to estrogen levels since the frequency of the wet form is reduced in postmenopausal women on estrogen-only replacement therapy. Cardiovascular disease, especially factors relating to hypertension, are also linked to AMD, as are high levels of HDL cholesterol, cigarette smoking, exposure to sunlight [104] and low ocular melanin (melanin itself being both a generator and potent quencher of free radicals). The latter three risk factors are of particular relevance in oxidative situations.

The etiology of AMD is recognized as being multifactorial. However, the concept of oxidative insult as one of the primary events is well substantiated. The retina is highly active metabolically with a respiratory quotient near unity and a much higher blood flow than other tissues. In such an environment, the oxidative nature of retinal functions, high oxygen tension, and simultaneous presence of light can ultimately produce singlet oxygen and numerous free radicals with the potential to induce peroxidation of polyunsaturated fatty acids, including that of docosahexaenoic acid, the most highly unsaturated naturally occurring fatty acid and major lipid constituent of vertebrate photoreceptors [71].

It is also possible that the selective distribution of the retinal carotenoids (and possibly vitamin E [84]) impinges on susceptibility to AMD. As pointed out by Snodderly [15], the foveal crest and immediately surrounding retina are the first areas to show degenerative changes in AMD. They are the site of maximal age-related rod photoreceptor loss even in healthy retinae, and of the gradual accumulation of lipofuscin, a product of lipid peroxidation. Snodderly suggested that the relatively low concentrations of both vitamin E and retinal carotenoids in the foveal crest (in contrast to the center of the fovea) may make it particularly susceptible to the development of AMD.

Differences in macular carotenoid levels have been identified in association with retinal damage, AMD and certain risk factors for AMD. In 1988, Haegerstrom-Portnoy [103] reported a faster decrease in short-wavelength (blue) cone sensitivity in older individuals with lower macular pigment concentrations. Acceleration of blue cone loss with aging is thought to be a form of direct retinal damage and perhaps a precursor of AMD. These results suggest that increased macular pigment density may be protective against such damage. Using HPLC in a study on postmortem eyes from 12 normal subjects and 12 subjects with AMD, Landrum et al. [105] found that average total carotenoid levels in the AMD retinae were approximately 30 % lower than in normal controls. The decrease was not restricted to the macula but found throughout the retina. In this case, however, it is not clear whether the lower carotenoid content is a consequence or the cause of the disease.

Clinical studies of the association between carotenoids and AMD have broadly been either epidemiological or interventional (Tables 5 and 6). Epidemiological surveys have tried to correlate the intake of antioxidant active substances from food (dietary intake) or micronutrient supplements (supplemental intake) with risk reduction for AMD. Serum levels of these agents have also been compared between subjects with healthy retinae and those in various stages of AMD. Such epidemiological studies, however, can never establish a causal relationship but only furnish circumstantial evidence. The situation is different with interventional studies, in which the agents are administered on a double-blind randomized basis vs placebo and the results compared using predefined efficacy parameters. In the case of supplementation with lutein and zeaxanthin, where only small to moderate responses can be expected, only studies such as these are likely to provide a definite answer as to the effect of lutein and zeaxanthin on AMD as was pointed out by Seddon and Hennekens [106]. However, the specific time-course and nature of the disease will make the design of such trials very difficult.

B. EPIDEMIOLOGICAL STUDIES

Although there is recently increasing interest in epidemiological studies of carotenoids and their effects, only a few studies as yet have been so specific as to deal with the issue of lutein and zeaxanthin with respect to their potential to reduce the risk of diseases of the macula such as AMD.

Those studies either studied the effect of dietary or supplemental intake. However, because of the current limited availability of lutein and/or zeaxanthin supplements, no supplemental intake studies for these carotenoids are reported. Another type of epidemiological studies evaluated the correlation of serum values of the micronutrients in question with the risk of AMD. In Table 5 those studies are listed giving information whether lutein or zeaxanthin or other micronutrients have been studied. Already in 1985, nutritional status had been proposed as a potential risk factor in AMD [130]. Subsequently, results from the first epidemiological investigation of the correlation of nutritional factors and the risk of AMD were reported [111]. This study was a case-control study comparing 26 AMD patients with 23 age- and sex-matched controls. The use of vitamin supplements and serum levels of vitamins A, C, and E did not differ significantly between the two groups. However, the sample size was small and as control spouses were used, which may have biased against detecting any dietary effect. Another early epidemiological study reevaluated AMD and nutritional data from NHANES I and suggested that subjects who ingested fruits and/or vegetables rich in vitamin A and C for 7 times per week or more had a statistically significant reduced risk for AMD [107]. Lutein or zeaxanthin, however, have not been assessed in this study. Another dietary intake study assessed past intake of carotenoids, antioxidants, and zinc but did not

Table 5[a]
Vitamins/Carotenoids and Reduction of Risk for AMD[b], Compilation of 14 Epidemiological Studies

Number of Subjects (n), or of Cases vs. Controls	Results (high. vs. low*), Odds Ratios (CI) * except where indicated		Reference
	Lutien/zeaxanthin	**Other micronutrients**	
	Dietary Intake Studies		
n = 3,082 (> 45 yrs old) NHANES I	not reported	fruit/vegs. rich in A or C 7x per week: rr: 0.59 (0.37-0.99)	[107]
55 vs. 67	not reported	β-C, C, E: no rr	[108]
356 vs. 520	L + Z: rr, 0.43 (0.2-0.7) Spinach (5-6+/wk): rr: 0.12 (0.01-0.9)	β-C: rr: 0.59 (0.4-0.96) Carrots (5-6+/wk): no rr: 0.72 (0.4-1.4)	[109]
n = 1,968	L + Z: no rr: 1.0 (0.7-1.5), early AMD	AO index: no rr: 01 (0.4-1.1), early AMD Zn: some effect	[110]
	Supplemental Intake Studies		
26 vs. 23	not reported	Multivitamins: no rr: 0.3 (0.1-0.6)	[111]
n = 2,152	not reported	C: no rr: 0.7 (0.5-1.0) Zn: rr: 0.4 (0.2-0.9)	[112]
n = 520	not reported	Any vitamin use: no rr 0.51 (0.11-2.36)	[113]
	Serum Level Studies		
26 vs. 23	not reported	A, C, E: no rr	[111]
80 vs. 86	not reported	E: no rr: 1.0 (0.95-1.03) Se: rr: 0.2 (0.03-1)	[114]
421 vs. 615	L + Z: rr: 0.3 (0.2-0.6)	all carotenoids: rr 0.3 (0.2-0.6) AO ind.: rr: 0.3 (0.1-0.7)	[115]
65 vs. 65	Lutein: no rr: 1.37 (0.57-3.38)	β-, α-carotene, lycopene, β-cryptoxanthin: no rr	[116]
n = 976	not reported	E: rr: 0.43 (0.25-0.73) AO ind.: rr: 0.43 (0.26-0.70)	[117]
71 vs. 61	Lutein: no rr, higher levels in cases	β-C: no rr: higher levels in cases	[118]
167 vs. 167	L + Z: no rr: 0.7 (0.4-1.4) low vs. high	Higher risk with lower lycopene levels: 2.2 (1.1-45), low vs. high	[119]

[a]: adapted from various sources as indicated, abbreviations see Table 6;
[b]: and related maculopathies.

produce statistically significant results for the carotenoids studied including lutein and zeaxanthin, while the intake of zinc was correlated with lower risk [110]. However, problems in accurately defining and assessing past nutritional intake contribute to questions about the significance of this finding. There are some smaller studies which did not report any correlation between serum levels of lutein and or zeaxanthin and the risk of AMD [116,118,119].

In contrast, interesting results were reported from the Beaver Dam Study [119] which had examined a largely Caucasian community in south central Wisconsin, comparing 167 subjects with retinal pigment epithelial abnormalities, soft drusen and exudative AMD with an equal number of normal controls. This study addressed the individual serum concentrations of lutein and zeaxanthin. While not statistically significant, serum lutein and zeaxanthin concentrations were slightly lower in the cases with exudative macular degeneration. Individuals with serum concentrations of lycopene in the lowest quintile were twice as likely to have AMD as compared to all others combined. Since lycopene does not occur in the retina, the investigators postulated that, because this carotenoid is a potent antioxidant, its presence could indirectly affect the establishment of AMD by reducing atherogenesis.

These results regarding lycopene were not confirmed by the largest and probably most powerful study which has assessed the effect of carotenoid serum levels regarding risk reduction of AMD. This study has investigated 421 subjects with advanced AMD and 615 controls. A reduced risk (OR 0.3, CI 0.2-0.6) of AMD was found in subjects with higher serum levels of carotenoids [115]. Carotenoids for which, statistically, risk reduction was strongest were lutein and zeaxanthin grouped together, β-carotene, and cryptoxanthin. Neither β-carotene nor cryptoxanthin, however, have so far been reported to occur in the retina. Therefore, their effects may either be indirect or they merely are markers of lutein and zeaxanthin.

Subsequently, in an investigation into the relationship between dietary intake of carotenoids, vitamins A, C, and E and the risk of neovascular AMD in 356 patients *vs* 520 controls, Seddon et al. reported that the highest quintile of carotenoid ingestion was associated with a 43% lower risk of AMD when compared with the lowest quintile [109]. Furthermore, it was the macular carotenoids, i.e., lutein and zeaxanthin, ingested predominantly in the form of spinach (for L and Z content see Table 2), which were most strongly associated with a lower risk for AMD. In contrast, no correlation was found with the ingestion of retinol, pre-vitamin A carotenoids, or vitamins C and E. In examining the relationship between smoking, carotenoids and AMD, the study also suggested that while current smokers were at greatest risk of AMD, the risk was somewhat reduced for those with the greater lutein and zeaxanthin intakes.

While the epidemiological evidence regarding the potential of lutein and zeaxanthin to reduce the risk of AMD may appear to be conflicting, it has to be appreciated that AMD is a difficult multifactorial disease to study. It also has a long time-course and etiologically may have its initiation much earlier than currently reported. Serum levels seem to be a good parameter to delineate the influence of nutrition on its development and progression. But they rather give information on the current intake, while long-term dietary history may be of particular significance especially since AMD is a disease of senescence. There are also other conditions, such as skin cancer and cataractogenesis, where exposure to radiation, relative presence of melanin, photosensitization conditions or antioxidant behavior at one point in time contribute to the expression of a condition decades later. Certainly there is sufficient evidence to indicate the need for other types of studies: some that address the effect of various concentrations and/or depletion of one or more carotenoids on cellular and physiological effects of macular tissue; some that specifically address the long-term clinical effects of such manipulations and some that pursue the need for additional epidemiological studies. In this context, interesting populations to study might be those in the South Pacific. Men from the Fiji islands are reported to have dietary lutein intakes up to 25.7 mg per day [129] *vs* an average intake of 1-6 mg per day in the US [26]. The implications of this elevated intake level in terms of potential retinal protection against light exposure could be evaluated by studying members of this population, who presumably have had a life-long high carotenoid intake, vs a control population with a lower and shorter lutein intake but comparable degree of light exposure.

C. INTERVENTION TRIALS

Unfortunately, there are no results of human intervention trials to date using lutein and/or zeaxanthin since these are of limited availability for human consumption. Also neither carotenoid is being used in the ongoing major clinical study called Age-Related Eye Disease Study (AREDS) initiated by the National Eye Institute [123]. Four intervention trials using related micronutrients and studying ophthalmologic parameters are tabulated in Table 6.

The only intervention data with zeaxanthin so far available were obtained in animals [124]. For three months quails were fed carotenoid free diets or diets supplemented with 5 mg/kg 3R,3′R-zeaxanthin. The animals were then exposed to intermittent white light (3200 lux) for 28 hours in order to induce general photic damage to the retina. After 14 hours in the dark, the eyes were excised for the determination by HPLC of zeaxanthin in the retina and the measurement of the extent of apoptosis, which was confirmed by TUNEL stain. The number of light-induced apoptoses of rod and cone photoreceptor cells was drastically reduced in treated *vs* untreated animals. Furthermore, the retinae containing more zeaxanthin as assessed by HPLC seemed to be better protected than those with less. This is the first direct preclinical demonstration of the efficacy of zeaxanthin for the prevention of one important consequence of light-induced retinal damage. It complements older data showing loss of macular pigment and more drusen and other indicators of increased photic damage in monkeys raised on a carotenoid-depleted diet for 5 years [125].

Table 6[a]
Vitamins/Carotenoids and Reduction of Risk for AMD, Results in Four Intervention Trials

Number of Subjects, duration	Results		Reference
	Lutein/zeaxanthin	Other micronutrients	
n = 278 7 - 12 yrs	not administered	β-C, C E, Se: Stabilization or improvement in 53% of subjects	[120]
n = 260 6 yrs	not administered	β-C or E; no rr	[121]
39 vs. 32 placebo, 1.5 yrs	not administered	AOs incl. β-C, C and E: no rr	[122]
n = 4,700 10 yrs[c]	not being studied	β-C, C, E, Zn: ongoing	[123][b]

[a]: adapted from various sources as indicated;
[b]: AREDS, Age-Related Eye Disease Study, ongoing NEI study, investigating β-C, C, E, and Zn;
[c]: projected duration.
Abbreviations: rr = risk reduction suggested; CI = confidence interval; AOs = antioxidants; AO ind. = antioxidant index; A, C, E, = vitamins A, C, E; β-C = β-carotene; Zn = zinc.

VII. MODULATION OF MACULAR PIGMENT BY SUPPLEMENTATION OR DIET

Given the possible relationship between retinal carotenoids and AMD, attempts have been made to enhance the retinal densities of lutein and zeaxanthin by diet or supplementation. Khachick et al. [126] purified lutein from marigold flowers and zeaxanthin from *Lycium chinense,* a berry used in Chinese traditional medicine, and administered suspensions in olive oil to three volunteers. Daily doses of 10 mg were given for 18 (lutein) or 21 (zeaxanthin) days. HPLC showed that the serum levels of both carotenoids peaked after one week: lutein at 0.9 μmol/L, and zeaxanthin considerably lower at 0.1 μmol/L. No explanation was offered for this large difference and the relevance of these findings is therefore unclear, partly because macular pigment density was not measured in this study.

This was different in the following work. Landrum et al. reported a supplementation study in two subjects receiving 30 mg lutein (as a marigold lutein ester extract suspended in canola oil) daily for 140 days [127]. Serum lutein levels rapidly increased 10-fold to 1.4-2.0 μmol/L in the first week and held that level for the remainder of the study. Noninvasive macular pigment estimation using heterochromatic flicker photometry showed a slower response than the serum levels, increasing after 200 days in one subject by an average of 41% and 37% in the right and left eye, respectively, and by only 21% bilaterally in the other subject. These results were expanded in a follow-up study in 5 subjects with the same daily dose [128], demonstrating that macular yellow pigment density could either plateau or continue to increase throughout the duration of supplementation. The authors concluded that increase in macula yellow pigmentation appears to be a slow process, with considerable interindividual variation.

The response of macular pigment density to dietary administration of lutein and zeaxanthin was investigated by Hammond et al. [51]. They found that the majority of subjects whose diets for 6 or 14-15 weeks had been supplemented with daily portions of spinach (containing 10.8 mg lutein and 0.3 mg zeaxanthin) and corn (containing 0.4 mg lutein and 0.3 mg zeaxanthin) or spinach alone responded with mean serum lutein increases of 33% and a mean increase in macular pigment density of 19%. Two subjects had decreases in macular pigment density despite increases in serum lutein and one subject had virtually unchanged serum and macular pigment density. Where elevations in macular pigment densities occurred, these were sustained for some months even after the subjects resumed their non-supplemented diet.

While there seems to be considerable variability, these findings demonstrate that macular pigment can indeed be altered by supplementation as well as by diet. This may be important, because macular pigment appears to be very stable over time when analyzed chemically postmortem [43] or psychophysically *in vivo* [52]. In this respect, Hammond et al. [51] reported a subject whose macular pigment was very stable over 5 years, yet increased by 50% after only 14 weeks of a test diet rich in lutein and zeaxanthin, and remained elevated for 9 months after the diet was discontinued.

VIII. CONCLUSIONS

There are two main putative functions of the carotenoids lutein, 3R, 3′S-(*meso*)-zeaxanthin and 3R,3′R-zeaxanthin comprising the macular yellow pigment that are particularly attractive in terms of macular health: antioxidant activity and blue-light filtration. Since the macula receives the bulk of incident light within the highly oxygenated environment of the retina, it is subjected to higher levels of photooxidative stress than other parts of the retina. The macular carotenoids can be presumed to filter the transmittance of blue light to the photoreceptors, lessening the overall incidence of photon energy and thus decreasing phototoxicity by quenching free radicals and singlet oxygen-driven oxidation.

We now have potent techniques for measuring the amount of macular yellow pigment *in vitro* and, noninvasively, *in vivo*. The resulting data, when tested against a number of environmental and genetic factors, show a consistent correlation between lower macular pigment density and the presence of risk factors for AMD, e.g., gender, smoking, and blue iris color. The same techniques have also shown that ingested lutein and 3R,3′R-zeaxanthin can reach the macula and that their amount can be increased by diet or supplementation. Either means can therefore be used to correct deficient or augment normal macular pigment.

Of all ophthalmologic diseases, AMD is of particular interest. It is a significant cause of irreversible blindness in old age, and a multifactorial disease with a long time course and a still uncertain etiology. Two powerful epidemiological studies have indicated that increases in the dietary intake and serum levels of lutein and zeaxanthin are statistically significantly correlated with a lower risk of AMD. This has not been confirmed in other (smaller and less powerful) epidemiological studies. Whether this apparent lack of concordance is due to a real lack of effect or to the difficulties in revealing it because of the complexity of AMD can only be determined in intervention trials which are of sufficient duration and well controlled for all possible levels of confounding. Such trials, if very carefully designed, would have the potential to demonstrate the small to moderate contribution to risk reduction of AMD that can be expected for lutein and zeaxanthin on experimental grounds. However, in view of the sound scientific rationale and the epidemiological and animal data already available, some additional pivotal animal experiments and some additional epidemiological studies may well settle the question of the quantitative contribution of lutein and zeaxanthin to the health of the retina and macula without the need for lengthy and costly human intervention trials. After all, we should keep in mind that nature expends very much effort in specifically concentrating specific carotenoids in the macula. One reason for this, viewed teleologically, may be to provide the retina with effective protection against the light damage which ultimately is one of several factors that trigger the initiation of AMD.

IX. REFERENCES

1. **Nussbaum JJ**, Pruett RC, Delori FC, Macular yellow pigment, the first 200 years, *Retina,* 1, 296-310, 1981.
2. **Wald GL**, Human vision and the spectrum, *Nature (London),* 101, 653-658, 1945.
3. **Hogan MJ**, Alvarado JA, Weddell JP, in *Histology of the Human Eye*, Hogan MJ, Ed., W.B. Saunders, Philadelphia, 1971, p. 491.
4. **Vingerling JR**, Klaver CW, Hofman A, de Jong PTVM, Epidemiology of age-related maculopathy, *Epidemiol. Rev.*, 17, 347-360, 1995.
5. **Snodderly DM**, Brown PK, Delori FC, Auran JD, The macular pigment. I. Absorbance spectra, localization, and discrimination from other yellow pigments in primate retinas, *Invest. Ophthalmol. Vis. Sci.*, 25, 660-673, 1984.
6. **Snodderly DM**, Auran JD, Delori FC, The macular pigment - II. Spatial

distribution in primate retinas, *Invest. Ophthalmol. Vis. Sci.*, 25, 674-685, 1984.

7. **Snodderly DM**, Handelman GJ, Adler AJ, Distribution of macular pigment carotenoids in central retina of macaque and squirrel monkeys, *Invest. Ophthalmol. Vis. Sci.*, 32, 268-279, 1991.
8. **Bone RA**, Landrum JT, Tarsis SL, Preliminary identification of the human macular pigment, *Vision Res.*, 25, 1531-1535, 1985.
9. **Handelman GJ**, Dratz EA, Reay CC, van Kuijk FJGM, Carotenoids in the human macula and whole retina, *Invest. Ophthalmol. Vis. Sci.*, 29, 850-855, 1988.
10. **Bone RA**, Landrum JT, Hime GW, Cains A, Zamor J, Stereochemistry of the human macular carotenoids, *Invest. Ophthalmol. Vis. Sci.*, 34, 2033-2040, 1993.
11. **Werner JS**, Donnelly SK, Kliegl R, Aging and human macular pigment density, *Vision Res.*, 27, 257-268, 1987.
12. **Ham WT**, Mueller WA, The photopathology and nature of the blue-light and near-UV retinal lesion produced by lasers and other optical sources, in *Laser Applications in Medicine and Biology,* Wolbarsht ML, Ed., Plenum Press, New York, 1989, pp. 191-246.
13. **Schalch W**, Dayhaw-Barker P, Barker FM, The photo-protective role of the macular yellow pigment - an update, in *Proceedings of the 12th International Congress on Photobiology*, Hönigsmann H, Knobler R, Eds., OEMF, Milan, 1997, in press.
14. Schalch W, Carotenoids in the retina - a review of their possible role in preventing or limiting damage caused by light and oxygen, in *Free Radicals and Aging,* Emerit I, Chance B, Eds., Birkhäuser Verlag, Basel, 1992, pp. 280-298.
15. **Snodderly DM**, Evidence for protection against age-related macular degeneration by carotenoids and antioxidant vitamins, *Am. J. Clin. Nutr.*, 62 (suppl.), 1448S-1461S, 1995.
16. **Zhang L-X**, Cooney RV, Bertram JS,Carotenoids enhance gap junctional communication and inhibit lipid peroxidation in C3H/10T1/2 cells: Relationship to their cancer chemopreventive action, *Carcinogenesis*, 12, 2109-2114, 1991.
17. **Weiser H**, Kormann AW, Provitamin A activities and physiological functions of carotenoids in animals, *Ann. NY Acad. Sci.*, 691, 213-215, 1993.
18. **Weiser H**, Kormann A,Provitamin A activities of carotenoids in animal models, poster at the *10th International Symposium on Carotenoids* in Trondheim/Norway, June 20-25, 1993.
19. **Weiser H**, Somorjai G, Bioactivity of cis and dicis isomers of vitamin A esters, *Int. J. Vitam. Nutr. Res.*, 62, 201-208, 1992.
20. **Gerster H**,Vitamin A - functions, dietary requirements and safety in humans, *Int. J. Vitam. Nutr. Res.*, 67, 71-90, 1997.
21. **dePee S**, West CE,Dietary carotenoids and their role in combating vitamin A

deficiency: a review of the literature, *Eur. J. Clin. Nutr.*, 50 (Suppl. 3), S38-S53, 1996.

22. **Mangels AR**, Holden JM, Beecher GR, Forman MR, Lanza E,Carotenoid content of fruits and vegetable: an evaluation of analytic data, *J. Am. Diet. Assoc.*, 93, 284-296, 1993.
23. **Hart DJ**, Scott KJ,Development and evaluation of an HPLC method for the analysis of carotenoids in foods, and the measurement of the carotenoid content of vegetables and fruits commonly consumed in the UK, *Food Chem.*, 54, 101-111, 1995.
24. Müller H, Die tägliche Aufnahme von Carotinoiden (Carotine und Xanthophylle) aus Gesamtnahrungsproben und die Carotinoidgehalte ausgewählter Gemüse- und Obstarten, *Z. Ernährungswiss.*, 35, 45-50, 1996.
25. Deutsch MJ, Vitamins and other nutrients, in *Methods of Analysis by the Association of Official Analytical Chemistry*, Williams S, Ed., AOAC International, Arlington, 1984, pp. 830-836.
26. **Ascherio A**, Stampfer MJ, Colditz GA, Rimm EB, Litin L, Willett WC, Correlation of vitamin A and E intakes with the plasma concentrations of carotenoids and tocopherols among American men and women, *J. Nutr.*, 122, 1792-1801, 1992.
27. **Buchecker R**, Hamm P, Eugster CH,Absolute Konfiguration von Xanthophyll (Lutein), *Helv. Chim. Acta*, 57, 631-656, 1974.
28. **Maoka T**, Arai A, Shimizu M, Matsuno T,The first isolation of enantiomeric and *meso*-zeaxanthin in nature, *Comp. Biochem. Physiol.*, 83B, 121-123, 1986.
29. van Vliet T, Absorption of β-carotene and other carotenoids in humans and animal models, *Eur. J. Clin. Nutr.,* 50 (Suppl. 3), S32-S37, 1996.
30. **White WS**, Stacewicz-Sapuntzakis M, Erdman JW, Bowen PE,Pharmacokinetics of β-carotene and canthaxanthin after ingestion of individual and combined doses by human subjects, *J. Am. Coll. Nutr.*, 13, 665-671, 1994.
31. **Erdmann JW**, Bierer TL, Gugger ET, Absorption and transport of carotenoids, *Ann. NY Acad. Sci.*, 691, 76-85, 1993.
32. **Gärtner C**, Stahl W. Sies H, Preferential increase in chylomicron levels of the xanthophylls lutein and zeaxanthin compared to β-carotene in the human, *Int. J. Vitam. Nutr. Res.,* 66, 119-125, 1996.
33. **Micozzi MS**, Brown ED, Edwards BK, Bieri JG, Taylor PR, Khachik F, Beecher GR, Smith JC, Plasma carotenoid response to chronic intake of selected foods and β-carotene supplements in men, *Am. J. Clin. Nutr.,* 55, 1120-1125, 1992.
34. **Albanes D**, Virtamo J, Taylor PR, Rautalahti, Pietinen P, Heinonen OP, Effects of supplemental β-carotene, cigarette smoking, and alcohol consumption on serum carotenoids in the α-tocopherol, β-carotene cancer prevention study, *Am. J. Clin. Nutr.*, 66, 366-372, 1997.
35. **Chylack LT Jr**, Wolfe JK, Friend J, Tung W, Singer DM, Brown NP, Hurst MA, Köpcke W, Schalch W, Validation of methods for the assessment of cataract progression in the Roche European-American Anticataract Trial

(REACT), *Ophthalmic Epidemiol.*, 2, 59-75, 1995.

36. **Schalch W**, Koepcke W, Chylack LT Jr, and the REACT group, Carotenoid serum levels in the REACT study, in preparation.
37. **Olmedilla B**, Granado F, Gil-Martinez E, Blanco I, Rojas-Hidalgo E. Reference values for retinol, tocopherol, and main carotenoids in serum of control and insulin-dependent diabetic Spanish subjects, *Clin. Chem.*, 43, 1066-1071, 1997.
38. **Khachik F**, Spangler CJ, Smith JC. Identification, quantification, and relative concentrations of carotenoids and their metabolites in human milk and serum, *Anal. Chem.*, 69, 1873-1881, 1997.
39. **Bone RA**, Landrum JT, Friedes LM, Gomez C, Kilburn MD, Menendez E, Vidal I, Wang W, Distribution of lutein and zeaxanthin stereoisomers in the human retina, *Exp. Eye Res.*, 64, 211-218, 1997.
40. **Crabtree DV**, Adler AJ, A step toward the isolation of a macular protein that binds endogenous carotenoids, *Invest. Ophthalmol. Vis. Sci.*, 38 (Suppl.), S4, 1997.
41. **Balashov NA**, Bernstein PS, Purification of a carotenoid binding protein from human retina, *Invest. Ophthalmol. Vis. Sci.*, 38 (Suppl.), S5, 1997.
42. **Bernstein PS**, Balashov NA, Tsong ED, Rando RR, Retinal tubulin binds macular carotenoids, *Invest. Ophthalmol. Vis. Sci.,* 38, 167-175, 1997.
43. **Bone RA**, Landrum JT, Fernandez L, Tarsis SL, Analysis of the macular pigment by HPLC: Retinal distribution and age study, *Invest. Ophthalmol. Vis. Sci.,* 29, 843-849, 1988.
44. **Ross MA**, Crosley LK, Brown KM, Duthie SJ, Collins AC, Arthur JR, Duthie GG, Plasma concentrations of carotenoids and antioxidant vitamins in Scottish males, *Eur. J. Clin. Nutr.*, 49, 861-865, 1995.
45. **Chan LI**, Lam KW, Tso MOM, Vitamin A and carotenoids in human subretinal fluid, *Invest. Ophthalmol. Vis. Sci.*, 38 (Suppl.), S305, 1997.
46. **van Kuijk FJGM**, Siems WG, Sommerburg O, Carotenoid localization in human eye tissues, *Invest. Ophthalmol. Vis. Sci.*, 38 (Suppl.), S1030, 1997.
47. **Bone RA,** Sparrock JMB, Comparison of macular pigment densities in human eyes, *Vision Res.*, 11, 1057-1064, 1971.
48. **Hammond BR**, Curran-Celentano J, Judd S, Fuld K, Krinsky NI, Wooten BR, Snodderly DM, Sex differences in macular pigment optical density: relation to plasma carotenoid concentrations and dietary patterns, *Vision Res.*, 36, 2001-2012, 1996.
49. **Hammond BR**, Wooten BR, Snodderly MR, Cigarette smoking and retinal carotenoids: implications for age-related macular, *Vision Res.,* 36, 3003-3009, 1996.
50. **Hammond BR**, Fuld K, Snodderly DM, Iris color and macular pigment optical density, *Exp. Eye Res.*, 62, 293-297, 1996.
51. **Hammond BR**, Johnson EJ, Russel RM, Krinsky NI, Yeum K-J, Edwards RB, Snodderly DM, Dietary modification of human macular pigment density, *Invest. Ophthalmol. Vis. Sci.*, 38, 1795-1801, 1997.

52. **Hammond BR**, Wooten BR, Snodderly DM, Individual variations in the spatial profile of human macular pigment, *J. Opt. Soc. Am. A.*, 14, 1187-1196, 1997.
53. **Sarks SH**, Sarks JP, Age-related macular degeneration: atrophic form, in *Retina. Vol. 2. Medical retina*, Ryan SJ, Schachat AP, Murphy RM, Eds., Mosby, St. Louis, 1994, pp.1071-1102.
54. **Bone RA**, The role of the macular pigment in the detection of polarised light, *Vision Res.*, 20, 213-220, 1979.
55. **Delori FC**, Goger DG, Hammond BR, Sodderly DM, Burns SA, Foveal lipofuscin and macular pigment, *Invest. Ophthalmol. Vis. Sci.*, 38 (Suppl.), S355, 1997.
56. **Delori FC**, Dorey CK, Staurenghi G, Arend O, Goger DG, Weiter JJ, In vivo fluorescence of the ocular fundus exhibits retinal pigment epithelium lipofuscin characteristics, *Invest. Ophthalmol. Vis. Sci.*, 36, 718-729, 1995.
57. **Bernstein PS**, Balashov NA, Yoshida M, McClane RW, Gellermann W, Raman spectroscopy of macular carotenoids in intact human retina, *Invest. Ophthalmol. Vis. Sci.*, 38 (Suppl.), S303, 1997.
58. **Hammond BR,** Fuld K, Curran-Celentano J, Macular pigment density in monozygotic twins, *Invest. Ophthalmol. Vis. Sci.*, 36, 2531-2541, 1995.
59. **Handelman GJ,** Snodderly DM, Krinsky NI, Russett MD, Adler AJ, Biological control of primate macular pigment, biological and densitometric studies, *Invest. Ophthalmol. Vis. Sci.*, 32, 257-267, 1991.
60. **Hammond BR**, Fuld K, Interocular differences in macular pigment density, *Invest. Ophthalmol. Vis. Sci.*, 33, 350-355, 1992.
61. **Seddon JM**, Samelson LJ, Page WF, Neale MC, Twin study of macular degeneration: methodology and application to genetic epidemiologic studies, *Invest. Ophthalmol. Vis. Sci.*, 38 (Suppl.), S676, 1997.
62. **Putting BJ**, Zweypfenning RCVJ, Vrensen GFJM, Osterhuis JA, van Best JA, Blood-retinal barrier dysfunction at the pigment epithelium induced by blue light, *Invest. Ophthalmol. Vis. Sci.*, 33, 3385-3393, 1992.
63. **Wihlmark U**, Wrigstad A, Roberg K, Nilsson SEG, Brunk UT, Lipofuscin accumulation in cultured retinal pigment epithelial cells causes enhanced sensitivity to blue light irradiation, *Free Radic. Biol. Med.*, 22, 1229-1234, 1997.
64. **Boettner EA**, Wolter JR, Transmission of the ocular media, *Invest. Ophthalmol. Vis. Sci.*, 1, 776-783, 1962.
65. **Barker FM,** Brainard GC, The direct spectral transmittance of the excised human lens as a function of age, FDA report, 1991.
66. **Hammond BR**, Wooten BR, Snodderly DM, Density of the human crystalline lens is related to the macular pigment carotenoids, lutein and zeaxanthin, *Optom. Vis. Sci.*, 74, 499-504, 1997.
67. **Yeum K-J**, Taylor A, Tang G, Russell RM, Measurement of carotenoids, retinoids and tocopherols in human lenses, *Invest. Ophthalmol. Vis. Sci.*, 36, 2756-2761, 1995.

68. **Bates CJ**, Chen S, Macdonald A, Holden R, Quantitation of vitamin E and a carotenoid pigment in cataractous human lenses, and the effect of a dietary supplement, *Int. J. Vitam. Nutr. Res.*, 66, 316-321, 1996.
69. **Landrum JT**, Bone RA, Kenyon E, Sprague K, Maya A, A preliminary study of the stereochemistry of human lens zeaxanthin, *Invest. Ophthalmol. Vis. Sci.*, 38 (Suppl.), S1026, 1997.
70. **Marshall J**, Radiation and the ageing eye, *Ophthalmic Physiol. Opt.*, 5, 241-263, 1985.
71. **Stone WL**, Farnsworth CC, Dratz EA, A reinvestigation of the fatty acid content of bovine, rat and frog photoreceptor outer segments, *Exp. Eye Res.*, 28, 387-397, 1979.
72. **De La Paz MA**, Anderson RE, Region and age-dependent variation in susceptibility of the human retina to lipid peroxidation, *Invest. Ophthalmol. Vis. Sci.,* 33, 3497-3499, 1992.
73. **Wang N**, Anderson RE, Enrichment of polyunsaturated fatty acids from rat retinal pigment epithelium to rod outer segments, *Curr. Eye Res.*, 11, 783-791, 1992.
74. **di Mascio P**, Kaiser S, Sies H, Lycopene as the most efficient biological carotenoid singlet oxygen quencher, *Arch. Biochem. Biophys.*, 274, 532-538, 1989.
75. **Conn PF**, Lambert C, Land EJ, Schalch W, Truscott TG, Carotene - oxygen radical interactions, *Free Radic. Res. Commun.*, 16, 401-408, 1992.
76. **Devasagayam TPA**, Ippendorf H, Werner T, Martin H-D, Sies H, Carotenoids, novel polyene polyketones and new capsorubin isomers as efficient quenchers of singlet molecular oxygen, in *Lipid-soluble Antioxidants: Biochemistry and Clinical Applications,* Ong ASH, Packer L, Eds., Birkhäuser Verlag, Basel, Switzerland, pp. 255-264, 1992.
77. **Burton GW**, Ingold KU, β-carotene - an unusual type of lipid antioxidant, *Science*, 224, 569-573, 1984.
78. **Conn PF**, Schalch W, Truscott GT, The singlet oxygen - carotenoid interaction, *J. Photochem. Photobiol. B-Biology*, 11, 41-47, 1991.
79. **Liebler DC**, Stratton SP, Kaysen KL. Antioxidant actions of β-carotene in liposomal and microsomal membranes: Role of carotenoid-membrane incorporation and α-tocopherol, *Arch. Biochem. Biophys.*, 338, 244-250, 1997.
80. **Foote CS**, Denny RW, Weaver L, Chang Y, Phil D, Peters J, Quenching of singlet oxygen, *Ann. NY Acad. Sci.,* 171, 139-148, 1970.
81. **Stahl W**, Nicolai S, Briviba K, Hanusch M, Broszeit G, Peters M, Martin HD, Sies H, Biological activities of natural and synthetic carotenoids: Induction of gap junctional communication and singlet oxygen quenching, *Carcinogenesis*, 18, 89-92, 1997.
82. **Truscott G,** Personal communication, 1997.
83. **Böhm F**, Edge R, Land EJ, McGarvey DJ, Truscott TG, Carotenoids enhance vitamin E antioxidant efficiency, *J. Am. Chem. Soc.*, 119, 621-622, 1997.
84. **Friedrichson T**, Kalbach HL, Buck P, van Kuijk FJGM, Vitamin E in macular

and peripheral tissues of the human eye, *Curr. Eye Res.*, 14, 693-701, 1995.

85. **Lai YL**, Fong D, Lam KW, Wang HM, Tsin ATC, Distribution of ascorbate in the retina, subretinal fluid and pigment epithelium, *Curr. Eye Res.,* 5, 933-938, 1986.
86. **Edge R**, McGarvey DJ, Truscott TG, The carotenoids as antioxidants: a review, *J. Photochem. Photobiol. B-Biology*, 41, 189-200, 1997.
87. **Crabtree DV**, Adler AJ, Is β-carotene an antioxidant?, *Med. Hypotheses*, 48, 183-187, 1997.
88. **Daicker B**, Schiedt K, Adnet JJ, Bermond P, Canthaxanthin retinopathy - an investigation by light and electron microscopy and physicochemical analysis, *Graefe's Arch. Clin. Exp. Ophthalmol.*, 225, 189-197, 1987.
89. **Mathews-Roth MM**, Carotenoids and photoprotection, *Photochem. Photobiol.*, 65S, 148S-151S, 1997.
90. **Lim BP**, Nagao A, Terao J, Tanaka K, Suzuki T, Takama K, Anti-oxidant activity of xanthophylls on peroxyl radical-mediated phospholipid peroxidation, *Biochim. Biophys. Acta,* 1126, 178-184, 1992.
91. **Dayhaw-Barker P**, Barker FM II, Photoeffects on the eye, in *Photobiology of Skin and Eye,* Jackson EM, Ed., Marcel Dekker, New York, 1986, pp. 117-147.
92. **Castorina C**, Campisi A, Di Giacomo C, Sorrenti V, Russo A, Vanella A, Lipid peroxidation and antioxidant enzymatic systems in rat retina as a function of age, *Neurochem. Res.*, 17, 599-604, 1992.
93. **De La Paz MA**, Zhang J, Fridovich I, Antioxidant enzymes of the human retina: effect of age on enzyme activity of macula and periphery, *Curr. Eye Res.*, 15, 273-278, 1996.
94. **Khachik F**, Bernstein PS, Garland DL, Identification of lutein and zeaxanthin oxidation products in human and monkey retinas, *Invest. Ophthalmol. Vis. Sci.*, 38, 1802-1811 , 1997.
95. **Mitchell P**, Smith W, Attebo K, Wang JJ, Prevalence of age-related maculopathy in Australia. The Blue Mountain Eye Study, *Ophthalmology,* 102, 1450-1460, 1995.
96. **Leibowitz HM,** Kreuger DE, Maunder LR, Milton RC, Kini MM, Kahn HA, Nickerson RJ, Pool J, Colton TL, Ganley JP, Loewenstein JI, Dawber TR, The Framingham Eye Study Monograph. An ophthalmological and epidemiological study of cataract, glaucoma, diabetic retinopathy, macular degeneration, and visual acuity in a general population of 2361 adults, 1973-1975, *Surv. Ophthalmol.,* 24 (Suppl.), 335-610, 1980.
97. **Klein R**, Klein BE, Jensen SC, Meuer SM, The five year incidence and progression of age-related maculopathy: the Beaver Dam Eye Study, *Ophthalmology*, 104, 7-21, 1997.
98. **Hirvela H**, Luukinen H, Laara E, Laatikainen L, Risk factors of age-related maculopathy in a population 70 years of age or older, *Ophthalmology,* 103, 871-877, 1996.
99. **Cruickshanks KJ**, Hamman RF, Klein R, Nondahl DM, Shetterly SM, The

prevalence of age-related maculopathy by geographic region and ethnicity. The Colorado-Wisconsin Study of Age-Related Maculopathy, *Arch. Ophthalmol.*, 115, 242-250, 1997.

100. **Hyman LG**, Lilienfeld AM, Ferris FL III, Fine SL, Senile macular degeneration: a case-control study, *Am. J. Epidemiol.*, 118, 213-227, 1983.
101. **Hyman LG**, Epidemiology of AMD, in *Age-related Macular Degeneration: Principles and Practice,* Hampton GR and Nelson DT, Eds., Raven Press, New York, 1992, pp. 1-35.
102. **Hyman LG**, Grimson R, Oden N, Schachhat AP, Leske MC, Risk factors for age-related maculopathy, *Invest. Ophthalmol. Vis. Sci.,* 33 (Suppl.), S801, 1992.
103. **Haegerstrom-Portnoy G**, Short-wavelength-sensitive-cone sensitivity loss with aging: a protective role for macular pigment?, *J. Opt. Soc. Am. A,* 5, 2140-2144, 1988.
104. **Taylor HR**, West S, Munoz B, Rosenthal FS, Bressler SB, Bressler NM, The long-term effects of visible light on the eye, *Arch. Ophthalmol.*, 110, 99-104, 1992.
105. **Landrum JT**, Bone RA, Kilburn MD, The macular pigment: A possible role in protection from age-related macular degeneration, in *Advances in Pharmacology,* Vol 38, Sies H, Ed., Academic Press, London, 1996, pp. 537-556.
106. **Seddon JM**, Hennekens CH, Vitamins, minerals, and macular degeneration, promising but unproven hypotheses, *Arch. Ophthalmol.*, 112, 176-179, 1994.
107. **Goldberg J**, Flowerdew G, Smith E, Brody JA, Tso MOM, Factors associated with age-related macular degeneration - Analysis of data from NHANES I, *Am. J. Epidemiol*, 128, 700-711, 1988.
108. **Drews CD**, Sternberg P, Samiec PS, Jones DP, Reed RL, Flagg E, Boddie A, Tinkelman R, Dietary antioxidants and age related macular degeneration (ARMD), *Invest. Ophthalmol. Vis. Sci.*, 34 (Suppl.), 1153S, 1993.
109. **Seddon JM**, Ajani UA, Sperduto RD, Hiller R, Blair N, Burton TC, Farber MD, Gragoudas ES, Haller J, Miller DT, Yannuzzi LA, Willett W, Dietary carotenoids, vitamins A, C and E and advanced age-related macular degeneration, *J. Am. Med. Assoc.*, 272, 1413-1420, 1994.
110. **Mares-Perlman JA**, Klein R, Klein BEK, Greger JL, Brady WE, Palto M, Ritter LL, Association of zinc and antioxidant nutrients with age-related maculopathy, *Arch. Ophthalmol.*, 114, 991-997, 1996.
111. **Blumenkranz MS**, Russell SR, Robey MG, Kott-Blumenkranz R, Penneys N, Risk factors in age-related maculopathy complicated by choroidal neovascularisation, *Ophthalmology*, 96, 552-558, 1986.
112. **Mares-Perlman JA**, Klein R, Klein BEK, Ritter LL, Relationships between age-related maculopathy and intake of vitamin and mineral supplements, *Invest. Ophthalmol. Vis. Sci.*, 34 (Suppl.), 1133S, 1993.
113. **Vitale S**, West S, Munoz B, Maguire M, Schein O, Taylor HR, Bressler N, Vitamin supplement use, age-related macular degeneration and cataract in

Chesapeake Bay watermen, *Invest. Ophthalmol. Vis. Sci.*, 34 (Suppl.), 1066S, 1993.

114. **Tsang NCK**, Penfold PL, Snitch PJ, Billson F, Serum levels of antioxidants and age-related macular degeneration, *Doc. Ophthalmol.*, 81, 387-400, 1992.

115. **EDCC (Eye Disease Case-Control) Study Group**, Antioxidant status and neovascular age-related macular degeneration, *Arch. Ophthalmol.*, 111, 104-109, 1993.

116. **Sanders TAB**, Haines AP, Wormland R, Wright LA, Obeid O, Essential fatty acids, plasma cholesterol, and fat-soluble vitamins in subjects with age-related maculopathy and matched control subjects, *Am. J. Clin. Nutr.*, 57, 428-433, 1993.

117. **West S**, Vitale S, Hallfrisch J, Munoz B, Muller D, Bressler S, Bressler NM, Are antioxidants or supplements protective for age-related macular degeneration?, *Arch. Ophthalmol.*, 112, 222-227, 1994.

118. **Alpers JR**, Gorla MSR, Singerman LJ, Serum carotenoids and age-related macular degeneration, *Invest. Ophthalmol, Vis. Sci.* 36 (Suppl.), S9, 1995.

119. **Mares-Perlman JA**, Brady WE, Klein R, Klein BEK, Bowen P, Stacewicz-Sapuntzakis M, Palta M, Serum antioxidants and age-related macular degeneration in a population based case-control study, *Arch. Ophthalmol.*, 113, 1518-1523, 1995.

120. **Crary EJ**, Antioxidant treatment of macular degeneration of the aging and macular edema in diabetic retinopathy, *South. Med. J.*, 80, 38, 1987.

121. **Teikari JM**, Laatikainen L, Virtamo J, Haukka J, Rautalahti M, Liesto K, Heinonen OP, α-tocopherol and β-carotene in age-related macular degeneration, *Invest. Ophthalmol. Vis. Sci.*, 36 (Suppl.), S9, 1995.

122. **Age-related Macular Degeneration Study Group**, Multicenter ophthalmic and nutritional age-related macular degeneration study - part 2: antioxidant intervention and conclusions, *J. Am. Optom. Assoc.*, 67, 30-49, 1996.

123. **AREDS (Age-related Eye Disease Study)**, Manual of procedures, National Eye Institute, Bethesda, MD, 1992.

124. **Dorey CK**, Toyoda Y, Thomson L, Garnett KM, Sapunzatkis M, Craft N, Nichols C, Cheng K, Light induced photoreceptor apoptosis is correlated with dietary and retinal levels of 3R,3′R-zeaxanthin, *Invest. Ophthalmol. Vis. Sci.*, 38 (Suppl.), S355, 1997.

125. **Malinow MR**, Feeney-Burns L, Peterson LH, Klein M, Neuringer M, Diet-related macular anomalies in monkeys, *Invest. Ophthalmol. Vis. Sci.*, 19, 857-863, 1980.

126. **Khachick F**, Beecher GR, Smith JC, Lutein, lycopene, and their oxidative metabolites in chemoprevention of cancer, *J. Cell Biochem. Suppl.*, 22, 236-246, 1995.

127. **Landrum JT**, Bone RA, Joa H, Kilburn MD, Moore LL, Sprague KE, A one year study of the macular pigment: the effect of 140 days of a lutein supplement, *Exp. Eye Res.*, 65, 57-62, 1997.

128. **Bone RA**, Landrum JT, Rosenfeld PJ, Moore LL, Sprague KE, Giraldo C,

Gomez C, One year study of macular pigment enhancement by a lutein supplement, *Invest. Ophthalmol. Vis. Sci.*, 38 (Suppl.), S90, 1997.

129. **Le Marchand L**, Hankin JH, Bach F, Kolonel LN, Wilkens LR, Stacewicz-Sapuntzakis M, Bowen PE, Beecher GR, Laudon F, Baque P, Daniel R, Servatu L, Henderson BE, An ecological study of diet and lung cancer in the South Pacific, *Int. J. Cancer*, 63, 18-23, 1995.

130. **Tso MOM**, Pathogenetic factors of aging macular degeneration, *Ophthalmology*, 92, 628-635, 1985.

Chapter 13

IN VIVO PSYCHOPHYSICAL ASSESSMENT OF NUTRITIONAL AND ENVIRONMENTAL INFLUENCES ON HUMAN OCULAR TISSUES: LENS AND MACULAR PIGMENT

D. Max Snodderly and Billy R. Hammond, Jr.

I. INTRODUCTION

Psychophysics is a hybrid field of science encompassing study of the perceptual (psychological) responses of subjects to sensory stimuli that are carefully controlled and measured by the methods of physics. For the visual system, light is the sensory stimulus. When light is absorbed by the photoreceptors of the retina, a neural response is generated that results in detection of the stimulus by the subject. For the studies to be discussed here, the ocular tissues can be considered a set of optical filters through which the light must pass. By careful choice of the wavelength and the mode of presentation of the stimulus, the subjects' responses can reveal the optical properties of these ocular filters. In the eye, light must pass through the lens and most of the retina before reaching the photoreceptors. In essence, the visual system of our subjects is used as an intricate photosensory apparatus to measure the optical density spectrum of these human ocular tissues.

The optical density (OD) of a filter is calculated from the transmittance T(λ), which is the ratio of the energy that is transmitted through the filter to the energy of the incident light at the wavelength λ. The formula [1] is

$$OD(\lambda) = \log_{10} [1/T(\lambda)], \text{ or } OD(\lambda) = -\log_{10} T(\lambda)$$

Conversely, $T(\lambda) = 10^{-OD(\lambda)}$

If the light is only absorbed and not scattered, as it would be in a clear solution, then OD(λ) is equivalent to the absorbance spectrum. However, in biological structures, such as the lens, the tissue usually scatters light in addition to absorbing it, so OD(λ) values include contributions from both scattering and absorption. Because T(λ) is always less than 1, its log is negative and OD(λ) is always positive. The smaller the amount of light transmitted, the larger the OD. Using OD as a measure has the advantage that the shape of the spectrum does not change with the concentration of the pigments involved [2], and the total OD of tissues through which light passes in succession is simply the sum of the individual ODs. [1] Here we describe the principles underlying psychophysical techniques to measure ODs of the lens and of the yellow macular pigment of the retina, which are the major ocular filters that affect the light detected by the photoreceptors.

This approach is possible because of the extensive body of knowledge of the spectral properties of ocular components. The eye lens of young people is nearly transparent to visible light, but in older people, the lens becomes noticeably yellow,

0-8493-8565-2/99/$0.00+$.50

largely because of changes in the lens proteins that cause absorption and scattering of light. [3] The OD of the lens as a function of wavelength can therefore be measured to characterize the alterations in optical properties that signify changes in functional status.

A nutrition-related feature of the retina that can be assessed by psychophysics is the density of the carotenoid pigments lutein and zeaxanthin [4,5] that accumulate in the central depression called the fovea. These pigments absorb blue light and confer a yellow color that has given the fovea and the immediately surrounding region the name, "macula lutea," or yellow spot. This yellow macular pigment is derived from the diet [6,7] and can be monitored as an indicator of ocular nutritional status. [8,9]

The advantage of psychophysical methodology is that it is noninvasive, yet extremely sensitive. An individual can be followed over time, and the same tissue can be repeatedly measured. Psychophysical methods are therefore well suited to studying the effects of nutritional and environmental influences on the aging process. Nevertheless, psychophysical methodology has distinct limitations. The measurements usually require relatively prolonged testing by a skilled examiner. They cannot be used with very young children, infirm or gravely handicapped individuals, or persons with dense cataracts that severely obscure vision. Furthermore, the subject must clearly understand the task and must be able to give reliable reports of sensory experience. This reliance on the participation and performance of the subject always introduces a risk of misunderstanding, with the need for careful cross-checking by the experimenter, as described later.

In the past, psychophysical methods have been used primarily in laboratories that have specialized and complex optical systems. However, the integration of modern electronic components into visual stimulus systems is making them cheaper and simpler to operate, so the methodology is becoming accessible to a wider community.

In this chapter we describe the principles underlying two psychophysical methods that have been used successfully with hundreds of naive subjects to measure the OD of the lens and the OD of the retinal macular pigment. These ocular parameters are linked to nutritional and environmental factors important for preventing two leading causes of visual disability–cataract and age-related macular degeneration (see other chapters in this volume).

II. PRESENTATION OF VISUAL STIMULI FOR PSYCHOPHYSICAL MEASUREMENTS

Our stimuli are specified in terms of location on the retina and size of the stimulus. The reference for retinal location is the specialized region called the fovea where we have the greatest density of photoreceptors and the best acuity. We use the fovea when we look directly at an object to scrutinize it. If instructed to fix our gaze on a point of light (the fixation point), most people turn their eyes to place the image of that point on a subregion of the fovea called the fixation locus. This fixation locus is usually near the center of the fovea [10] and it becomes the reference location for stimulus position on the retina.

Other, eccentric locations on the retina are tested by placing the stimulus at specified distances from the fixation point. The stimulus location can be expressed in terms of the angle by which the stimulus is displaced from the fixation point. Similarly, stimulus size is specified in terms of visual angle subtended at the eye. For most subjects, 1 deg of visual angle is subtended by an object 1 cm in diameter at a distance of 57.3 cm from the subject (about the width of a thumbnail held at arm's length), which forms an image on the retina approximately 300 μm wide. [11]

Visual stimuli can be presented to the subject in two different modes [1]. Free viewing, or Newtonian view, simply permits subjects to look at a stimulus display, using their normal corrective lenses. This procedure is most comfortable for the subject and involves the least preparation. However, it is sometimes desirable to control the absolute intensity of light reaching the retina, or the path of the light through the lens, and free viewing has the disadvantage that fluctuations in pupil size conflict with control of these parameters. Improved control during free viewing can be achieved by using a small artificial pupil placed in front of the eye so that light passes only through the center of the lens and variations in the subject's own pupil do not affect the light entering the eye. Unfortunately, an artificial pupil reduces the amount of light reaching the retina, which may render the stimulus conditions unsuitable for older subjects, particularly those with dense lenses.

To avoid the limitations of free viewing, much past work has used Maxwellian view optical systems. [1,11,12] In Maxwellian view, the stimulus is imaged on the retina by an external lens that has a focal point centered in the subject's pupil. The beam of light that enters the eye is very small so that it only traverses the center of the subject's lens and does not intersect the subject's pupil. Aligning the subject's eye with the external Maxwellian lens, however, requires that the position of the head be precisely controlled. It is customary to make a "bite bar" with an impression of the subject's teeth so that when the subject rests the upper jaw on the bite bar, the head can be positioned to align the eye with the optical system. Once this is done, stimuli can be presented with the techniques of classical optics, to control a wide range of parameters, including size, wavelength, and intensity. In fact, precautions must be taken to avoid damage to the eye from overexposure.

The choice of the mode of stimulus presentation often involves compromises among competing factors. Some of those factors will be considered below in the context of measuring lens and macular pigment OD. For both types of measurements, stimuli of different wavelengths are compared. The bandwidths of the stimuli are less critical than the center wavelength and total energy. In our system, monochromator and filter bandwidths are generally 15-20 nm full width at half the energy of the peak wavelength.

III. PSYCHOPHYSICAL MEASUREMENT OF LENS OPTICAL DENSITY

A. IMPORTANCE OF EARLY ASSESSMENT

A wide body of evidence has shown increasing visual impairment as a function of age (reviewed by Kline [13]). For most people, this visual disability is primarily due to increased OD of the crystalline lens. [14,15] Even among subjects with no discernible lens opacities, lens OD can vary dramatically. For example, our past measurements at 440 nm have a range of lens OD values from 0.06 to 0.98 for younger subjects (mean OD = 0.74 +/- 0.24, age = 24-36 yrs). [9] Both the mean OD and the standard deviation increase with age (mean OD = 1.06 +/- 0.53, age = 48-65 yrs).

A dense lens is particularly pernicious when optimal vision is required in dim light, such as driving a vehicle at dusk. [13,16] In addition to affecting visual performance by decreasing the amount of light reaching the retina, a dense lens also increases forward scattering of light, which reduces contrast by producing a veiling illumination over retinal images. [17] Since insurance companies typically do not fund lens removal until a cataract is relatively advanced, elderly people with a dense lens may suffer many years of decreased visual performance before their vision is improved by removal of the lens.

Age-related cataracts develop slowly over a lifetime and epidemiologic studies that focus only on patients with well-established cataracts may miss factors important in the early development of cataract. Information is needed regarding changes in the lens that begin the process of loss of transparency but precede frank cataract. Lenticular transparency is the result of the short-range order of crystallin proteins. [18] Modification in the ordering of these proteins causes reduced transparency, resulting in higher OD. One type of disruption is aggregation and insolubilization of crystallin proteins, which is considered a primary event in the development of cataract. [19] Mota et al. [20] have shown that lens OD measured *in vivo* is highly correlated with the accumulation of these protein aggregates.

In addition to *morphological* changes, age-related changes in lens *physiology* also occur and can be tracked by monitoring lens OD. For example, lens membrane potential and resistance decreases with age, while Na^+ and free Ca^{2+} content within the lens increases. [21] Such changes are thought to signal approaching cataract since they are most extreme in the cataractous lens. [22,23] Duncan et al. [21] have shown that these changes in cation concentrations are well correlated with *in vivo* measurements of lens OD. The combination of evidence suggests that measurements of lens OD early in life may signal important changes in the health of the lens.

Although no longitudinal data are available showing that increased lens OD early in life predicts risk for later cataract development, cross-sectional data indicate this possibility. For example, Sample et al. [24] have shown that the lens OD of individuals with cataract is higher than lens OD of age-matched individuals who do not have cataract. Moreover, diabetics, who have a higher risk of developing age-related cataract than normal individuals [25], also have higher than average lens OD prior to developing cataract. [26-29] In fact, cataract classification systems (e.g., densitometric analysis of Scheimpflug photography; autofluorophotometry) often use high lens OD to establish cataractous status. For example, cataract has been quantified by measuring back-scattered light, [30] a method that is significantly correlated ($p<0.001$) with psychophysical measurements of lens OD. [31] Cataract has also been quantified by Scheimpflug photography [32], which is also significantly correlated ($p<0.001$) with psychophysical measurements of lens OD. [33]

B. PRINCIPLES OF THE MEASUREMENT

The sensitivity of a subject at each wavelength is conventionally specified as the reciprocal of the energy needed to reach threshold [1]. To measure the OD of the lens, we take advantage of the fact that the dark-adapted (scotopic) sensitivity of observers whose lens has been surgically removed is determined by the visual pigment of the rod photoreceptors, rhodopsin. [34] Thus, for individuals with an intact lens, deviations from the rhodopsin spectrum in their scotopic sensitivity are due primarily to the OD of the lens. Results from studies of excised lenses suggest that most of the variation in OD with wavelength is due to the properties of the lens nucleus. [35] Lens OD is greatest at short wavelengths and it increases with aging, although for normal subjects the OD at long wavelengths remains low at all ages. [36] Lens OD can therefore be estimated by selecting as a reference a long wavelength light where lens OD is minimal, and comparing the sensitivity of the observer at that reference wavelength to the sensitivity at shorter wavelengths. Because the form of the dependence of the OD of the lens on wavelength is well established [36-38], the measurements need only be made at a few wavelengths to estimate the full curve. The correlation between lens OD measured in the left and right eyes is relatively high, $r = 0.75$, $p<0.01$ [24]; so, measurements of one eye are an adequate indicator of lens status for most people.

C. SELECTING STIMULUS PARAMETERS

1. Reference wavelength

The selection of the reference wavelength is dependent upon two factors. The reference wavelength needs to be long enough so that the OD of the lens is minimal, yet short enough to minimize the possibility that cone photoreceptors will contribute to detection of the stimulus. The peak sensitivity of rods (ca. 500 nm) occurs at shorter wavelengths than the peak sensitivity of the major cone types (ca. 540-570 nm). Thus, as the wavelength of the reference is increased, lens OD is minimized, but the risk that cones will contribute to the measurement increases. As a compromise, we have used 550 nm as our reference wavelength [9], and others have used 560 nm. [24] Choosing these wavelengths accepts a small amount of lens OD at the reference wavelength [36] and hence slightly underestimates total lens OD. If a longer wavelength is chosen as reference to achieve lower lens OD, a control experiment should be conducted to ensure that only rods are contributing to detection of the stimulus.

The period when rods control the sensitivity of the subject can be identified by tracking the time course of dark-adaptation using the reference wavelength. In brief, subjects are exposed to an intense (about 5 log Tds) broad band light for about two minutes, followed by repeated threshold measurements obtained as rapidly as possible. These determinations can be made by experienced subjects who adjust the intensity of the test stimulus themselves. A smooth dark adaptation curve with two time constants should be obtained, with a break indicating the transition from cone vision to rod vision at around six minutes (see examples in Wyszecki and Stiles [11], pp 519-520). This control experiment demonstrates that the rods are determining visual sensitivity under the conditions of the experiment, and also ensures that enough stray light has been eliminated so that true scotopic thresholds are obtained. Note that stimulus size and location on the retina also influence the probability of detection by rods vs cones; so, the effects of any changes in stimulus parameters must be checked by this type of control experiment.

2. Measuring wavelengths

When selecting wavelengths at which to measure lens OD, several points need to be considered. Because the OD of the lens is inversely related to wavelength, the experimenter can maximize differences among subjects by using a short measuring wavelength. This consideration is of particular importance when measuring the lenses of subjects with low OD, such as adolescents. Typically a limiting factor when using shorter wavelengths is the energy output of most optical systems. Given the relatively low sensitivity of the visual system from 400-440 nm, relatively high energy is required if a wavelength near 400 nm is selected as the measuring wavelength. The energy available may be of particular concern if older subjects with high lens OD are to be tested with the same wavelength.

Another consideration is ease of computing lens OD. If the reference wavelength and the measuring wavelength are selected to be equally well absorbed by rhodopsin, then any difference in visual sensitivity at the two wavelengths can be taken directly as due to lens OD. Furthermore, no assumptions need to be made about the amount of rhodopsin present in order to correct for self screening (explained below). As an example of this approach, Sample et al. [24] have used a reference wavelength of 560 nm and a measuring wavelength of 410 nm to locate their measurements at equal absorption values on the rhodopsin spectrum.

Because of age-related differences and small individual differences in shape of the density spectrum of the lens, measurements of lens OD used to estimate light reaching the photoreceptors will be more precise if done at the specific wavelengths of interest. For example, if an investigator wishes to determine how much light reaches the retina at the absorption peaks of specific cone types, [39] the data are more precise if OD at the wavelengths corresponding to the absorption peaks is measured rather than estimating from interpolated values using a standard spectral curve of lens OD. [11] If more complete information is desired, measurements at additional wavelengths allow spectral curves to be constructed for individual subjects that can be checked against standard, age-referenced, spectral density curves. [11,17,37]

3. Procedure for obtaining scotopic sensitivity values

The psychophysical detection task is explained using suprathreshold stimuli, and then the subject is given 30-40 minutes of dark adaptation. About 95% of maximum dark-adapted sensitivity is reached by this time. During testing, subjects are instructed to stare directly at a small (~20 min), illuminated fixation point that can be located 6-8 degrees eccentric to the test stimulus (Fig. 1). It is important to remind subjects frequently to maintain fixation and not to look directly at the test stimulus so that the test stimulus falls outside the retinal region with the highest number of cones and is detected by rods. The size of the test stimulus is typically 2-3 degrees (i.e., large enough to be detected easily with peripheral vision). A check that subjects are detecting the stimulus with their rods may be incorporated by asking subjects to report the color of the test flash. Near threshold, subjects should report that the test flash appears colorless.

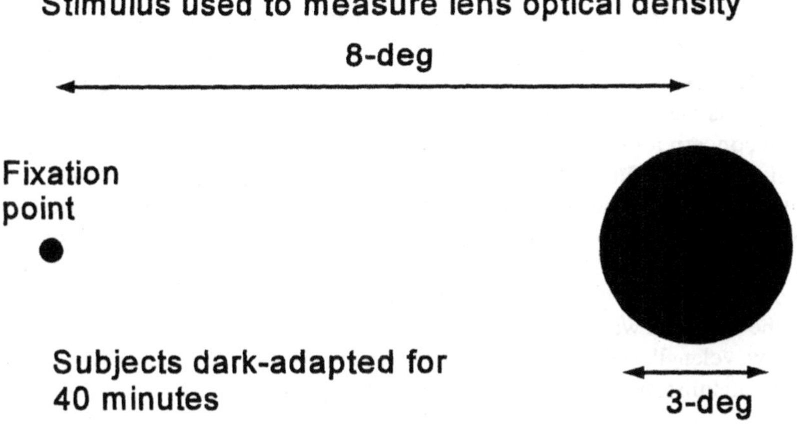

Figure 1. Stimulus arrangement for measuring lens optical density. Subjects are dark adapted for 40 min. They are then instructed to stare at the small fixation point while a test stimulus is flashed repeatedly at the eccentric test location. The fixation point is a long wavelength that is yellow or red and is designed to be detected by the cones of the fovea. The test stimulus is moderately large and is a shorter wavelength designed to stimulate the rods of the parafovea.

A quantitative measure of the absolute threshold of each subject to the flashed test stimulus can be obtained using a variety of techniques. In a typical protocol, subjects are warned of a coming test flash by the experimenter. The test stimulus is then flashed for 500 msec or less, and the subject indicates whether it was seen or not. The intensity of the flash is varied progressively in 0.05 log increments or decrements over a 1.5 log unit range (method of limits) or the intensity is randomly varied within a fixed range (method of constant stimuli). The percentage of time the subjects report seeing the test flash can be plotted against intensity to produce a psychometric function. Absolute thresholds are then defined as the intensity at which the flash is seen 50% of the time. Although reasonably accurate, this process is fairly slow.

We have found that a more expeditious method is to present the subject with the flashing test stimulus repeatedly (e.g., in 300 msec exposures at 1.5 sec intervals) and then allow the subject to identify the intensities for which the stimulus is visible 100% of the time, none of the time, and half the time. The subject's performance is aided by providing an auditory cue each time the stimulus is flashed. This cue can be as simple as the click of a shutter that controls the stimulus flash. With this procedure, the entire range from 100% detection to 100% nondetection is typically limited to about 0.5 log units, and the subject is able to estimate the 50% detection value with good reliability. For example, when five repeat determinations are made, the standard deviation of the threshold is about 0.08 log units at 550 nm and about 0.15 log units at 410 nm.

After the psychophysical session, the radiant power at each stimulus wavelength should be measured (e.g., in nanowatts) using a calibrated radiometer placed at the usual location of the subject's pupil. The energy then is the power times the temporal duration of the stimulus. Because we are comparing different wavelengths we can consider only the relative energies in the discussion below, without concern for stimulus durations or absolute calibrations.

If attenuating filters are used to adjust the light intensity, each of them should be calibrated in the optical system in which the filter is used. [1] The most accurate measurement is obtained by measuring the maximum output of the optical system with no filters present. Then the attenuation of the light needed to reach the subject's threshold is given by the sum of the ODs of all the filters in the system when the threshold was measured. The relative energy reaching the subject's eye at each wavelength is the product of the maximum output of the optical system and the net transmission ($T = 10^{-OD\ filters}$) of the filters present so that

$$\text{Threshold energy} = \text{Maximum output x } 10^{-OD\ filters} \qquad (1)$$

Because the excitation of the photoreceptors is a function of the number of photons (quanta) that are absorbed, the threshold values should be recorded in quantum units. If the output of the optical system is measured in energy units, the energy/quantum is proportional to $1/\lambda$; so the relative number of quanta at threshold for different wavelengths is threshold energy multiplied by λ.

D. CALCULATION OF LENS DENSITY

We assume that light reaches the threshold of visibility when rhodopsin absorbs a sufficient number of quanta at the wavelength being presented. The spectral properties of rhodopsin are usually summarized in its absorbance, or optical density spectrum, $OD(\lambda)$. Data on human rhodopsin are available in graphical form in Wald and Brown (1958) [34]; other authors [24] have used tables in reference 11. The fraction of the incident photons absorbed at each wavelength is called the absorptance, J [2], which is (1 - the fraction of photons transmitted,T), or equivalently:

$$J(\lambda) = 1 - 10^{-OD(\lambda)} \qquad (2)$$

If balanced wavelengths are chosen so that the OD of rhodopsin at the reference and the measuring wavelengths, is equal, then J, the fraction of photons absorbed at the two wavelengths will also be equal. At the reference wavelength, light absorption by the lens is assumed to be negligible, which is equivalent to assuming that the light transmitted through the lens is equal to the incident light. In other words, the light sufficient to reach threshold at the reference wavelength is the light incident on the eye that was measured in quantal units. Because the same number of quanta are required to reach threshold at the measuring wavelength, it follows that the number of quanta transmitted through the lens at the measuring wavelength equals the threshold number of quanta incident on the eye at the reference wavelength. So the transmittance of the lens at the measuring wavelength is the ratio of transmitted light to incident light or

$$T\text{ (lens)} = \text{Threshold quanta, ref } \lambda \text{ / Threshold quanta, meas } \lambda \qquad (3)$$

and because OD (lens) = $\log_{10} 1/T$,

$$OD\text{ (lens)} = \log_{10} \text{Threshold quanta, meas } \lambda \text{ / Threshold quanta, ref } \lambda. \qquad (4)$$

If balanced wavelengths are not chosen, and the rhodopsin OD at the measuring wavelength is not the same as the OD at the reference wavelength, another factor, known as self-screening, must be considered. Because the fraction of photons absorbed, J, is a nonlinear function of OD, the relative values of J at two wavelengths that are not at equal ODs will vary in different ways with the overall density of rhodopsin (see reference 2 for a detailed discussion of this effect). Consequently, to estimate J at the wavelengths of interest, we must assume an appropriate value of OD for rhodopsin in the retina, then multiply the published absorbance spectrum by the appropriate factor, and calculate J at that wavelength. Then equation (3) must be modified to take into account the different quantum catch of rhodopsin at the two wavelengths. For this purpose, in our work [9] using a 440 nm measuring wavelength and a 550 nm reference we have assumed that rhodopsin has a maximum OD of 0.3 at 500 nm in human retinas. Because these wavelengths are not grossly out of balance, the exact density assumed for rhodopsin has only a small effect [40] compared to the differences in lens OD measured between subjects.

IV. PSYCHOPHYSICAL MEASUREMENT OF MACULAR PIGMENT OPTICAL DENSITY

The macular pigment (MP) is an accumulation of the two carotenoids lutein and zeaxanthin in the fovea and in the immediately surrounding retina. Extensive evidence indicates that these carotenoids and/or dietary factors with which they are associated contribute to preservation of normal retinal function. They protect the retina from damage by light [41], retard the loss of visual sensitivity with age [39], and may reduce the risk of age-related macular degeneration. [41] Both *in vitro* and *in vivo* studies have shown that MP density varies by more than a factor of ten between individuals and is probably the most variable feature of the fovea. [8, 42-44] Given the putative protective functions of MP, and the wide individual variations in OD, measurements of MP may provide information regarding both ocular nutritional status and risk for ocular disease.

A. GENERAL APPROACH

The ability to measure MP density by psychophysical methods is dependent both upon its spatial distribution and its spectral absorption characteristics. The density of MP is greatest at the fixation locus and declines approximately exponentially with eccentricity to a baseline at about 6-8 deg eccentricity where it is no longer optically detectable. [45,46] To a first approximation, nutritional and environmental influences probably affect the entire pigment distribution, either increasing or decreasing the OD. [7] For most purposes, it is therefore only necessary to determine the OD at the fixation locus relative to the baseline at an eccentric location. If a more detailed spatial profile of pigment density is desired, then separate determinations must be made at additional retinal locations as described elsewhere. [46]

The basic approach is to present a small test stimulus that alternates between a wavelength absorbed by MP and a wavelength outside the MP absorption band. For best signal to noise ratio, the stimulus alternates between 460 nm (blue) at the wavelength of maximal absorption of MP and 550 nm (green) which is a reference wavelength that is not absorbed by MP. To the subject, this alternating stimulus appears as a small flickering light. The subject is given control of the intensity of the blue light and the subject's task is to adjust it to minimize the flicker. This flicker task provides an easy way for the subject to match the visual effectiveness of the blue and the green light.

Settings are made at two retinal loci, one at the reference locus of 6 deg eccentricity (the parafovea), and one at the fixation locus (in the fovea). The underlying assumption is that the relative sensitivity of the retina to blue and to green light is the same at the two loci (see later). The energy of the blue light necessary to minimize flicker at the test locus in the fovea (B fov) compared to the energy needed at the reference locus in the parafovea (B ref) is a measure of the density of MP. As long as the lens is not so cataractous as to cause degradation of the borders of the stimulus, moderate differences in lens OD between subjects have no effect because the MP density value for each subject is derived by comparing the settings at the two retinal loci.

We assume that at minimum flicker, the same amount of light must be absorbed by the visual pigment of the photoreceptors at the test locus as at the reference locus. However, at the test locus, the light must pass through MP, which allows us to derive its OD. Because we are comparing the same wavelength in the fovea and at the reference location, the intensity of blue light incident at minimum flicker can be expressed in energy or quantum units. The blue light absorbed by the photoreceptors in each case is then the product of the incident light times the transmission of the lens (T_{lens}) and the transmission of MP (T_{MP}). Algebraically, the computation of the OD of MP reduces to the following:

$$B\ fov \times T_{lens} \times T_{MP} = B\ ref \times T_{lens} \tag{5}$$

then

$$T_{MP} = B\ ref / B\ fov \tag{6}$$

and

$$MP\ OD = \log_{10} 1/T_{MP} = \log (B\ fov / B\ ref) \tag{7}$$

To avoid response bias, the experimenter sets the intensity of the blue light to an unpredictable value before each trial. Because of the rapidity of the stimulus flicker, the subjects cannot easily judge the amount of the offset and they must attend to the flicker instead of attempting to repeat some 'desired' brightness setting. Five trials at each retinal location are averaged for each data point.

B. SELECTION OF STIMULUS CONDITIONS

1. Spatial parameters and stimulus intensity

One determinant of task difficulty for naive or elderly subjects is the size of the test stimulus. Most subjects find the task comfortable with test stimuli 0.75 to 1 degree in diameter. A typical stimulus configuration seen by the subject when performing the task is illustrated in Fig. 2. The small test field is superimposed on an intense blue (460 nm, 2.2 log troland or brighter) background about 10 degrees in diameter for reasons described later. The green reference stimulus that alternates with the blue test stimulus is set to a constant value that provides a retinal illumination of 2.6 log Td. This value was selected to be 1 log unit above the threshold for detection of the green stimulus when it is flickered alone on the blue background at 1 Hz.

The subject only has to attend to the small flickering stimulus; the larger background is constant throughout the measurement. To set the minimum flicker at the fixation locus, the subject looks directly at the test stimulus. To make the baseline determination in the parafovea, the subject looks at the fixation point at the left edge of the field, which places the flickering test stimulus at an eccentric location. The subject then must make the settings for minimum flicker while paying attention to the test stimulus but not looking directly at it.

2. Effects of optics of the eye

For some subjects chromatic aberration of the eye causes slight differences in the position or size of the blue and the green test stimuli, so that it is impossible to eliminate flicker in the narrow arcs where the two stimuli fail to superimpose. When the stimulus is presented in Maxwellian view, we use an achromatizing lens (placed at the last focal point before the pupil and after the beams providing the blue and the green stimuli had been combined) and we adjust the horizontal and

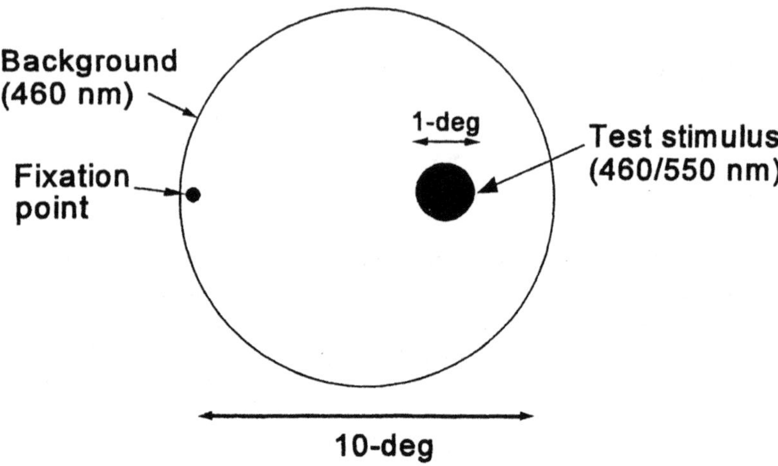

Figure 2. Typical stimulus configuration for psychophysical measurement of MP density. The small test stimulus alternates at about 12-15 Hz between a blue light (460 nm) absorbed by MP and a green light (550 nm) not absorbed by MP. The test stimulus is superimposed on a larger blue background to minimize the contribution of the short-wavelength cone system to the measurement. To obtain a value for the fovea, the subject looks directly at the test stimulus. To obtain a value for the parafovea, the subject looks at the fixation point illustrated at the left edge of the background field while attending to the flickering test stimulus, which is now in the periphery. The MP density is computed from the difference between the foveal and the parafoveal values. Note that *the density that is measured is the sum of the densities of lutein, zeaxanthin, and meso-zeaxanthin* [47] *that together form the yellow macular pigment*. The absorbance spectra of these carotenoids are so similar [48] that they cannot be distinguished *in vivo*.

vertical positions of the achromatizing lens until the two colors are in best superposition for each individual. However, achromatizing lenses are not standard optical components, and may not be available in all laboratories. A suitable approach is to be sure that the test aperture is in good focus for emmetropic subjects and to add supplementary lenses for subjects who need optical correction. Usually the chromatic aberration is just a minor nuisance, and does not prevent the subject from successfully executing the task. In any case, if the stimulus is not presented in Maxwellian view, correction of chromatic aberration is difficult to implement, and does not appear to be essential.

3. Flicker Rate

Because thresholds for critical flicker frequency vary with age and other factors [49], appropriate frequencies of alternation of the colors of the test stimulus must be chosen for each individual. Choice of the best temporal frequency is the most challenging part of the procedure for the experimenter. When the conditions are properly chosen, subjects should perceive distinct changes in the degree of flicker as they vary the energy of the blue light. Ideally there should be a narrow range of settings that correspond to minimum flicker, which we call the null range. If the flicker rate is too low, the null range will be very broad, the subject's settings will have high variance, and the precision of the measurement will be poor. If the flicker rate is too high, no setting produces strong flicker, causing the subject to have difficulty locating the null region, again resulting in variable settings. The maximum flicker rate we have used for both fovea and parafovea is 18 Hz, and the minimum rate is 10 Hz.

For most people, it is useful to demonstrate the variation of flicker strength with the energy of the blue light by starting with the parafoveal measurement using 12 Hz alternation. If the subject continues to see no flicker over a broad range of settings, the flicker rate should be raised until the null range is sufficiently narrow to produce settings of acceptable variance. At the correct flicker rate, it should be possible for the subject to adjust the energy of the blue test light to achieve a complete null, that is, the perception that flicker has ceased entirely. Either increasing or decreasing the energy of the blue light from this null point should cause perception of increased flicker.

Some subjects who have very steady eye position experience perceptual (Troxler) fading of the parafoveal stimulus, which confuses them and makes determination of the flicker null difficult. To avoid this problem it is useful to remind subjects to blink at a normal rate and it may be helpful to periodically turn the test stimulus off entirely. To be sure that the subject has not confused fading of the stimulus with a flicker null, we ask the subject to rate the flicker magnitude, from 0 for no flicker to 10, lots of flicker. Then the subject takes a rest without changing the settings. (They may close their eyes or get off the bite bar.) We resume testing and ask the subject to rate the flicker again with the same settings. If the flicker now appears much stronger, it suggests that fading had occurred or the subject simply became fatigued and the setting needs to be redone.

Once the subject is able to make reliable settings for the parafoveal location, the foveal measurement can be added. Usually the flicker rate for the foveal determination can be around 15 Hz or higher. In the fovea, the fact that MP declines so rapidly with eccentricity means that the amount of flicker at different points within the test stimulus can be different. Consequently, the null may not be complete, but a clear range of minimum flicker is nevertheless attainable. One cue that sometimes helps the subject is the occurrence of an apparent shift in the flicker frequency when approaching the minimum. In a narrow zone around the null point, the stimulus appears to flicker more rapidly, even though the actual flicker rate has not changed. This is apparently a sign that the stimulus is activating only a subset of the visual neurons and the setting is close to the point of minimum flicker.

C. CHECKS FOR INTERNAL CONSISTENCY OF THE DATA

From our experience, we estimate that 95% of healthy adults can successfully measure their own MP. Nevertheless, this is a foreign experience for most people, and one must always be alert to the possibility that the subject is doing the task incorrectly. In particular, if data show extreme values or high variability, it is prudent to check that subjects are doing the task correctly. One way to check this is to change the wavelength of the test stimulus. The settings should change by the amount predicted by the absorbance spectrum of MP. For example if the 460 nm test is replaced by a 500 nm test, the measured OD should decrease by about 45%. If the wavelength can not easily be changed, then the size or configuration of the test stimulus can be changed instead. The dependence of MP density on test stimulus geometry can be predicted from our published data. [46] As an additional check, MP density estimates can be compared for the two eyes. For most people, the densities should not differ by more than about 0.1 absorbance units. [50] The similarity of the two eyes also means that only one eye of reliable subjects need be monitored to follow changes over time or to compare with population ranges.

For subjects in past studies the standard deviation of MP density from repeat sessions with well-motivated subjects was 0.05-0.08 absorbance units. [46,50] Thus, the variability from session to session for a given subject is small compared to the range of MP across subjects, which can be more than 1.0 absorbance units. [8,51] Furthermore, with practice the variability of subjects' settings decreases; so, long-term studies could be conducted with greater precision.

D. EVIDENCE FOR VALIDITY OF THE MACULAR PIGMENT MEASUREMENT TECHNIQUE

We have selected the flicker method (known in the vision literature as 'heterochromatic flicker photometry') for three main reasons: 1) most naive subjects can do the task with minimal training, 2) the method has been rigorously validated by varying the test wavelength [42,50] and showing that the pigment being measured has the spectrum of MP as measured directly in excised retinal tissue by microspectrophotometry, [4] and 3) very small stimuli can be used, which makes it possible to map out the spatial distribution of MP in any subject. [46]

Psychophysical methods for measuring MP density are based on the crucial assumption that the foveal patch of retina underlying the pigment has the same relative spectral sensitivity as the parafoveal patch of retina that provides the baseline value. This means that the ratio of the sensitivity to blue light to the sensitivity to green light should be the same at the two retinal loci. Note that this does not require the same absolute sensitivity to light at different retinal loci. Even so, it is not a trivial condition to satisfy, because neural organization varies dramatically with distance from the center of the fovea.

For normal observers, the retinal photoreceptors consist of the rods and three cone types whose responses peak in the short-, middle-, and long-wavelength parts of the visible spectrum. Two of these four types of photoreceptors, the rods and the short-wave sensitive cones, are known to be distributed in a very nonuniform manner. [52,53] However, the long-wave and mid-wave sensitive cones are present in a fairly constant ratio across the central retina. [54] Thus our strategy is to establish stimulus conditions that minimize the contributions of the rods and the short-wave cone system to the flicker determinations, while favoring detection by the mid- and long-wave cone systems.

To minimize the contribution of the short-wave cone system and the rods to the flicker determinations, the wavelength of the background adapting field is selected to be more strongly absorbed by those photoreceptors than by the mid- and long-wave cone systems. In addition, the flicker rate is a temporal frequency near the fusion frequency for the short-wave cone system, but well below fusion frequency for the mid- and long-wave cone systems. [55] (The fusion frequency is the flicker rate at which a light appears steady because the visual system can not resolve the flicker.) Both the adapting field and the flicker rate contribute to accomplishing the desired goal of biasing detection toward the mid- and the long-wave cone systems.

At this writing, we do not know how wide a range of subjects can be studied without violating the assumption of a uniform relative spectral sensitivity across the retina. A more detailed description of the types of evidence needed to answer this question is currently in preparation (B.R. Wooten et al.). At present the evidence indicates that normal subjects of any age who can behaviorally accomplish the task should be appropriate. Healthy subjects with inherited color vision anomalies also give valid measurements of MP. However, the psychophysical method has not yet been validated for disease states such as age-related macular degeneration or retinitis pigmentosa that might cause selective loss of photoreceptor types or selective damage to neural pathways. The validation can be accomplished by using the psychophysical method to derive the MP absorption spectrum [42,50] of subjects with these clinical conditions and then comparing the derived spectrum to established norms. [4]

E. COMPARISONS WITH PHYSICAL METHODS FOR MEASURING MACULAR PIGMENT DENSITY

There are only limited data comparing MP measured psychophysically to MP measured using other techniques in the same subjects. A recent study compared

MP density measured psychophysically with MP measured by using the fluorescence of the retinal pigment epithelium. For the fluorescence technique, a subject's retina is exposed to wavelengths (470, 510, 550 nm) that are chosen to excite lipofuscin fluorophores in the retinal pigment epithelium, which then emit light that is measured by a detector. By comparing the fluorescence excited by wavelengths that are absorbed or not absorbed by MP, a noninvasive physical measure of MP density can be obtained. Delori et al. (1997)[56] used this technique for 22 subjects and found that the MP values derived by the psychophysical and the fluorescence methods were highly correlated ($p<0.0001$), suggesting that both methods are measuring MP as expected.

Other physical methods for measuring MP can be expected to evolve as electronic instrumentation and computer processing methods continue to improve. A recent example is Raman spectroscopy, which has been shown to provide a measure of MP in excised eyes [57], and is being modified for *in vivo* measurements.

Finally, light that traverses the retina and is reflected out of the eye can be used to derive the density of MP if two wavelengths that are differentially absorbed by MP are compared. [58-60] This method is known as reflection densitiometry and its relative simplicity is appealing. Unfortunately, reflection densitiometry can produce artifactually low values of MP due to scattering in the lens and the ocular media, and reflections from the surface of the retina. Consequently, MP densities obtained by reflectance measures have sometimes been implausibly low. It is likely that reflectance methods could be used with suitable precautions to eliminate spurious reflections as long as the subjects have very clear lenses and ocular media. However, the denser lenses and light scatter encountered in older subjects represent serious obstacles to the application of reflectance methods.

V. UTILIZATION OF THE *IN VIVO* MEASUREMENTS

Age-related macular degeneration (AMD) and cataract are conditions that take many years to develop. Most etiologic studies of these conditions, however, have focused on patients that already exhibit frank clinical symptoms. Yet efforts to prevent loss of visual function must emphasize retarding the aging process that precedes the disease. For preventive approaches to be successful, information is needed from *in vivo* measurements regarding the status of the lens and the retina before deleterious changes are far advanced and intervention may be too late.

A. LENS

Measurements of lens OD are essential for assessing the impact of nutrition and of lifestyle factors such as smoking and environmental exposures at different times in the life span. The results could be used to motivate subjects to change their lifestyle. For example, smokers who learn that they have high lens densities for their age group might feel added motivation to stop smoking in order to avoid cataract.

Because the psychophysical measurements are nontraumatic they can be repeated as frequently as needed to follow changes over time. Cross-sectional data on lens OD as a function of age [9,24,38,61] suggest that lens OD increases linearly from about 15-50 years, but there is a rapid acceleration in OD changes after age 50. If there are differences in the rate of lens OD changes in younger (<50 yrs) and older (>50 yrs) individuals (as is widely suggested), differences may also exist in their respective risk factor profiles. The factors that may be responsible for the putative acceleration in lens OD changes with age should be investigated by following individual subjects over time. Otherwise, one cannot distinguish between a common pattern that occurs in most individuals, and a break point where some subjects suddenly begin to get worse, while others age more gradually.

For older individuals, the lens may absorb and scatter enough light to limit their visual capacities. [15,62] In particular, increased lens OD probably is associated with poorer visual performance in dim light. Thus, lens OD is important to study, not just for predicting possible later disease, but also for understanding its immediate deleterious effects on normal vision. Prevention of visual handicaps due to increased lens density may require modification of unhealthy behavior patterns. To convince people to modify their behavior we need to demonstrate how the health of their lens affects their quality of life.

B. MACULAR PIGMENT

The fact that MP can be measured psychophysically provides the unusual opportunity to monitor noninvasively the concentration of a nutrient in tissue. By exploiting this opportunity, we have assembled evidence that the MP carotenoids protect against age-related losses in visual sensitivity [39] and age-related ocular disease. MP selectively absorbs "blue" light (ca. 400-500 nm), which is particularly harmful to ocular tissues [63, 64], and the MP carotenoids may have other protective roles as well. [41] Consistent with a protective role for MP, we have found that low MP density is associated with many risk factors for AMD (iris color [65], sex [8], smoking status [66], dietary patterns [8]). A protective role is also consistent with biochemical studies of postmortem eyes showing that MP density is lower in AMD eyes compared to matched controls. [67]

Utilization of *in vivo* measurements of MP might help to resolve some of the inconsistencies in the epidemiologic literature. For example, although some studies have indicated that dietary intake of lutein and zeaxanthin [68], and higher blood concentrations of carotenoids [69], protect against AMD, other studies have not found a relationship. [70,71] However, our data have shown that dietary intake and blood concentrations of lutein and zeaxanthin are only moderately related to retinal concentrations of lutein and zeaxanthin as measured by MP density. [8] The blood-retina relationship is particularly poor for women, who comprise the majority of subjects for most epidemiologic studies of AMD. Moreover, we also showed that, although most subjects respond to increased intake of lutein and zeaxanthin with increases in MP density, a minority did not respond. [7] If lutein and zeaxanthin protect the retina locally, measures of these nutrients in the blood may be imprecise predictors of the state of the retina.

Similar discrepancies between blood and tissue measures of nutrients have been encountered when characterizing the nutritional status of the lens. For example, in the Italian-American Cataract study [72] of risk factors for cataract, the antioxidant status of the lens was characterized by measuring the activity of antioxidant enzymes in erythrocytes. No relationship was found between these measures and cataract risk. A later analysis [73] of the lenses of these same patients, however, revealed that there was no correlation between the erythrocyte measures and the same enzyme activity measured in the lens epithelium.

The uncertainties inherent in using blood values of nutrients to predict tissue status have led us to suggest that measuring MP may provide a more precise estimate of long-term ocular nutritional status. As long as dietary patterns remain stable, MP density remains stable over much of the life span. [46] This stability probably reflects the tendency for individuals to maintain the same diet for long time periods. [74,75] When individuals change their intake of dietary carotenoids significantly, however, MP density of most subjects changes in tandem. [7] A generally healthy diet would be indicated by high intake of fruits and vegetables, which is usually associated with high serum concentrations of lutein and zeaxanthin [76], which in turn produces high MP density. [7] In addition high MP density signals the subject's ability to accumulate carotenoids from the diet into the retina.

Consideration of MP as a biomarker for the nutritional state of the eye is motivated in part by our recent investigations of lens OD. We found that high MP density is associated with low lens density. [9] One possible interpretation of this finding is that retinal lutein and zeaxanthin are correlated with lenticular lutein and zeaxanthin [77], which may protect the lens from age-related increases in density. The other interpretation is that MP is a biomarker for ocular nutritional status, and individuals with high MP are supplying other nutrients to the lens that are derived from the same foods as the MP carotenoids. These two interpretations will probably have to be distinguished by experimental manipulation. Nevertheless, the data suggest that good nutrition can help to prevent many cases of visual disability and reduce the number of cases requiring surgical intervention.

VI. REFERENCES

1. **Boynton, RM**, Vision, in *Experimental Methods and Instrumentation in Psychology*, Sidowski, JB, Ed., McGraw-Hill, New York, 1966, pp. 273-330, see especially pp 300-328.
2. **Knowles, A**, Dartnall, HJA, The photobiology of vision. in *The Eye*, 2nd ed., Vol 2B, Davson, H, Ed., Academic Press, New York, 1977, pp. 56-57.
3. **Pierscionek, BK**, Weale, RA, The optics of the eye and lenticular senescence, *Doc. Ophthalmol.*, 89, 321-25, 1995.
4. **Snodderly, DM**, Brown, PK, Delori, FC, Auran, JD, The macular pigment. I. Absorbance spectra, localization, and discrimination from other yellow pigments in primate retinas, *Invest. Ophthalmol. Vis. Sci.*, 25, 660-673, 1984.
5. **Bone, RA**, Landrum, JT, Tarsis, SL, Preliminary identification of the human macular pigment, *Vision Res.*, 25, 1531-1539, 1985.

6. **Malinow, MR**, Feeney-Burns, L, Peterson, LH, Klein, ML, Neuringer, M, Diet related macular anomalies in monkeys, *Invest. Ophthalmol. Vis. Sci.*, 19, 857-863, 1980.
7. **Hammond, BR**, Johnson, EJ, Russell, RM, Krinsky, NI, Yeum, K-J, Edwards, RB, Snodderly, DM, Dietary modification of human macular pigment density, *Invest. Ophthalmol. Vis. Sci.*, 38, 1795-1801, 1997.
8. **Hammond, BR**, Curran-Celentano, J, Judd, S, Fuld, K, Krinsky, NI, Wooten, BR, Snodderly, DM, Sex differences in macular pigment optical density: Relation to plasma carotenoid concentrations and dietary patterns, *Vision Res.*, 36, 2001-2012, 1996.
9. **Hammond, BR**, Wooten, BR, Snodderly, DM, Density of the human crystalline lens is related to the macular pigment carotenoids, lutein and zeaxanthin, *Optom. Vis. Sci.*, 74, 499-504, 1997.
10. **Zeffrin, BS**, Applegate, RA, Bradley, A, van Heuven, WA, Retinal fixation point location in the foveal avascular zone, *Invest. Ophthalmol. Vis. Sci.*, 31, 2099-2105, 1990.
11. **Wyszecki, G**, Stiles, WS, *Color Science*, 2nd ed., Wiley, New York, 1982.
12. **Westheimer, G**, The Maxwellian View, *Vision Res.*, 6, 669-82, 1966.
13. **Kline, D**, Light, Ageing and Visual Performance, in *Vision and Visual Dysfunction: The Susceptible Visual Apparatus*, Marshall, J, Ed., CRC Press, Boca Raton, 1991, pp. 150-161.
14. **Mangione,** CM, Phillips, RS, Seddon, JM, Lawrence, MG, Cook, EF, Dailey, R, Goldman, L, Development of the 'Activities of Daily Vision Scale,' *Med. Care.*, 30, 1111-1126, 1992.
15. **Klein, BEK**, Klein, R, Jensen, SC, Visual sensitivity and age-related eye diseases. The Beaver Dam Eye Study, *Ophthal. Epidemiol.*, 3, 47-55, 1996.
16. **Kosnik, W**, Winslow, L, Kline, D, Rasinski, K, Sekuler, R, Visual changes in daily life through adulthood, *J. Gerontol. Psychol. Sci.*, 43, 63-70, 1988.
17. **Van Den Berg, TJTP**, Depth-dependent forward light scattering by donor lenses, *Invest. Ophthalmol. Vis. Sci.*, 37, 1157-66, 1996.
18. **Delaye, M**, Tardieu, A, Short-range order of crystallin proteins accounts for eye lens transparency, *Nature*, 302, 415-17, 1983.
19. **Berman, E**, Biochemistry of the Eye,. Plenum Press, New York, 1991, pp. 201-274.
20. **Mota, MC**, Ramalho, JS, Carvalho, P, Quadrado, J, Baltar, AS, Monitoring *in vivo* lens changes: A comparative study with biochemical analysis of protein aggregation, *Doc. Ophthalmol.*, 82, 287-96, 1992.
21. **Duncan, G**, Hightower, KR, Gondolfi, SA, Tomlinson, J, Maraini, G, Human lens membrane cation permeability increases with age, *Invest. Ophthalmol. Vis. Sci.*, 30, 1855-59, 1989.
22. **Duncan, G**, Bushell, AR, Ion analyses of human cataractous lenses, *Exp. Eye Res.*, 20, 223-229, 1975.
23. **Maraini, G**, Mangili, R, Differences in proteins and in the water balance of the lens in nuclear and cortical types of senile cataract, in *The Human Lens in Relation to Cataract.* CIBA Symposium 19. Associated Science Pub., Amsterdam, 1973.

24. **Sample, PA**, Esterson, FD, Weinreb, RN, Boynton, RM, The aging lens: *In vivo* assessment of light absorption in 84 human eyes, *Invest. Ophthalmol. Vis. Sci.,* 29, 1306-1311, 1988.
25. **Leske, MC**, Chylack, LT, Wu, S-Y, The Lens Opacity Case Control Study Group, The lens opacity case control study: Risk factors for cataract, *Arch. Ophthalmol.*, 109, 244-251, 1991.
26. **Lutze, M**, Bresnick, GH, Lenses of diabetic patients "yellow" at an accelerated rate similar to older individuals, *Invest. Ophthalmol. Vis. Sci.,* 32, 194-199, 1991.
27. **Olbert, D**, Hockwin, O, Baumgartner, A, Wahl, P, Hasslacher, C, Laser, H, Eschenfelder, V, Long-term follow up of the lenses of diabetic patients using Scheimpflug photography linear densitometry, *Klinische Monatsblatter fur Augenheilkunde*, 189, 363-366, 1986.
28. **Cotlier, E**, Senile cataracts: Evidence for acceleration by diabetes and deceleration by salicylate, *Can. J. Ophthalmol.*, 16, 113-118, 1981.
29. **Hardy, KJ**, Scarpello, JH, Foster, DH, Moreland, JD, Effect of diabetes associated increases in lens optical density on colour discrimination in insulin dependent diabetes, *Br. J. Ophthalmol.*, 78, 754-756, 1994.
30. Ben-Sira, I, Weinberger, D, Bodenheimer, J, Yassur, Y, Clinical method for measurement of light back scattering from the *in vivo* human lens, *Invest. Ophthalmol. Vis. Sci.*, 19, 435-437, 1980.
31. **Sample, PA**, Quirante, JS, Weinreb, RN, Age-related changes in the human lens, *Acta Ophthalmologica*, 69, 310-314, 1991.
32. **Muller-Breitenkamp, U**, Hockwin, O, Scheimpflug photography in clinical ophthalmology: A review, *Ophthalmic Res*., 24 (Suppl.), 47-54, 1992.
33. **Bosem, ME**, Sample, PA, Martinez, GA, Lusky, M, Weinreb, RN, Age-related changes in human lens: A comparison of Scheimpflug photography and lens density index, *J. Cataract Refract. Surg.,* 20, 70-73, 1994.
34. **Wald, G,** Brown, PK, Human rhodopsin, *Science*, 127, 22-226, 1958.
35. **Mellerio, J**, Yellowing of the human lens: Nuclear and cortical contributions, *Vision Res.*, 27, 1581-1587, 1987.
36. **Van Norren, D**, Vos, JJ, Spectral transmission of the human ocular media, *Vision Res*, 14, 1237-1244, 1974.
37. **Pokorny, J**, Smith, VC, Lutze, M, Aging of the human lens, *Applied Optics*, 26, 1437-40, 1987.
38. **Johnson, CA**, Howard, DW, Marshall, D, Shu, H, A noninvasive video-based method of measuring lens transmission properties of the human eye, *Opt. Vis. Sci.*, 70, 944-955, 1993.
39. **Hammond, BR,** Wooten, BR, Snodderly, DM, Preservation of visual sensitivity of older subjects: Association with macular pigment density, *Invest. Ophthalmol. Vis. Sci.,* 39, 397-406, 1998.
40. **Werner, JS**, Development of scotopic sensitivity and the absorption spectrum of the human ocular media, *J. Opt. Soc. Am.,* 72, 247-258, 1982.
41. **Snodderly, DM**, Evidence for protection against age-related macular degeneration by carotenoids and antioxidant vitamins, *Am. J. Clin. Nutr.*, 62S, 1448S-1461S, 1995.

42. **Werner, JS**, Donnelly, SK, Kliegl, R, Aging and human macular pigment density, *Vision Res.*, 27, 257-268, 1987.
43. **Snodderly, DM**, Handelman, GJ, Adler, AJ, Distribution of individual macular pigment carotenoids in central retina of macaque and squirrel monkeys, *Invest. Ophthalmol. Vis. Sci.*, 32, 268-279, 1991.
44. **Bone, RA**, Landrum, JT, Fernandez, L, Tarsis, SL, Analysis of the macular pigment by HPLC: Retinal distribution and age study, *Invest. Ophthalmol. Vis. Sci.*, 29, 843-849, 1988.
45. **Snodderly, DM**, Auran, JD, Delori, FC, The macular pigment. II. Spatial distribution in primate retinas, *Invest. Ophthalmol. Vis. Sci.*, 25, 674-685, 1984.
46. **Hammond, BR**, Wooten, BR, Snodderly, DM, Individual variations in the spatial profile of human macular pigment, *J. Opt. Soc. Am. A.,* 14, 1187-1196, 1997.
47. **Bone, RA**, Landrum, JT, Hime, GW, Cains, A, Zamor, J, Stereochemistry of the human macular carotenoids, *Invest. Opthalmol. Vis. Sci.*, 34, 2033-2040, 1993.
48. **Handelman, GJ**, Snodderly, DM, Krinsky, NI, Russett, MD, Adler, AJ, Biological control of primate macular pigment: Biochemical and densitometric studies, *Invest. Ophthalmol. Vis. Sci.*, 32, 257-267, 1991.
49. **Curran, S**, Critical fusion flicker techniques in psychopharmacology, in *Human Psychopharmacology: Methods and Measures*. Vol. 3, Hindmarch, I, Stonier, PD, Eds., John Wiley, Chichester, 1990, pp. 21-38.
50. **Hammond, BR**, Fuld, K, Interocular differences in macular pigment density, *Invest. Ophthalmol. Vis. Sci.*, 33, 350-355, 1992.
51. **Pease, PL**, Adams, AJ, Nuccio, E, Optical density of human macular pigment, *Vision Res.*, 27, 705-710, 1987.
52. **Curcio, CA**, Sloan, KR, Kalina, RE, Hendrickson, AE, Human photoreceptor topography, *J. Comp. Neurol.*, 292, 497-523, 1990.
53. **Curcio, CA**, Allen, KA, Sloan, KR, Lerea, CL, Hurley, JB, Klock, IB, Milam, AH, Distribution and morphology of human cone photoreceptors stained with anti-blue opsin, *J. Comp. Neurol.*, 312, 610-624, 1991.
54. **Nerger, JL**, Cicerone, CM, The ratio of L cones to M cones in the human parafoveal retina, *Vision Res.*, 32, 879-888, 1992.
55. **Brindley, GS**, DuCroz, J, Rushton, WAH, The flicker fusion frequency of the blue-sensitive mechanism of colour vision, *J. Physiolol.*, 183, 497-500, 1966.
56. **Delori, FC**, Goger, DG, Hammond, BR, Snodderly, DM, Burns, SA, Foveal lipofuscin and macular pigment, *ARVO Abstracts, Invest. Ophthalmol. Vis. Sci.,* 38, S355, 1997.
57. **Bernstein, PS**, Balashov, NA, Yoshida, M, McClane, RW, Gellerman, W, Raman spectroscopy of macular carotenoids in intact human retina, *ARVO Abstracts, Invest. Ophthalmol. Vis. Sci.,* 38, S303, 1997.
58. **Kilbride, PE**, Alexander, KR, Fishman, M, Fishman, GA, Human macular pigment assessed by imaging fundus reflectometry, *Vision Res.*, 29, 663-673, 1989.

59. **Delori, FC**, Staurenghi, G, Goger, D, Weiter, JJ, Macular pigment density measured by reflectometry and flourophotometry, *Noninvasive Assessment of the Visual System. OSA Technical Digest*, 3, 240-243, 1993.
60. **Van Norren, D**, Tiemeijer, LF, Spectral reflectance of the human eye, *Vision Res.*, 26, 313-320, 1986.
61. **Coren, S**, Girgus, JS, Density of human lens pigmentation: *In vivo* measures over an extended age range, *Vision Res.*, 12, 343-346, 1972.
62. **Attebo, K**, Mitchell, P, Smith, W, Visual acuity and the causes of visual loss in Australia, *Ophthalmology,* 103, 357-364, 1996.
63. **Ham, WT**, Mueller, HA, Retinal sensitivity to damage by short-wavelength light, *Nature*, 260, 153-154, 1976.
64. **Ham, WT**, Ruffolo, JJ, Mueller, HA, Clarke, AM, Moon, ME, Histologic analysis of photochemical lesions produced in rhesus retina by short wavelength light, *Invest. Ophthalmol. Vis. Sci.*, 17, 1029-1035, 1978.
65. **Hammond, BR**, Fuld, K, Snodderly, DM, Iris color and macular pigment optical density, *Exp. Eye Res.*, 62, 715-720, 1996.
66. **Hammond, BR**, Wooten, BR, Snodderly, DM, Cigarette smoking and retinal carotenoids: Implications for age-related macular degeneration, *Vision Res.,* 36, 3003-3009, 1996.
67. **Landrum, JT**, Bone, RA, Kilburn, MD, The macular pigment: A possible role in protection from age-related macular degeneration, in *Advances in Pharmacology,* Sies, H, Ed., Academic Press. New York. 1996, pp. 537-556.
68. **Seddon, JM**, Ajani, UA, Sperduto, RD, Hiller, R, Blair, N, Burton, TC, Farber, MD, Gragoudas, ES, Haller, J, Miller, DT, Yannuzzi, LA, Willet, W, Dietary carotenoids, vitamins A, C, and E, and advanced age-related macular degeneration, *J.A.M.A.*, 272, 1413-1420, 1994.
69. **Eye Disease Case-Control Study Group**, Antioxidant status and neovascular age-related macular degeneration, *Arch. Ophthalmol.*, 111, 104-109, 1993.
70. **Mares-Perlman, JA**, Brady, WE, Klein, R, Klein, BE, Bowen, P, Stacewicz-Sapuntzakis, M, Palta, M, Serum antioxidants and age-related macular degeneration in a population-based case-control study, *Arch. Ophthalmol.*, 113, 1518-1523, 1995.
71. **Mares-Perlman, JA**, Brady, WE, Klein, R, VandenLangenberg, GM, Klein, BE, Palta, M., Dietary fat and age-related maculopathy, *Arch. Ophthalmol.*, 113, 743-748, 1995.
72. **Italian Cataract Study Group**, Risk factors for age-related cortical, nuclear, and posterior subcapsular cataracts, *Am. J. Epidemiol.*, 133, 541-553, 1991.
73. **Belpoliti, M**, Maraini, G, Alberti, G, Corona, R, Crateri, S, Enzyme activities in human lens epithelium age-related cataract, *Invest. Ophthalmol. Vis. Sci.*, 34, 2843-2847, 1993.
74. **Jensen, OM**, Wahrendorf, J, Rosenqvist, A, Geser, A, The reliability of questionnaire-derived historical dietary information and temporal stability of food habits in individuals, *Am. J. Epidemiol.*, 120, 281-290, 1984.

75. **Thompson, FE**, Mezner, HL, Lamphiear, DE, Hawthorne, VM, Characteristics of individuals and long term reproducibility of dietary reports: The Tecumseh diet methodology study, *J. Clin. Epidemiol.*, 43, 1169-1178, 1990.
76. **Martini, MC**, Campbell, DR, Gross, MD, Grandits, GA, Potter, JD, Slavin, JL, Plasma carotenoids as biomarkers of vegetable intake: The University of Minnesota Cancer Prevention Research Unit Feeding Studies, *Cancer Epidemiol. Biomark. Prev.*, 4, 491-496, 1995.
77. **Yeum, K-J**, Taylor, A, Tang, G, Russell, RM, Measurement of carotenoids, retinoids and tocopherols in human lenses, *Invest. Ophthalmol. Vis. Sci.*, 36, 2756-2761, 1995.
78. **Cornsweet, TN**, *Visual Perception*, Academic Press, New York, 1972. This is an introductory text that readers unfamiliar with visual psychophysics may find helpful.

INDEX

B

C

D

E

V

W

X

Z

9 780367 399849